Advances in Neuromodulation

Editors

WON KIM
ANTONIO DE SALLES
NADER POURATIAN

NEUROSURGERY CLINICS OF NORTH AMERICA

www.neurosurgery.theclinics.com

Consulting Editors
RUSSELL LONSER
ISAAC YANG

January 2014 • Volume 25 • Number 1

ELSEVIER

1600 John F. Kennedy Boulevard • Suite 1800 • Philadelphia, Pennsylvania, 19103-2899

http://www.theclinics.com

NEUROSURGERY CLINICS OF NORTH AMERICA Volume 25, Number 1
January 2014 ISSN 1042-3680, ISBN-13: 978-0-323-26400-6

Editor: Jennifer Flynn-Briggs
Developmental Editor: Donald Mumford

Neurosurgery Clinics of North America (ISSN 1042-3680) is published quarterly by Elsevier Inc., 360 Park Avenue South, New York, NY 10010-1710. Months of issue are January, April, July, and October. Business and Editorial Offices: 1600 John F. Kennedy Blvd., Suite 1800, Philadelphia, PA 19103-2899. Customer Service Office: 11830 Westline Industrial Drive, St. Louis, MO 63146. Periodicals postage paid at New York, NY, and additional mailing offices. Subscription prices are $380.00 per year (US individuals), $572.00 per year (US institutions), $415.00 per year (Canadian individuals), $711.00 per year (Canadian institutions), $525.00 per year (international individuals), $711.00 per year (international institutions), $185.00 per year (US students), and $255.00 per year (international students). International air speed delivery is included in all *Clinics* subscription prices. All prices are subject to change without notice. **POSTMASTER:** Send address changes to *Neurosurgery Clinics of North America*, Elsevier Periodicals Customer Service, 11830 Westline Industrial Drive, St. Louis, MO 63146. **Customer Service: 1-800-654-2452 (US and Canada). From outside the US and Canada, call: 1-314-453-7041. Fax: 1-314-453-5170. E-mail: JournalsCustomerService-usa@elsevier.com (for print support) and journalsonlinesupport-usa@elsevier.com (for online support).**

Reprints. For copies of 100 or more, of articles in this publication, please contact the Commercial Reprints Department, Elsevier Inc., 360 Park Avenue South, New York, NY 10010-1710. Tel. 212-633-3874; Fax: 212-633-3820; E-mail: reprints@elsevier.com.

Neurosurgery Clinics of North America is covered in *MEDLINE/PubMed (Index Medicus), EMBASE/Excerpta Medica, and Current Contents/Clinical Medicine (CC/CM).*

Printed and bound by CPI Group (UK) Ltd, Croydon, CR0 4YY

Transferred to digital print 2012

Contributors

EDITORS

WON KIM, MD
Resident Physician, Department of Neurosurgery, University of California, Los Angeles, Los Angeles, California

ANTONIO DE SALLES, MD, PhD
Head of Stereotactic Surgery Section, Professor of Neurosurgery, Departments of Neurosurgery and Radiation Oncology, David Geffen School of Medicine, University of California, Los Angeles, Los Angeles, California; Chief, HCor Neuroscience, Hospital do Coração, São Paulo, Brazil

NADER POURATIAN, MD, PhD
Assistant Professor of Neurosurgery, Departments of Neurosurgery and Bioengineering; Brain Research Institute; Director, UCLA Neuromodulation Program, David Geffen School of Medicine, University of California, Los Angeles, Los Angeles, California

AUTHORS

JOSHUA P. ARONSON, MD
Neurosurgical Resident, Department of Neurosurgery, Massachusetts General Hospital, Boston, Massachusetts

NICHOLAS AUYONG, MD, PhD
Department of Neurosurgery, University of California, Los Angeles, Los Angeles, California

AUSAF BARI, MD, PhD
Department of Neurosurgery, Geffen School of Medicine, University of California, Los Angeles, Los Angeles, California

HOWARD JAY CHIZECK, ScD
Electrical Engineering, University of Washington, Seattle, Washington

IAN A. COOK, MD
Director, UCLA Depression Research and Clinic Program, Semel Institute for Neuroscience and Human Behavior at UCLA, Professor of Psychiatry and Biobehavioral Sciences, David Geffen School of Medicine at UCLA, Professor of Bioengineering, Henry Samueli School of Engineering at UCLA, Los Angeles, California

ROB DALLAPIAZZA, MD, PhD
Department of Neurosurgery, University of Virginia School of Medicine, Charlottesville, Virginia

ANTONIO DE SALLES, MD, PhD
Head of Stereotactic Surgery Section, Professor of Neurosurgery, Departments of Neurosurgery and Radiation Oncology, David Geffen School of Medicine, University of California, Los Angeles, Los Angeles, California; HCor Neuroscience, Hospital do Coração, São Paulo, Brazil

MILIND DEOGAONKAR, MD
Associate Professor, Department of Neurological Surgery, Ohio State University, Columbus, Ohio

ANGELA DOWNES, MD
Department of Neurosurgery, Morsani College of Medicine, University of South Florida, Tampa, Florida

W. JEFF ELIAS, MD
Associate Professor of Neurosurgery, University of Virginia School of Medicine, Charlottesville, Virginia

EMAD N. ESKANDAR, MD
Director of Stereotactic and Functional Neurosurgery, Department of Neurosurgery, Massachusetts General Hospital, Professor, Harvard Medical School, Boston, Massachusetts

RANDALL ESPINOZA, MD, MPH
Medical Director, Electroconvulsive Therapy Program, Resnick Neuropsychiatric Hospital at UCLA, Associate Director, UCLA Longevity Center, Semel Institute for Neurosciences and Human Behavior at UCLA; Clinical Professor, Department of Psychiatry and Biobehavioral Sciences, David Geffen School of Medicine at UCLA, Los Angeles, California

ITZHAK FRIED, MD, PhD
Department of Neurosurgery, Geffen School of Medicine, University of California, Los Angeles, Los Angeles, California

ALESSANDRA A. GORGULHO, MD, MSc
Departments of Neurosurgery and Radiation Oncology, David Geffen School of Medicine, University of California, Los Angeles, Los Angeles, California; HCor Neuroscience, Hospital do Coração, São Paulo, Brazil

ADAM O. HEBB, MD, FRCSC, FAANS
Visiting Assistant Professor, Electrical and Computer Engineering, Neurosurgeon, Colorado Brain and Spine Institute, Member, Colorado Neurological Institute, University of Denver, Englewood, Colorado

KATHRYN L. HOLLOWAY, MD
Professor and Director of Movement Disorders, Department of Neurosurgery, Parkinson's Disease Research, Education, and Clinical Care Center, McGuire VA Medical Center, Virginia Commonwealth University, Richmond, Virginia

FORREST JELLISON, MD
Fellow in Division of Pelvic Medicine and Reconstructive Surgery, Department of Urology, UCLA School of Medicine, Los Angeles, California

HUSAM A. KATNANI, PhD
Research Fellow, Department of Neurosurgery, Massachusetts General Hospital, Boston, Massachusetts

JA-HONG KIM, MD
Assistant Professor, Division of Pelvic Medicine and Reconstructive Surgery, Department of Urology, UCLA School of Medicine, Los Angeles, California

WON KIM, MD
Resident Physician, Department of Neurosurgery, University of California, Los Angeles, Los Angeles, California

SCOTT KRAHL, PhD
Departments of Neurosurgery, David Geffen School of Medicine, University of California, Los Angeles; VA Great Los Angeles Healthcare Hospital, Los Angeles, California

JEAN-PHILIPPE LANGEVIN, MD, PhD
Department of Neurosurgery, Greater LA VA Healthcare, Geffen School of Medicine, University of California, Los Angeles, Los Angeles, California

PAUL S. LARSON, MD
Associate Professor and Vice Chair, Department of Neurological Surgery, University of California, San Francisco; Chief, Neurosurgery, San Francisco VA Medical Center, San Francisco, California

AARON LAVIANA, MD
Resident Physician in Department of Urology, UCLA School of Medicine, Los Angeles, California

JEAN-JACQUES LEMAIRE, MD, PhD
Service of Neurosurgery, University Hospital, Clermont-Ferrand; EA 7292 (Image-Guided Clinical Neuroscience and Connectomics), Auvergne University, France

SCOTT F. LEMPKA, PhD
Center for Neurological Restoration, Neurological Institute, Cleveland Clinic, Cleveland, Ohio

ANDREW F. LEUCHTER, MD
Director, Laboratory of Brain, Behavior, and Pharmacology, Semel Institute for Neuroscience and Human Behavior, Professor of Psychiatry and Biobehavioral Sciences, David Geffen School of Medicine at UCLA, Los Angeles, California

ROBERT M. LEVY, MD, PhD
Department of Neurological Surgery, University of Florida College of Medicine, Jacksonville, Florida

DANIEL C. LU, MD, PhD
Department of Neurosurgery, University of California, Los Angeles, Los Angeles, California

ANDRE MACHADO, MD, PhD
Department of Neurosurgery, Center for Neurological Restoration, Neurological Institute, Cleveland Clinic, Cleveland, Ohio

MOHAMMAD H. MAHOOR, PhD
Electrical and Computer Engineering, University of Denver, Englewood, Colorado

CHARLES MATLACK, MS
Electrical Engineering, University of Washington, Seattle, Washington

M. SEAN MCKISIC, MD
Department of Neurosurgery, University of Virginia School of Medicine, Charlottesville, Virginia

KELLY A. MILLS, MD
Movement Disorders Fellow, UCSF Department of Neurology, PADRECC, San Francisco VA Medical Center, San Francisco, California

NINA Z. MOORE, MD, MSE
Department of Neurosurgery, Center for Neurological Restoration, Neurological Institute, Cleveland Clinic, Cleveland, Ohio

TIANYI NIU, MD
Department of Neurosurgery, Geffen School of Medicine, University of California, Los Angeles, Los Angeles, California

JILL L. OSTREM, MD
Associate Professor of Neurology and Medical Director, Surgical Movement Disorders Center, UCSF Department of Neurology, PADRECC, San Francisco VA Medical Center, San Francisco, California

JULIO L.B. PEREIRA, MD
Departments of Neurosurgery and Radiation Oncology, David Geffen School of Medicine, University of California, Los Angeles, Los Angeles, California

NADER POURATIAN, MD, PhD
Assistant Professor of Neurosurgery, Departments of Neurosurgery and Bioengineering; Brain Research Institute; Director, UCLA Neuromodulation Program, David Geffen School of Medicine, University of California, Los Angeles, Los Angeles, California

BINIT SHAH, MD
Assistant Professor of Neurology, University of Virginia School of Medicine, Charlottesville, Virginia

KONSTANTIN V. SLAVIN, MD, FAANS
Professor, Department of Neurosurgery, University of Illinois at Chicago, Chicago, Illinois

PHILIP A. STARR, MD, PhD
Professor in Residence of Neurological Surgery; Dolores Cakebread Endowed Chair, UCSF Department of Neurosurgery; Surgical Director, PADRECC, San Francisco VA Medical Center, San Francisco, California

DARYOUSH TAVANAIEPOUR, MD
Department of Neurological Surgery, University of Florida College of Medicine, Jacksonville, Florida

CHRISTOS TSIOKOS, MS
Department of Biomedical Engineering, University of California, Los Angeles, California

RAFAEL A. VEGA, MD, PhD
Resident, Department of Neurosurgery, Virginia Commonwealth University, Richmond, Virginia

JUN JASON ZHANG, PhD
Electrical and Computer Engineering, University of Denver, Englewood, Colorado

ZION ZIBLY, MD
Fellow, Department of Neurological Surgery, Ohio State University, Columbus Ohio

Contents

Erratum xiii

Preface xv

Won Kim, Antonio De Salles, and Nader Pouratian

Peripheral Nerve and Spinal Cord Stimulation

Peripheral Nerve/Field Stimulation for Neuropathic Pain 1

Milind Deogaonkar and Konstantin V. Slavin

Peripheral nerve stimulation and peripheral nerve field stimulation are emerging as a viable neuromodulatory therapy in the treatment of refractory pain. Although the technology of percutaneous stimulation has been available for decades, recent advancements have broadened the number of indications. Success of treatment revolves around identifying the correct patient population, and the selection and placement of the appropriate electrodes and implantable pulse generators. Most results to date have come from case reports and retrospective studies. However, given the promising outcomes in reducing otherwise medically refractory pain, future randomized controlled studies are needed to assess this emerging technology.

Peripheral Neuromodulation for Treatment of Chronic Migraine Headache 11

Daryoush Tavanaiepour and Robert M. Levy

Chronic migraines (CM) affect approximately 2% of the population, resulting in significant disability, economic burden, and impairments in quality of life. Historical neurosurgical procedures, such as lesioning of the trigeminal dorsal root entry zone or neurolysis of the occipital nerve, have not gained favor because of procedural morbidity and poor durability, respectively. Occipital nerve stimulation is emerging as a potentially promising modality for the treatment of CM, with greater than 50% pain reduction in approximately 80% of patients in open-label trials and ~40% of patients in randomized controlled trials. Mechanisms of neuromodulation remain unclear.

Neuromodulation of the Lumbar Spinal Locomotor Circuit 15

Nicholas AuYong and Daniel C. Lu

The lumbar spinal cord contains the necessary circuitry to independently drive locomotor behaviors. This function is retained following spinal cord injury (SCI) and is amenable to rehabilitation. Although the effectiveness of task-specific training and pharmacologic modulation has been repeatedly demonstrated in animal studies, results from human studies are less striking. Recently, lumbar epidural stimulation (EDS) along with locomotor training was shown to restore weight-bearing function and lower-extremity voluntary control in a chronic, motor-complete human SCI subject. Related animal studies incorporating EDS as part of the therapeutic regiment are also encouraging. EDS is emerging as a promising neuromodulatory tool for SCI.

Spinal Cord Stimulation for the Treatment of Vascular Pathology 25

Milind Deogaonkar, Zion Zibly, and Konstantin V. Slavin

Multiple studies have shown proved efficacy of spinal cord stimulation (SCS) in peripheral vascular disease (PVD). The exact mechanism by which SCS acts in the treatment of PVD is not completely understood, and may include stimulating the release of nitric oxide, modulation of the sympathetic nervous system, or modulation of prostaglandin production. Patient selection criteria have been well defined and SCS should be reserved for patients with end-stage lower limb PVD unresponsive to medical therapy and not amenable to surgical reconstruction but in whom disease has not caused inevitable limb loss. This article reviews the outcomes, techniques, patient selection criteria, and putative mechanisms of SCS for PVD.

Sacral Neuromodulation for Refractory Overactive Bladder, Interstitial Cystitis, and Painful Bladder Syndrome 33

Aaron Laviana, Forrest Jellison, and Ja-Hong Kim

Various pelvic floor conditions, including overactive bladder syndrome and chronic pelvic pain, have been successfully managed with the neuromodulation of sacral nerves. Sacral neuromodulation is a minimally invasive procedure involving the implantation of a programmable pulse generator that delivers low-amplitude electrical current via quadripolar tined leads through the S3 foramen. Durable efficacy has been demonstrated in retrospective studies, but questions regarding ideal patient candidacy and optimal technical considerations remain unanswered.

Central Neuromodulation

Neuromodulation for Movement Disorders 47

Rob Dallapiazza, M. Sean McKisic, Binit Shah, and W. Jeff Elias

Surgical neuromodulation has emerged as the primary method to treat the medically refractory symptoms of essential tremor and Parkinson disease. With reversible manipulation of CNS neurons, neuromodulation can be used to intraoperatively localize and verify a stereotactic target, and to chronically treat movement disorders. This article discusses the historical advances in stereotactic surgery using various modalities of neuromodulation leading to contemporary treatment. Electrical neuromodulation, or deep brain stimulation, is emphasized as the major surgical intervention with a discussion of the technique, surgical targets, and clinical outcomes. A comparison of neuromodulation techniques is presented.

Neuromodulation for Dystonia: Target and Patient Selection 59

Kelly A. Mills, Philip A. Starr, and Jill L. Ostrem

Treatment of dystonia refractory to oral medications or botulinum toxin injections includes the use of deep brain stimulation (DBS). Expectations should be established based on patient-related factors, including type of dystonia, genetic cause, target symptoms, age at the time of surgery, disease duration, or the presence of fixed skeletal deformities. Premorbid conditions such as psychiatric illness and cognitive impairment should be considered. Target selection is an emerging issue in DBS for dystonia. Although efficacy has been established for targeting the globus pallidus internus for dystonia, other brain targets such as the subthalamic nucleus, thalamus, or cortex may be promising alternatives.

Central Neuromodulation for Refractory Pain 77

Nina Z. Moore, Scott F. Lempka, and Andre Machado

Chronic neuropathic pain affects 8.2% of adults, extrapolated to roughly 18 million people every year in the United States. Patients who have pain that cannot be controlled with pharmacologic management or less invasive techniques can be considered for deep brain stimulation or motor cortex stimulation. These techniques are not currently approved by the Food and Drug Administration for chronic pain and are, thus, considered off-label use of medical devices for this patient population. Conclusive effectiveness studies are still needed to demonstrate the best targets as well as the reliability of the results with these approaches.

Neuromodulation for Obsessive-Compulsive Disorder **85**

Joshua P. Aronson, Husam A. Katnani, and Emad N. Eskandar

This article describes the basis for neuromodulation procedures for obsessive-compulsive disorder (OCD) and summarizes the literature on the efficacy of these interventions. Discussion includes neural circuitry underlying OCD pathology, the history and types of ablative procedures, the targets and modalities used for neuromodulation, and future therapeutic directions.

Neuromodulation for Depression: Invasive and Noninvasive (Deep Brain Stimulation, Transcranial Magnetic Stimulation, Trigeminal Nerve Stimulation) **103**

Ian A. Cook, Randall Espinoza, and Andrew F. Leuchter

Major depressive disorder is among the most disabling illnesses and, despite best practices with medication and psychotherapy, many patients remain ill even after several treatment trials. For many of these patients with treatment-resistant or pharmacoresistant depression, treatment with neuromodulation offers an alternative. Options range from systems that are implanted to others that are entirely noninvasive. This review surveys recent literature to update readers on 3 particular interventions: deep brain stimulation, transcranial magnetic stimulation, and trigeminal nerve stimulation. Additional comparative research is needed to delineate the relative advantages of these treatments, and how best to match individual patients to neuromodulation intervention.

Deep Brain Stimulation for Tourette Syndrome **117**

Won Kim and Nader Pouratian

Gilles de la Tourette syndrome is a movement disorder characterized by repetitive stereotyped motor and phonic movements with varying degrees of psychiatric comorbidity. Deep brain stimulation (DBS) has emerged as a novel therapeutic intervention for patients with refractory Tourette syndrome. Since 1999, more than 100 patients have undergone DBS at various targets within the corticostriatothalamocortical network thought to be implicated in the underlying pathophysiology of Tourette syndrome. Future multicenter clinical trials and the use of a centralized online database to compare the results are necessary to determine the efficacy of DBS for Tourette syndrome.

Limbic Neuromodulation: Implications for Addiction, Posttraumatic Stress Disorder, and Memory **137**

Ausaf Bari, Tianyi Niu, Jean-Philippe Langevin, and Itzhak Fried

Deep brain stimulation, a technique whereby electrodes are implanted into specific brain regions to modulate their activity, has been mainly used to treat movement disorders. More recently this technique has been proposed for the treatment of drug addiction, posttraumatic stress disorder (PTSD), and dementia. The nucleus accumbens, amygdala, and hippocampus, central nuclei within the limbic system, have been studied as potential targets for neuromodulation for the treatment of drug addiction, PTSD, and dementia, respectively. As the scope of neuromodulation grows to include disorders of mood and thought, new ethical and philosophic challenges that require multidisciplinary discussion and cooperation are emerging.

Neuromodulation for Eating Disorders: Obesity and Anorexia **147**

Alessandra A. Gorgulho, Julio L.B. Pereira, Scott Krahl, Jean-Jacques Lemaire, and Antonio De Salles

Extremes of eating disorders (ED) have become prevalent in both developed and developing countries. Available therapies, though largely effective, fail in a substantial number of patients and carry considerable side effects. Morbid obesity and anorexia nervosa (AN) represent important causes of morbidity and mortality among young adults. Morbid obesity affects disproportionate numbers of children. AN is also important for its high mortality in young adults. The challenges of effectively treating AN are well recognized. In this article, important aspects of ED are reviewed in detail and novel approaches to the treatment of ED are proposed.

Techniques in Neuromodulation

Image-Guided Deep Brain Stimulation **159**

Rafael A. Vega, Kathryn L. Holloway, and Paul S. Larson

Advances in deep brain stimulation (DBS) surgery have been achieved through the use of stereotactic targeting of key tracks in patients undergoing awake surgery. Intraoperative detection of track location has been useful in interpreting physiologic results, has limited the number of brain penetrations, and has decreased the incidence of reoperations. Alternatively, some centers are gaining experience with placement of the lead under general anesthesia using a purely anatomic approach, for which both computed tomography and magnetic resonance imaging have proved useful. In this article, the use of image guidance with both the anatomic and physiologic approaches is described.

Advanced Neuroimaging Techniques for Central Neuromodulation **173**

Angela Downes and Nader Pouratian

Deep brain stimulation an effective treatment of many neurologic conditions such as Parkinson disease, essential tremor, dystonia, and obsessive-compulsive disorder. Structural and functional neuroimaging studies provide the opportunity to visualize the dysfunctional nodes and networks underlying neurologic and psychiatric disease, and to thereby realize new targets for neuromodulation as well as personalize current therapy. This article reviews contemporary advances in neuroimaging in the basic sciences and how they can be applied to redirect and propel functional neurosurgery toward a goal of functional localization of targets with individualized maps and identification of novel targets for other neuropsychiatric diseases.

Creating the Feedback Loop: Closed-Loop Neurostimulation **187**

Adam O. Hebb, Jun Jason Zhang, Mohammad H. Mahoor, Christos Tsiokos, Charles Matlack, Howard Jay Chizeck, and Nader Pouratian

Current DBS therapy delivers a train of electrical pulses at set stimulation parameters. This open-loop design is effective for movement disorders, but therapy may be further optimized by a closed loop design. The technology to record biosignals has outpaced our understanding of their relationship to the clinical state of the whole person. Neuronal oscillations may represent or facilitate the cooperative functioning of brain ensembles, and may provide critical information to customize neuromodulation therapy. This review addresses advances to date, not of the technology per se, but of the strategies to apply neuronal signals to trigger or modulate stimulation systems.

Index **205**

NEUROSURGERY CLINICS OF NORTH AMERICA

FORTHCOMING ISSUES

April 2014
Minimally Invasive Spine Surgery
Richard Fessler, MD and Zachary Smith, MD, *Editors*

July 2014
Endovascular Management of Cerebrovascular Disease
Ricardo Hanel, MD, Ciaran Powers, MD, and Eric Sauvageau, MD, *Editors*

October 2014
Pain Management
Andre Machado, MD, PhD, Milind S. Deogaonkar, MD, and Ashwini D. Sharan, MD, *Editors*

RECENT ISSUES

October 2013
Intracranial Stereotactic Radiosurgery
Bruce E. Pollock, MD, *Editor*

July 2013
Neurocritical Care in Neurosurgery
Paul A. Nyquist, MD, Marek A. Mirski, MD, and Rafael J. Tamargo, MD, *Editors*

April 2013
Spinal Deformity Surgery
Christopher P. Ames, MD, Brian Jian, MD, and Christopher I. Shaffrey, MD, *Editors*

RELATED INTEREST

Neurologic Clinics, February 2013
Spinal Cord Diseases
Alireza Minagar and Alejandro A. Rabinstein, *Editors*

Erratum

An error was made in the October 2003 issue of Neurosurgery Clinics of North America (Volume 14, number 1) on pages 25–39. Figures 17 and 18 (electron photomicrographs) were reversed in the article, "Pathology of Pituitary Tumors," by Naoko Sanno, Akira Teramoto, R. Yoshiyuki Osamura, Eva Horvath, et al.

Neurosurg Clin N Am 25 (2014) xiii
http://dx.doi.org/10.1016/j.nec.2013.10.004

Preface

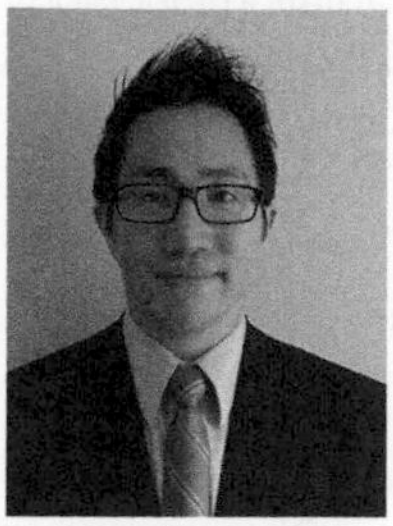

Won Kim, MD

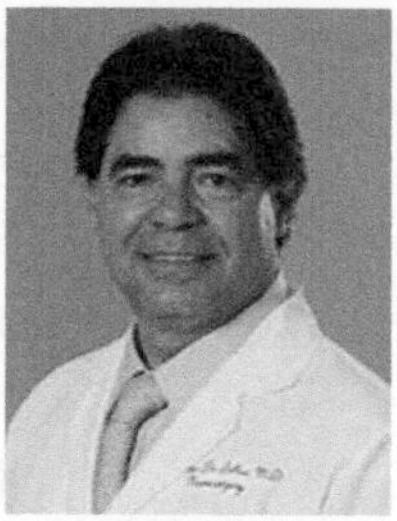

Antonio De Salles, MD, PhD

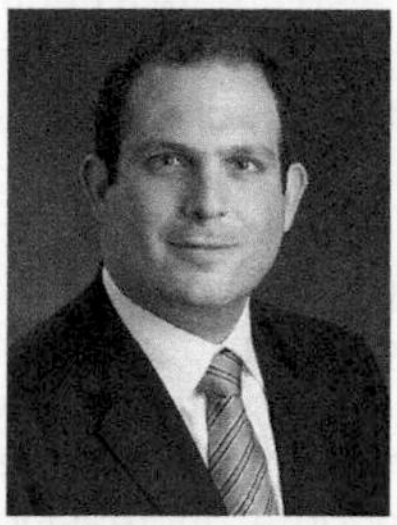

Nader Pouratian, MD, PhD

Editors

The field of neurosurgery has been one of the leaders in medicine in integrating advances in technology into everyday clinical practice. From intraoperative image-guided stereotaxy and endovascular techniques to molecular and individualized therapies, the synergy of engineering and neuroscience has allowed for neurosurgeons to maximize clinical outcomes in diseases with traditionally poor prognoses.

Functional neurosurgery as a subspeciality within neurological surgery stands to experience many great advances. With an ever-increasing understanding of the intricate cortical and subcortical networks interconnecting the human brain, we are continuing to increase our understanding of the mechanisms that underlie movement, sensation, memory, pain, and even consciousness. With this knowledge, our applications and indications for neuromodulation through both central and peripheral stimulation of neurons and nerves continue to expand. Deep brain stimulation, for example, is proving to be efficacious for numerous other neurologic and psychiatric conditions beyond movement disorders including obsessive compulsive disorder, depression, Tourette syndrome, pain, posttraumatic stress disorder, and addiction, to name a few. Spinal cord and peripheral nerve stimulators are emerging as novel therapeutics in pain management as well as gait reanimation and incontinence. Many of these technologies are still in their infancy and have not been recognized as a suitable adjuvant therapy to the current standards of care. Forward-thinking innovation is necessary to identify opportunities to intervene and modulate diseases that have previously been beyond the realm of neurosurgery. Such innovation will arise from increasing our understanding of the various intricate neural circuits mediating function and pathophysiology. Advances in neuroimaging, circuit modeling, pharmacotherapy, and surgical techniques provide unparalleled opportunities to accelerate neuromodulation as a field.

This issue of the *Neurosurgery Clinics of North America* aims to comprehensively review many of these novel advances in neuromodulation. Through the scientific analysis of the current literature by numerous experts in the field of functional

Neurosurg Clin N Am 25 (2014) xv–xvi
http://dx.doi.org/10.1016/j.nec.2013.10.003
1042-3680/14/$ – see front matter

neurosurgery, we hope to not only provide a handbook of the current state of neuromodulation from the periphery to the brain, but also create a central resource that clinicians interested in integrating these treatment modalities into their clinical practice may reference.

As the advancements in neuroscience and technology continue to refine neurosurgery to allow us to not only save lives from devastating neurologic diseases, but to also improve lives from functionally debilitating ones, the field of neuromodulation will become increasingly invaluable. It is our sincere hope that this volume will inspire further research and innovation in neuromodulation such that neurosurgery will advance beyond the confines of medicine to become a genuine force in improving the human condition.

Won Kim, MD
Department of Neurosurgery
University of California, Los Angeles
10945 Le Conte Ave Suite 2120
Los Angeles, CA 90095, USA

Antonio De Salles, MD, PhD
Departments of Neurosurgery and Radiation Oncology
David Geffen School of Medicine
University of California, Los Angeles
10945 Le Conte Ave Suite 2120
Los Angeles, CA 90095, USA

Chief of HCor Neuroscience
Sao Paulo, Brazil

Nader Pouratian, MD, PhD
Departments of Neurosurgery and Bioengineering
University of California, Los Angeles
10945 Le Conte Ave Suite 2120
Los Angeles, CA 90095, USA

UCLA Neuromodulation Program
University of California, Los Angeles
10945 Le Conte Ave Suite 2120
Los Angeles, CA 90095, USA

E-mail addresses:
wonkim@mednet.ucla.edu (W. Kim)
afdesalles@yahoo.com (A. De Salles)
NPouratian@mednet.ucla.edu (N. Pouratian)

Peripheral Nerve and Spinal Cord Stimulation

Peripheral Nerve/Field Stimulation for Neuropathic Pain

Milind Deogaonkar, MD[a], Konstantin V. Slavin, MD[b,*]

KEYWORDS

• Peripheral neuromodulation • Field stimulation • Chronic pain • Nerve stimulation • Neuropathic pain • Headache • Occipital neuralgia • Post-herpetic neuralgia

KEY POINTS

- Peripheral nerve stimulation and peripheral nerve field stimulation are emerging as viable neuromodulatory therapies in the treatment of refractory pain.
- Although the technology of percutaneous stimulation has been around for decades, recent advancements have broadened the number of indications to include neuropathic pain disorders (eg, post-herpetic neuralgia, trigeminal neuralgia, occipital neuralgia, posttraumatic neuralgia), complex regional pain syndrome, various cephalgias, axial pain syndromes, musculoskeletal pain, and fibromyalgia.
- Success of treatment revolves around identifying the correct patient population, and the selection and placement of the appropriate electrodes and implantable pulse generators.
- Most of the results to date have been in the form of case reports and retrospective studies.
- Given the promising outcomes in reducing otherwise medically refractory pain, future randomized controlled studies are needed to assess this emerging technology.

INTRODUCTION

Chronic neuropathic pain syndromes are frequently very difficult to treat. Various surgical, medical, and physical therapy modalities have been used to relieve such pain. One of the surgical options is direct electrical stimulation of the affected nerve by placing a stimulating electrode over the nerve or under the skin in the area of pain. Peripheral nerve stimulation (PNS) or peripheral nerve/field stimulation (PNFS), as such subcutaneous stimulation has been called in the literature, has been used for the treatment of chronic neuropathic pain for many years. The practice of using electrical stimulation for pain control has ancient roots. In the modern era, Wall and Sweet[1] first demonstrated the use of peripheral electrical stimulation for the abolition of pain. In later years, better understanding of the physiology and anatomy of pain and pain pathways allowed for the development of multiple therapeutic options. The improvement in the tools, techniques, and paradigms of neuromodulation in recent years has resulted in a resurgence of interest in this surgical modality. PNS remains an attractive option because of its minimally invasive nature and an ability to provide focal neuromodulation. PNFS is a surgical intervention whereby procedural pain is minimal, and the area of stimulation and area of pain converge without the need for any complex programming. It provides an excellent modality for the treatment of various neuropathic[2,3] and musculoskeletal[4] and, at times, intractable visceral

[a] Department of Neurosurgery, Ohio State University, Columbus, 480 Medical Center Drive, Columbus, OH 43210, USA; [b] Department of Neurosurgery, University of Illinois, Chicago, IL, USA
* Corresponding author.
E-mail address: kslavin@uic.edu

Neurosurg Clin N Am 25 (2014) 1–10
http://dx.doi.org/10.1016/j.nec.2013.10.001
1042-3680/14/$ – see front matter

pain[5] conditions. It may be used to complement other electrical neuromodulation procedures such as spinal cord stimulation (SCS) whereby a hybrid of PNFS and SCS can be used.[6,7] It may also be used in place of other neuromodulation procedures such as SCS when the pain is focal or predominantly truncal or axial.[8] Although the mechanisms of action of PNFS are not clear, it is thought to have a somewhat peripheral action, similar to that of SCS, based on the gate-control theory of pain.[9] In addition, it probably works by a more central neuromodulation of medial pain pathways[10] or by inhibiting the central nociceptive processing of painful stimuli.[11]

Despite its proven efficacy in multiple indications,[6,12–14] PNS/PNFS is still considered novel or experimental. However, this is far from the truth. Although a resurgence of this technique has been witnessed in the last few years, the use of electroanalgesia is many decades old.[15] When in 1967 Wall and Sweet tried to find a new approach to suppress neuropathic pain, they inserted an electrode first into their own infraorbital foramina and then implanted devices in the extremities of 8 patients.[1] The stimulation resulted in temporary pain suppression lasting half an hour after a stimulation period of 2 minutes.[1] In a later larger series of 69 patients studied by Sweet,[16] 17 had permanent relief and 13 had temporary but sustained relief. In the subsequent 5 decades, multiple reports have been published expanding the indications, refining the techniques, and consistently showing increased efficacy of this modality.

In recent years, the focus of stimulation has moved from identifying individual nerves and stimulating them directly to placing an electrode under the skin in the area of pain for certain indications.[17–19] In addition, a discussion has started on whether to name the technique subcutaneous field stimulation, or continue with the term peripheral nerve stimulation.[20] PNFS seems an acceptable intermediate option.

INDICATIONS AND PATIENT SELECTION

The common indications of PNFS can be classified based on the pain type and pain location. However, certain common factors underlie all of these indications. Whatever the type or location of pain may be, the pain has to be chronic, severe, negatively affecting the patient's functionality, and refractory to the usual medical treatments, including opioid and nonopioid medications, physical therapy, trigger-point injections, injections of botulinum toxin, application of transcutaneous electrical nerve stimulation (TENS), and somatic and sympathetic nerve blocks.

There are 4 main pillars of patient selection for PNFS that are almost universally accepted.

1. Intractable pain. As already described, the pain has to be treatment-resistant and disabling. It is important to make sure that the patient has tried all other noninvasive methods of pain control, and has either failed or had only transient or partial benefit.
2. Distribution of pain. Extent of the area of pain is an important factor in deciding on which neuromodulation approach will work better. For PNS, the pain must be in the distribution of a single nerve, whereas for PNFS it is more important for the pain to be in an area that can be covered by the commercially available length of electrodes. Larger areas of pain can be better treated by other neuromodulation modalities such as SCS, targeted brain stimulation (such as deep brain stimulation or motor cortex stimulation), or intrathecal drug-delivery systems.
3. Pain psychology testing. This factor is borrowed from the standard approach when using neuromodulation procedures such as SCS. Psychological characteristics play an important role in shaping responses to any neuromodulation approach in chronic pain including PNS, PNFS, and SCS, in addition to a variety of other pain treatments.[21] In SCS, the influence of psychological evaluation on outcomes has been noted by various groups.[21–23] The same holds true for PNFS. All patients must undergo pain psychology testing and should be treated adequately for any underlying or unresolved anxiety, depression, or other psychiatric disorders.
4. Successful trial. Again this is similar to the SCS procedure.[22,23] All patients need to undergo an externalized trial whereby the electrodes are placed percutaneously and are connected to an external stimulation generator. It is done exclusively on an outpatient basis. The length of the trial varies from 2 to 10 days. In most patients the response is seen within the first 48 hours. Some patients need outpatient reprogramming during the trial. A cutoff of 50% improvement in pain and concordant improvement in quality of life is generally accepted as a successful trial.

In addition to these criteria, some minor factors play a role in patient selection. These factors are PNFS specific and vary according to centers, but are generally agreed on by most implanters.

1. Sensory loss. Partial or complete sensory loss in the area of pain increases the chances of a failed trial, especially when performing field stimulation. For activation of the gait-control

mechanism of pain suppression, at least partially functioning vibrotactile inflow is necessary. Even in patients with postlaminectomy syndromes with truncal or axial pain, electrodes placed very close to the scar of previous spinal surgery tend to fail to give as much benefit as electrodes placed farther away from the scar.

2. Allodynia. Severe allodynia changes the strategy of implantation. An electrode underlying a patch of allodynia can sometimes aggravate the pain. It is better to bracket a patch of allodynia with electrodes placed on either side of it rather than directly in it while performing field stimulation.
3. Predictive value of TENS. Failure of TENS does not have any negative predictive value. If a patient fails to improve with TENS, it should not stand in the way of trying PNFS for pain control. On the other hand, if TENS provides improvement in pain, the location of the effective TENS electrodes can help guide the placement of PNFS electrodes. However, by no means should the use of TENS be considered as a trial for PNFS.
4. Diagnostic nerve blocks. Apart from patients with injury to specific nerves in whom a nerve block can delineate the extent of area covered by that specific nerve, the usefulness of nerve blocks as a predictive tool is doubtful. Most notably, in patients with cephalgias and occipital neuralgia (ON), nerve blocks have no predictive value.[3]

As in any surgical procedure, PNFS would be contraindicated in patients with bleeding disorders and those on anticoagulation that cannot be withheld in the perioperative period. Patients with severe immunosuppression or active infection are not candidates for any implantable device including PNFS. Patients with major cognitive impairment or untreated psychiatric conditions are not candidates for PNFS. Some centers will not offer neuromodulation for pain in patients who have ongoing litigation related to the cause of their pain. Patients who need routine magnetic resonance imaging (MRI) in conditions such as multiple sclerosis or metastatic disease have not been candidates for PNFS, as to date the implants have not been MRI compatible. Even with the recent introduction of MRI-compatible (conditionally safe) devices, MRI safety is only guaranteed for SCS applications and does not cover the use of PNFS.

Indications for PNFS have dramatically expanded in recent years. Ability to provide focused neuromodulation with minimal intervention has led to the more aggressive use of PNFS in various chronic pain conditions. Initially, neuropathic pain disorders along with complex regional pain syndrome (CRPS) were considered as some of the main indications for PNFS[24]; this was the followed by various cephalgias[14,25] and complex craniofacial pain.[14,26,27] Axial[8,13,28] and appendicular[4] musculoskeletal pain then became an indication for PNFS. Recently, intractable visceral pain[5] has also been treated by PNFS.

Indications of PNFS can be broadly classified as follows:

1. Neuropathic pain disorders. These pain disorders develop secondary to trauma, inflammation, neuropathy, or postintervention changes in a nerve. Sometimes, as in many cases of ON, this pain develops without obvious reasons (idiopathic). The specific neuropathic pain disorders that respond to PNFS are the following:
   a. Post-herpetic neuralgias (PHN). PHN patients have been treated by electrical neurostimulation from as early as 1974.[29] PNFS has been used with varying degrees of success for treating truncal[8,30] and ophthalmic/trigeminal PHN.[31,32]
   b. Posttraumatic neuralgias. Pain related to the nerve trauma resulting from either injury[33] or intervention[32] causing neuropathic pain also seems to reliably respond to PNFS.
   c. Complex craniofacial neuralgias. These neuralgias include trigeminal neuropathic pain, atypical face pain, supraorbital, infraorbital, or mandibular neuralgias, or a combination of these. These neuralgias may be secondary to repeated sinus or dental surgeries, or following interventions for trigeminal neuralgia, trauma, or facial fractures. Most of these neuralgias respond to very well to PNFS.[26,27,34,35]
   d. Occipital neuralgia. One of the most common neuralgias, this has been successfully treated by PNS/PNFS using a variety of leads and approaches.[3,36–41]
   e. Inguinal neuralgias. Ilioinguinal and genitofemoral neuralgias are an established indication for the use of PNFS. Most commonly, ilioinguinal neuralgia is seen after hernia repair, whereas genitofemoral neuralgias are generally a result of retroperitoneal or uterine and ovarian surgeries; both may be successfully treated with PNFS.[5,8,42]
   f. Other neuralgias. These neuralgias include suprascapular neuralgia, meralgia paresthetica, neuropathic pain in limbs following trauma, or nerve entrapment decompression surgeries. In the authors' experience, all of these may be successfully treated with PNFS in well-selected patients.

2. CRPS. CRPS can be treated by various neuromodulation modalities such as SCS, intrathecal drug delivery, or PNS/PNFS. Well-localized CRPS secondary to a nerve injury (type II) can be treated by PNFS, with excellent results.[43]
3. Cephalgias. A variety of headache syndromes can be successfully treated by PNFS[2,10,25,36,38,40,44–48]:
   a. Classic migraine, transformed migraine
   b. Hemicrania continua
   c. Occipital headaches
   d. Cervicogenic headaches
   e. Cluster headaches
   f. Chronic daily headaches

   A recent review summarized all of these indications in a systematic fashion.[44]
4. Axial pain syndromes. Axial pain in the neck and middle and low back is difficult to control with SCS. PNFS alone or in combination with SCS has shown promise in treating this type of pain. Isolated PNFS has shown improvement in axial low back and neck pain in various retrospective studies.[8] A recently published prospective, randomized, controlled, crossover study showed safety and effectiveness of PNFS as an aid in the management of chronic, localized back pain.[19] The study design consisted of 2 phases. During phase I, patients were divided into 4 stimulation groups (minimal, subthreshold, low frequency, and standard stimulation). Responders, classified as those who had a 50% reduction in pain during any of the 3 active stimulation groups, proceeded with phase II, which began with the implantation of the permanent system and lasted 52 weeks. The primary end point was the reduction in pain, assessed by the visual analog scale (VAS). During phase I, there were significant differences in mean VAS scores between minimal stimulation and subthreshold stimulation (P = .003), low-frequency stimulation (P<.001), and standard stimulation (P<.001). Twenty-four patients were classified as responders to the therapy, and 23 patients out of 44 trailed underwent permanent implant. Significant differences in VAS scores were observed between baseline and all follow-up visits during phase II (P<.001).[19] In addition, the combination of PNFS and SCS has been used in several studies.[6,7,49]
5. Musculoskeletal pain. This pain is one of the emerging indications for PNFS. PNFS applied directly to an affected knee was found to be extremely effective for the relief of knee pain.[4] In the authors' experience, this also holds true for shoulder and elbow pain.
6. Other emerging indications. Fibromyalgia is a condition marked by widespread chronic pain, accompanied by a variety of other symptoms, including sleep and fatigue disorders, headaches, disorders of the autonomic nervous system, and cognitive and psychiatric symptoms. Recent literature shows that PNFS is effective in treating fibromyalgia.[50–52]

SURGICAL TECHNIQUE

The surgical technique for PNFS is simple, and involves subcutaneous placement of stimulating electrodes, small incisions, and placement of an appropriate implantable pulse generator (IPG).

1. Type of electrodes. For PNFS the electrodes used are generally cylindrical leads implanted in the vicinity of the stimulated nerve or under the area of pain. Occasionally paddle electrodes are used for occipital nerve stimulation.[36] For true PNS, multicontact paddle electrodes may be used as an overlay or to sandwich the nerve (**Fig. 1**) after the nerve is surgically exposed.
2. Location of electrodes. In PNS the electrode leads are placed above or below the fascia close to the affected nerve, whereas in PNFS the course of the electrode lead is independent of the nerve path. The depth of placement is important, as electrodes that are too close to dermal layer will cause a stinging or burning sensation and, eventually, lead erosion, and electrodes that are too deep may cause unintended muscular stimulation and the twitching of muscles. A useful tool in the placement of PNFS electrodes is an ON-Q tunneler (I-Flow, Lake Forest, CA) (**Fig. 2**). By virtue of its blunt tip and flexibility, and adequate inner lumen to accommodate the electrodes without making a large tunnel, it helps to accommodate the body contours and reliably follows the subcutaneous plane. As an alternative, a

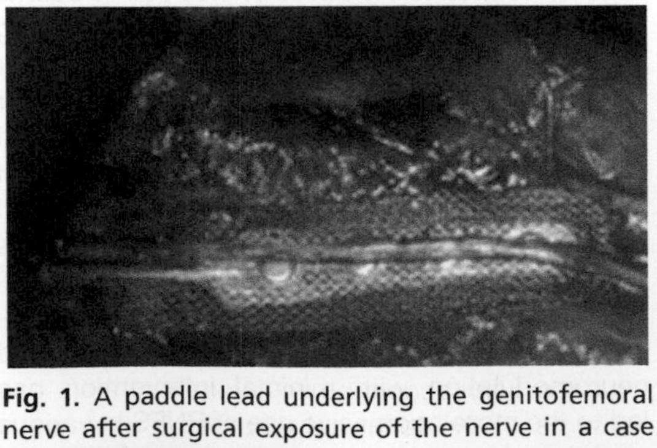

Fig. 1. A paddle lead underlying the genitofemoral nerve after surgical exposure of the nerve in a case of genitofemoral neuralgia.

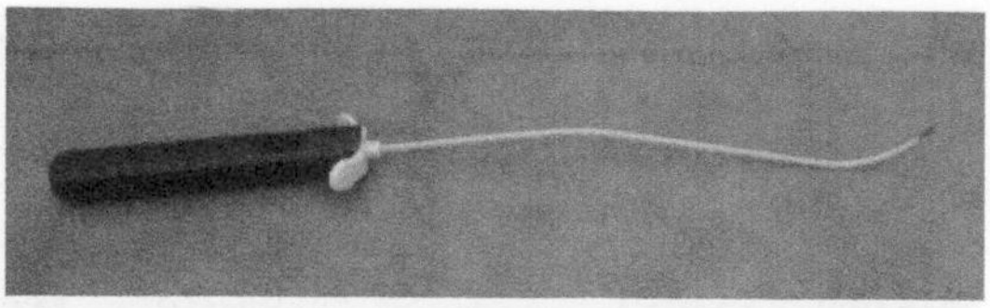

Fig. 2. ON-Q tunneler (I-Flow, Lake Forest, CA). Because of its blunt tip, flexibility, and adequate inner lumen to accommodate the electrodes without making a large tunnel, it helps to accommodate to body contours and always moves in the subcutaneous plane.

custom-made kit consisting of a curved needle and interchangeable stylets with sharp and blunt tips may be used for percutaneous PNFS electrode insertion (Deogaonkar, personal communication, 2013). Some centers use ultrasound guidance for identifying the right plane of placement or for identifying the nerve.[39,42,53]

3. Placement of electrodes in relation to the area of pain. The electrodes are generally placed close to the affected nerve (in the case of PNS) or underlying the area of pain (in the case of PNFS). In patients with severe allodynia, outcomes are better if the electrodes bracket the area of pain rather than cross it.
4. Anchors. Every center has its own opinion on which commercially available anchors to use and whether to use anchors at all. The general rule for craniofacial or limb electrode leads is that low-profile anchors are better suited because large anchors can themselves become a source of discomfort. Figure-of-8 sutures (nonabsorbable [silk or Dacron] but not monofilament, such as Prolene) work as effectively as any anchor.
5. IPG placement. With newer, smaller, rechargeable models, there is an abundance of choice regarding IPGs. For the authors' craniofacial cases including occipital nerve stimulators (ONS), an infraclavicular IPG placement is more efficient and has less chance of lead migration. In truncal PNFS placement, the IPG may be placed in the lower back, flank, or abdominal wall. In extremity PNFS placement, the IPG should be placed in such a way that the number of joints crossed by wires is minimized. The authors have placed IPGs in the thigh in cases of meralgia paresthetica and posterior thigh pain (**Fig. 3**), and in calf in cases of infrapatellar pain, with good results.
6. Technical considerations for individual indications. Incisions for the placement of electrode leads vary according to indication. Here are some of the technical nuances with each of the aforementioned indications:

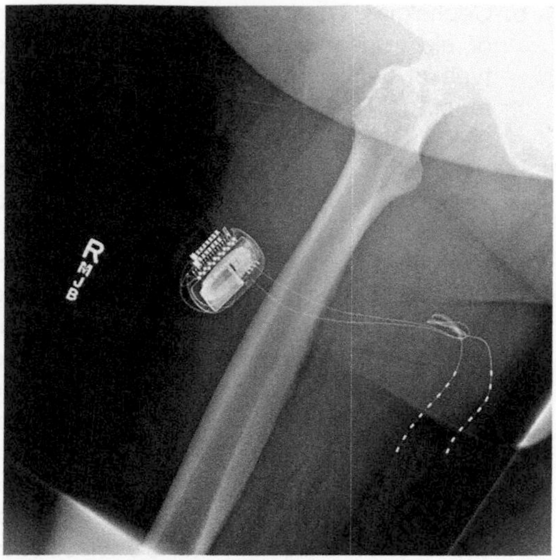

Fig. 3. A postoperative radiograph showing posterior thigh PNFS electrodes with an implantable pulse generator placed in the lateral thigh.

a. ONS. A variety of leads and approaches are used for ONS.[36,48,54–56] Incisions are either midline or laterally placed. The leads are either placed transversely at the level of C2 or directed laterally toward the ipsilateral mastoid process from the midline. Some centers use paddle leads, others use cylindrical leads. In all cases, however, the basic features of crossing the course of the occipital nerve and the subcutaneous placement of the leads remain (**Fig. 4**).

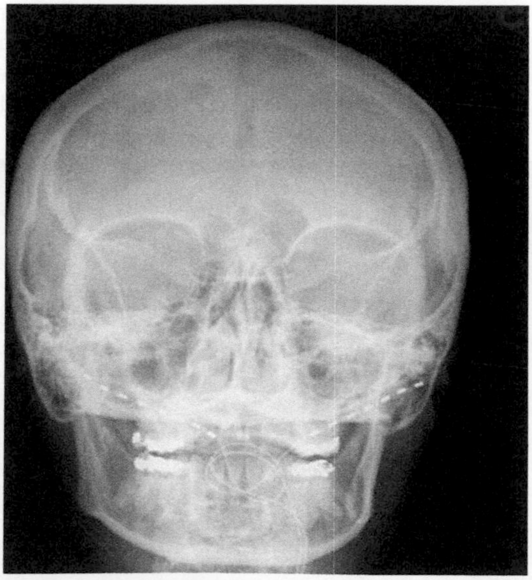

Fig. 4. An anteroposterior (AP) radiograph of an occipital nerve stimulator placed though the midline, using cylindrical leads going toward ipsilateral mastoid processes.

b. Cephalgias. The location and configuration of electrodes changes depending on the type of headache. For cluster headaches, most published experience suggests the use of ONS, but a combination of supraorbital (SO) and infraorbital (IO) electrodes seems to be fairly effective. For generalized intractable headaches or migraines, a combination of bilateral SO and ONS has been the most effective (**Fig. 5**).[55] The same combination can be used on one side for hemicrania continua. Depending on the number of electrodes used, 1 or 2 IPGs may be needed to power these electrodes. The incisions are kept behind the hairline.

c. Trigeminal neuropathic pain. The electrodes may be placed in each affected division of the trigeminal nerve. The SO electrodes should remain distant to the eyebrow, otherwise they tend to erode the skin. The IO electrodes should not be very close to the angle of the eye, otherwise they can cause eye twitching. The authors have not found any increased incidence of mandibular electrode migration as mentioned in a previous study.[32] Incisions are usually placed behind the hairline in the temporal or supra-auricular region, and the IPGs are placed in the infraclavicular area (**Fig. 6**).

d. Truncal pain. The most common indications for this are PHN or inguinal neuralgia.[8] The electrodes are generally placed parallel to the axis of pain, and because truncal PHN pain is mostly in an elongated shape, the electrode leads are placed in tandem around the area of pain (**Fig. 7**). For inguinal pain, the electrodes are placed close to the ilioinguinal nerve localized with ultrasound, or based on location of a positive Tinel sign near the herniorrhaphy scar.

e. Axial pain. Use of PNFS for axial back pain or neck pain is becoming more common. The electrodes are placed in a way to cover the maximum area of pain. In cases of greater pain distribution, the area of most severe pain is covered by the PNFS electrodes. The electrodes can be placed across or around the area of pain with small incisions placed at the periphery of the pain area (**Fig. 8**).[13]

f. Extremity pain. While placing the electrodes for joint pain they should be positioned or tunneled away from the flexor surfaces of joints, preferably on the lateral aspects. There is always a greater chance of electrode migration in distal limb areas, so anchoring becomes important (**Fig. 9**).[55]

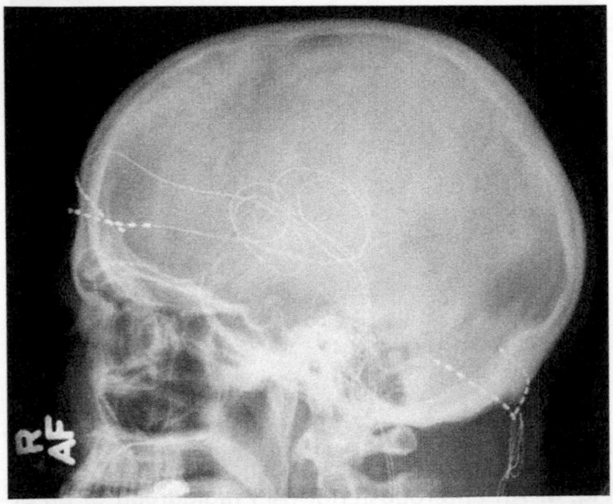

Fig. 5. A lateral radiograph of bilateral supraorbital and occipital nerve stimulators placed for intractable migraines.

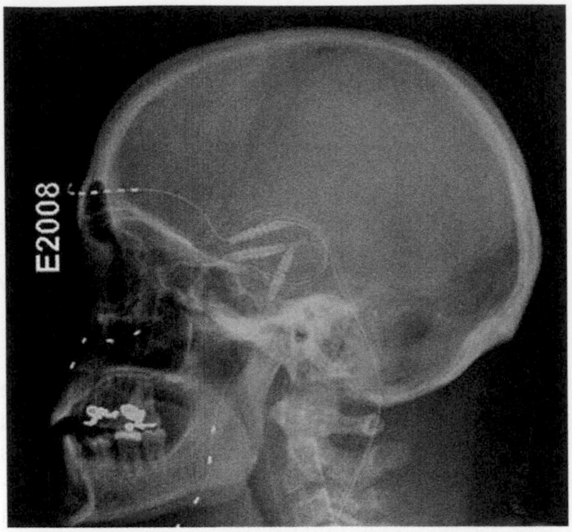

Fig. 6. A lateral radiograph of trigeminal nerve stimulators placed for intractable trigeminal neuropathic pain in all 3 divisions of the trigeminal nerve.

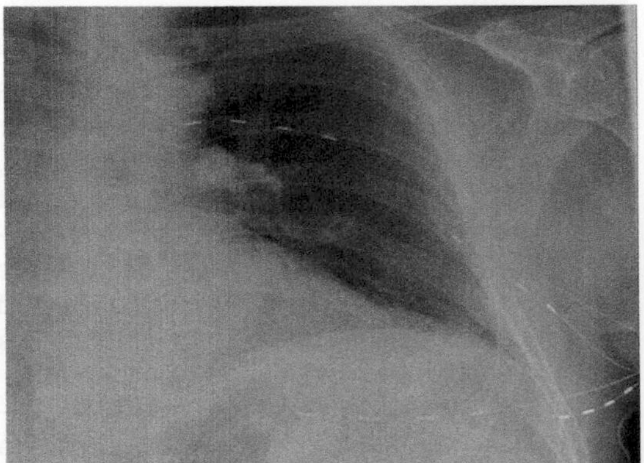

Fig. 7. An AP radiograph of the chest showing stimulators placed for post-herpetic neuralgia.

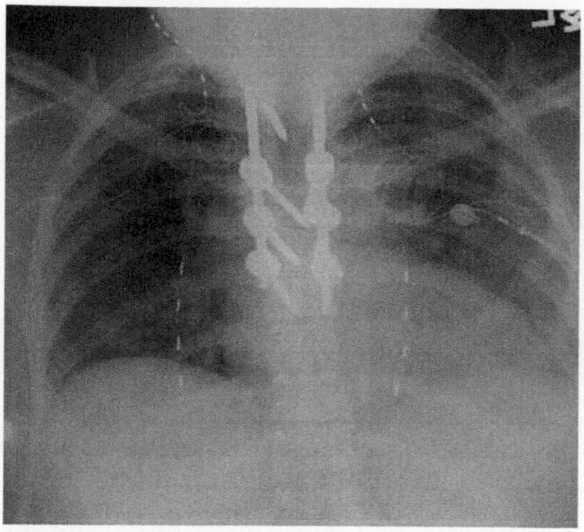

Fig. 8. An AP radiograph of the chest showing stimulators placed for axial cervicothoracic pain.

PROGRAMMING OF PNFS

Distinctive features of PNFS programming are lower rate, lower pulse width, and lower amplitude. As long as the electrodes are optimally placed, the programing of PNFS is very simple.

1. Rate. Most patients like the rate to be between 20 and 50 Hz. Anything higher than this may be felt as a very strong sensation, or cause burning or pinching.
2. Pulse width (PW). PW in the range of 90 to 250 milliseconds is best tolerated. Higher PW may cause a pinching or burning sensation of the skin. If the leads are placed too deep, a higher PW may be helpful. In hybrid stimulation[7] whereby anodes and cathodes are paired on epidural and PNFS leads, higher PW is generally used.
3. Amplitude. Optimally placed PNFS leads do not need more than 1.5 to 2 mA for adequate stimulation. Deeper leads will need higher stimulation amplitudes.
4. Contact polarity. Most often a simple bipolar setting is most effective. The number of cathodes should be limited, as it needs higher charge resulting in more frequent IPG recharging or, in the case of nonrechargeable IPGs, an earlier IPG replacement.

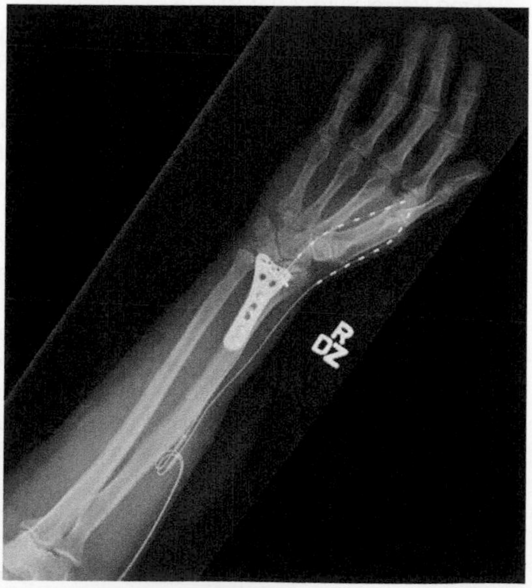

Fig. 9. A radiograph of the forearm and hand showing stimulators placed for wrist pain and neuropathic pain caused by medial nerve injury.

OUTCOMES AND COMPLICATIONS

Several case reports, case series, and retrospective studies, and one prospective trial show the efficacy of PNFS in reducing chronic pain.[3,19,28,49,55,57–59] On average, there is 50% reduction seen on VAS for pain that is sustained over an extended period (**Fig. 10**).[55] In the only published prospective, randomized, controlled, crossover study, a consistent 50% reduction in pain was obtained with PNFS with effective stimulation ($P = .003$).[19] A significant reduction in VAS scores was observed also between baseline and all follow-up visits during the stimulation phase with PNFS ($P<.001$). Most of the present published evidence supports the safety and effectiveness of PNFS as an aid in the management of chronic, localized pain, and shows around 50% improvement in pain scores.

Complications of PNFS include infection (up to 5%), erosion (5%), and migration of electrodes (5%). The rate of complications depends on implanter experience and optimal placement of the device. Adequate depth of electrode insertion, proper length of electrodes, appropriate selection of anchors, consideration of different angles and axes of force with movement of body parts, and strict aseptic precautions help minimize the rate of complications.

FUTURE DIRECTIONS

Neuromodulation is progressing toward simplicity and minimal invasiveness. This approach, coupled with smaller IPGs, novel smaller leads, and more experience with different indications, makes PNFS the apparent next frontier in neuromodulation. In addition, the ability to affect central neuromodulation processes with peripheral stimulation is a very attractive proposition. As with any

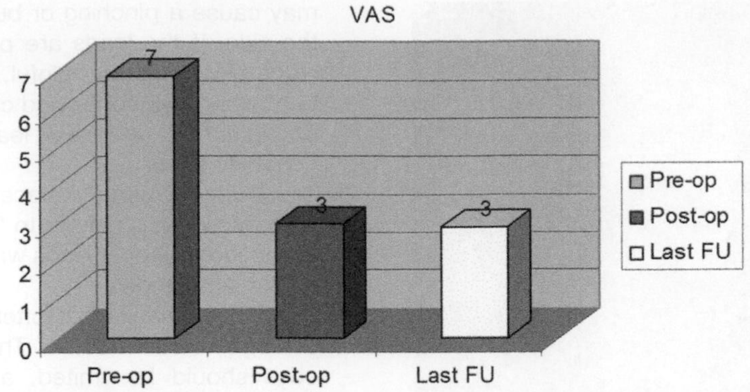

Fig. 10. Chart showing visual analog scale (VAS) scores in a cohort of 170 patients with PNFS with 1 to 5 years of follow-up (FU).

technology, it must be used wisely. Randomized, controlled, double-blind trials and evidence-based specific practice guidelines will help the field expand in a more orderly and scientific fashion.

REFERENCES

1. Wall PD, Sweet WH. Temporary abolition of pain in man. Science 1967;155:108–9.
2. Al-Jehani H, Jacques L. Peripheral nerve stimulation for chronic neurogenic pain. Prog Neurol Surg 2011;24:27–40.
3. Slavin KV. Peripheral nerve stimulation for neuropathic pain. Neurotherapeutics 2008;5:100–6.
4. McRoberts WP, Roche M. Novel approach for peripheral subcutaneous field stimulation for the treatment of severe, chronic knee joint pain after total knee arthroplasty. Neuromodulation 2010;13:131–6.
5. Paicius RM, Bernstein CA, Lempert-Cohen C. Peripheral nerve field stimulation in chronic abdominal pain. Pain Physician 2006;9:261–6.
6. Lipov EG. 'Hybrid neurostimulator': simultaneous use of spinal cord and peripheral nerve field stimulation to treat low back and leg pain. Prog Neurol Surg 2011;24:147–55.
7. Navarro RM, Vercimak DC. Triangular stimulation method utilizing combination spinal cord stimulation with peripheral subcutaneous field stimulation for chronic pain patients: a retrospective study. Neuromodulation 2012;15:124–31.
8. Cairns KD, McRoberts WP, Deer T. Peripheral nerve stimulation for the treatment of truncal pain. Prog Neurol Surg 2011;24:58–69.
9. Melzack R, Wall PD. Pain mechanisms: a new theory. Science 1965;150:971–9.
10. Bartsch T, Goadsby PJ. Central mechanisms of peripheral nerve stimulation in headache disorders. Prog Neurol Surg 2011;24:16–26.
11. Ellrich J, Lamp S. Peripheral nerve stimulation inhibits nociceptive processing: an electrophysiological study in healthy volunteers. Neuromodulation 2005;8:225–32.
12. Hegarty D, Goroszeniuk T. Peripheral nerve stimulation of the thoracic paravertebral plexus for chronic neuropathic pain. Pain Physician 2011;14:295–300.
13. Burgher AH, Huntoon MA, Turley TW, et al. Subcutaneous peripheral nerve stimulation with inter-lead stimulation for axial neck and low back pain: case series and review of the literature. Neuromodulation 2012;15:100–6 [discussion: 106–7].
14. Rasskazoff SY, Slavin KV. Neuromodulation for cephalgias. Surg Neurol Intl 2013;4(Suppl 3):S136–50.
15. Slavin KV. History of peripheral nerve stimulation. Prog Neurol Surg 2011;24:1–15.
16. Sweet WH. Control of pain by direct electrical stimulation of peripheral nerves. Clin Neurosurg 1976;23:103–11.
17. Yakovlev AE, Resch BE. Treatment of chronic intractable hip pain after iliac crest bone graft harvest using peripheral nerve field stimulation. Neuromodulation 2011;14:156–9.
18. Patil AA, Otto D, Raikar S. Peripheral nerve field stimulation for sacroiliac joint pain. Neuromodulation 2013. http://dx.doi.org/10.1111/ner.12030.
19. McRoberts WP, Wolkowitz R, Meyer DJ, et al. Peripheral nerve field stimulation for the management of localized chronic intractable back pain: results from a randomized controlled study. Neuromodulation 2013. http://dx.doi.org/10.1111/ner.12055.
20. Abejon D, Krames ES. Peripheral nerve stimulation or is it peripheral subcutaneous field stimulation; what is in a moniker? Neuromodulation 2009;12(1):1–4.
21. Campbell CM, Jamison RN, Edwards RR. Psychological screening/phenotyping as predictors for

spinal cord stimulation. Curr Pain Headache Rep 2013;17(1):307.

22. Mekhail NA, Mathews M, Nageeb F, et al. Retrospective review of 707 cases of spinal cord stimulation: indications and complications. Pain Pract 2011;11:148–53.
23. Kumar K, Hunter G, Demeria D. Spinal cord stimulation in treatment of chronic benign pain: challenges in treatment planning and present status, a 22-year experience. Neurosurgery 2006;58: 481–96.
24. Bittar RG, Teddy PJ. Peripheral neuromodulation for pain. J Clin Neurosci 2009;16:1259–61.
25. Ellens DJ, Levy RM. Peripheral neuromodulation for migraine headache. Prog Neurol Surg 2011;24: 109–17.
26. Slavin KV, Colpan ME, Munawar N, et al. Trigeminal and occipital peripheral nerve stimulation for craniofacial pain: a single-institution experience and review of the literature. Neurosurg Focus 2006;21(6):E5.
27. Slavin KV, Wess C. Trigeminal branch stimulation for intractable neuropathic pain: technical note. Neuromodulation 2005;8:7–13.
28. Krutsch JP, McCeney MH, Barolat G, et al. A case report of subcutaneous peripheral nerve stimulation for the treatment of axial back pain associated with postlaminectomy syndrome. Neuromodulation 2008;11:112–5.
29. Nathan PW, Wall PD. Treatment of post-herpetic neuralgia by prolonged electric stimulation. Br Med J 1974;3:645–7.
30. Mekhail NA, Cheng J, Narouze S, et al. Clinical applications of neurostimulation: forty years later. Pain Pract 2010;10:103–12.
31. Dunteman E. Peripheral nerve stimulation for unremitting ophthalmic postherpetic neuralgia. Neuromodulation 2002;5:32–7.
32. Johnson MD, Burchiel KJ. Peripheral stimulation for treatment of trigeminal postherpetic neuralgia and trigeminal posttraumatic neuropathic pain: a pilot study. Neurosurgery 2004;55:135–41 [discussion: 141–2].
33. Hsu E, Cohen SP. Postamputation pain: epidemiology, mechanisms, and treatment. J Pain Res 2013;6:121–36.
34. Stidd DA, Wuollet AL, Bowden K, et al. Peripheral nerve stimulation for trigeminal neuropathic pain. Pain Physician 2012;15:27–33.
35. Benoliel R, Zadik Y, Eliav E, et al. Peripheral painful traumatic trigeminal neuropathy: clinical features in 91 cases and proposal of novel diagnostic criteria. J Orofac Pain 2012;26:49–58.
36. Abhinav K, Park ND, Prakash SK, et al. Novel use of narrow paddle electrodes for occipital nerve stimulation—technical note. Neuromodulation 2012. http://dx.doi.org/10.1111/j.1525-1403.2012.00524.x.
37. Alo KM, Abramova MV, Richter EO. Percutaneous peripheral nerve stimulation. Prog Neurol Surg 2011;24:41–57.
38. Deshpande KK, Wininger KL. Feasibility of combined epicranial temporal and occipital neurostimulation: treatment of a challenging case of headache. Pain Physician 2011;14:37–44.
39. Eldrige JS, Obray JB, Pingree MJ, et al. Occipital neuromodulation: ultrasound guidance for peripheral nerve stimulator implantation. Pain Pract 2010;10:580–5.
40. Skaribas I, Alo K. Ultrasound imaging and occipital nerve stimulation. Neuromodulation 2010;13: 126–30.
41. Stojanovic MP. Stimulation methods for neuropathic pain control. Curr Pain Headache Rep 2001;5:130–7.
42. Carayannopoulos A, Beasley R, Sites B. Facilitation of percutaneous trial lead placement with ultrasound guidance for peripheral nerve stimulation trial of ilioinguinal neuralgia: a technical note. Neuromodulation 2009;12:296–301.
43. Monti E. Peripheral nerve stimulation: a percutaneous minimally invasive approach. Neuromodulation 2004;7:193–6.
44. Perini F, De Boni A. Peripheral neuromodulation in chronic migraine. Neurol Sci 2012;33(Suppl 1): S29–31.
45. Mammis A, Gudesblatt M, Mogilner AY. Peripheral neurostimulation for the treatment of refractory cluster headache, long-term follow-up: case report. Neuromodulation 2011;14:432–5.
46. Jenkins B, Tepper SJ. Neurostimulation for primary headache disorders: part 2, review of central neurostimulators for primary headache, overall therapeutic efficacy, safety, cost, patient selection, and future research in headache neuromodulation. Headache 2011;51:1408–18.
47. Broggi G, Messina G, Marras C, et al. Neuromodulation for refractory headaches. Neurol Sci 2010; 31(Suppl 1):S87–92.
48. Trentman TL, Rosenfeld DM, Vargas BB, et al. Greater occipital nerve stimulation via the Bion microstimulator: implantation technique and stimulation parameters. Clinical trial: NCT00205894. Pain Physician 2009;12:621–8.
49. Reverberi C, Dario A, Barolat G. Spinal cord stimulation (SCS) in conjunction with peripheral nerve field stimulation (PNfS) for the treatment of complex pain in failed back surgery syndrome (FBSS). Neuromodulation 2013;16:78–82 [discussion: 83].
50. Plazier M, Vanneste S, Dekelver I, et al. Peripheral nerve stimulation for fibromyalgia. Prog Neurol Surg 2011;24:133–46.
51. Thimineur M, De Ridder D. C2 area neurostimulation: a surgical treatment for fibromyalgia. Pain Med 2007;8:639–46.

52. Slavin KV. Peripheral neurostimulation in fibromyalgia: a new frontier?! Pain Med 2007;8:621–2.
53. Chan I, Brown AR, Park K, et al. Ultrasound-guided, percutaneous peripheral nerve stimulation: technical note. Neurosurgery 2010;67(3 Suppl Operative):ons136–9.
54. Trentman TL, Zimmerman RS, Dodick DW. Occipital nerve stimulation: technical and surgical aspects of implantation. Prog Neurol Surg 2011;24:96–108.
55. Vadera S, Machado A, Boulis NM, et al. Peripheral nerve stimulation for chronic pain: one institution's experience. Neurosurgery 2009;65:416–7.
56. Trentman TL, Slavin KV, Freeman JA, et al. Occipital nerve stimulator placement via a retromastoid to infraclavicular approach: a technical report. Stereotact Funct Neurosurg 2010;88:121–5.
57. Al Tamimi M, Davids HR, Barolat G, et al. Subcutaneous peripheral nerve stimulation treatment for chronic pelvic pain. Neuromodulation 2008;11:277–81.
58. Tamimi MA, Davids HR, Langston MM, et al. Successful treatment of chronic neuropathic pain with subcutaneous peripheral nerve stimulation: four case reports. Neuromodulation 2009;12:210–4.
59. Sator-Katzenschlager S, Fiala K, Kress HG, et al. Subcutaneous target stimulation (STS) in chronic noncancer pain: a nationwide retrospective study. Pain Pract 2010;10:279–86.

Peripheral Neuromodulation for Treatment of Chronic Migraine Headache

Daryoush Tavanaiepour, MD, Robert M. Levy, MD, PhD*

KEYWORDS

• Migraine • Neuromodulation • Occipital nerve stimulation • Headache

KEY POINTS

- Chronic migraine affects a large proportion of the population and is a significant source of disability and lost productivity.
- Traditional neurosurgical procedures that favor lesioning or decompressing the greater occipital nerve have not gained favor.
- Occipital nerve stimulation provides an attractive nondestructive alternative, but its degree of efficacy remains to be fully elucidated in randomized controlled trials.
- Mechanism of action is unknown but it has been attributed to the gate theory of pain or modulation of the trigeminocervical complex in the rostral spinal cord.

Between 25 and 45 million Americans experience migraine headaches; approximately 2.0% have chronic migraine (CM) headaches.[1,2] CM is characterized by a minimum of 15 headache days per month, and approximately half of the headache days meet the diagnostic criteria for migraine without aura or respond to a migraine-specific acute medication.[3] Individuals with CM are 4 times more likely to have major depression with more frequent suicide attempts than in the general population.[4–6] Furthermore, compared with episodic migraine, CM is associated with significantly greater disability, economic burden, and impairments in health-related quality of life.[7–10]

Pharmacotherapy for migraine headaches includes medications to relieve the acute pain (abortive agents) and medication to prevent the onset of headache (preventative agents). Abortive agents include nonsteroidal antiinflammatory agents, tryptans, opioids, ergot compounds, and sedatives. Preventative agents include anticonvulsants, antidepressants, β-adrenergic blockers, and serotonin antagonists. In addition, recognition and prevention of exposure to precipitating agents such as caffeine, many foods including cheeses and red wines, and stress can provide significant relief and reduce medication intake.

Historically, neurosurgical therapies for headache have included destructive procedures including dorsal root entry zone (DREZ) lesioning, dorsal root ganglionectomy, peripheral neurolysis, and neurectomy. These therapies, however, have not been effective for migraine headaches and such techniques may result in secondary neuropathic pain in the distribution of the surgically treated nerve(s). For example, ganglionectomy at the second cervical level has been reported to be 80% effective at 3 year follow-up in posttraumatic second cervical pain syndromes.[11] Nontraumatic pain in this region, however, was not significantly relieved by ganglionectomy. Ventrolateral DREZ lesioning at the first, second, or third cervical level has been variably effective for occipital neuralgia but is highly invasive and has

Department of Neurological Surgery, University of Florida College of Medicine, Jacksonville, FL, USA
* Corresponding author.
E-mail address: rlevy@neuromodulation.com

Neurosurg Clin N Am 25 (2014) 11–14
http://dx.doi.org/10.1016/j.nec.2013.08.010
1042-3680/14/$ – see front matter

significant risks.[12] Greater occipital nerve neurolysis has demonstrated short-term efficacy, however, there was a significant recurrence rate within 2 years.[13] In addition to neurolysis and neurectomy, fusion of the first and second cervical vertebrae has relieved pain in some patients with occipital neuralgia.[14]

Initially, peripheral nerve stimulation using a cuff electrode or direct stimulation of the greater occipital nerve was found to be effective for treating occipital neuralgia.[15,16] More recently, peripheral neuromodulation in the occipital region has emerged as a promising treatment modality for a variety of chronic headache disorders, including CM.[17–25] Weiner and Reed[26] first reported the use of occipital nerve stimulation (ONS) for the treatment of occipital neuralgia. However, positron emission tomography (PET) imaging of these patients demonstrated activation patterns more consistent with CM than with occipital neuralgia, leading Matharu and colleagues[17] to suggest that Weiner and Reed's patients suffered from CM. Since then, ONS has been reported to be efficacious for the treatment of several headache disorders including migraine headaches,[4,5] cluster headache,[6] hemicrania continua,[25] and true occipital neuralgia.[24]

An extensive literature search was performed with a specific focus on high-quality clinical trials of peripheral neuromodulation for the treatment of intractable CM. This search revealed 6 independent and 3 industry-sponsored clinical trials, the results of which are listed here.

INDEPENDENT CLINICAL TRIALS

- Weiner and Reed.[26] This open-label trial included 13 patients implanted with percutaneous occipital leads for CM. Twelve patients reported a good to excellent response and required minimal oral analgesic medications at follow-up ranging from 18 months to 6 years.
- Popeney and Alo.[25] This open-label trial included 25 patients implanted with percutaneous occipital leads for CM. At the 18-month follow-up, 88% of patients showed a positive response, with an overall 50% reduction in the number of headache days per month.
- Oh and colleagues.[27] This open-label trial included 20 patients with transformed migraine headaches implanted with paddle-type occipital nerve stimulating leads. At 6 months, 80% of patients reported greater than 75% pain relief and 95% reported improvement in their quality of life and their willingness to undergo the procedure again.
- Slavin and colleagues.[28] This open-label trial included 10 patients with CM implanted with percutaneous occipital nerve stimulating leads. At the 22-month follow-up, 70% of patients had pain reduction ranging from 60% to 90% with a corresponding decrease in the use of analgesics.
- Levy.[29] This open-label prospective trial included 45 patients treated with peripheral nerve stimulation for CM. At the 2-year follow-up, 83% of patients reported good to excellent (>50% relief) results with an additional 9% of patients reporting fair (30%–50%) results; 92% of the patients reported satisfaction with the therapy, a willingness to have the device implanted again based on their treatment experience, and their unwillingness to have the device removed even at no cost.
- Silberstein and colleagues.[30] This prospective, randomized, double-blind study included 157 patients with CM randomized 2:1 between active (n = 105) and sham (n = 52) ONS. At 12 weeks, there was no statistically significant difference between the groups in terms of responder rate, defined as greater than 50% pain reduction, which was their primary end point. There was, however, a statistically significant difference between groups at the level of 30% pain reduction. Furthermore, the active group had a statistically significant reduction in the number of headache days and in the degree of migraine-related disability.

INDUSTRY-SPONSORED CLINICAL TRIALS

In 2013, peripheral neurostimulation for the treatment of CM has been approved for use in the European Union and in Australia. However, it has not yet been approved by the US Food and Drug Administration (FDA). ONS for CM is therefore used by physicians in the United States on an off-label basis. Industry is not allowed to market or promote the use of their products for off-label indications. Because of this limitation and the significant potential of this therapy for the treatment of migraine headache, the 3 major device manufacturers in this sector (Medtronic, Boston Scientific, St. Jude Medical) have sponsored research trials to investigate the safety and efficacy of their neurostimulation products for the treatment of migraine headaches.

Medtronic ONSTIM Trial

The Occipital Nerve Stimulation for the Treatment of Intractable Migraine (ONSTIM) trial, sponsored by Medtronic, was a multicenter, randomized, blind, controlled feasibility study. Patients with CM were included if they responded to occipital nerve block and were randomized to 3 groups: adjustable stimulation (AS), preset (sham) stimulation (PS), or medical management (MM). Seventy-five of the 110 enrolled participants were assigned to a treatment group and complete data were available for 66 of these patients. The response rate, defined as greater than 50% pain reduction, was 39%, 6%, and 0% for the AS, PS, and MM groups, respectively. Lead migration occurred in 24% of patients and infections developed in 14%.[20]

Boston Scientific PRISM Trial

The Precision Implantable Stimulator for Migraine (PRISM) trial, sponsored by Boston Scientific, was a prospective, randomized, double-blind, placebo-controlled trial of ONS for medically intractable migraine. All 139 patients had 6 days or more per month of migraine headaches and had failed therapy with a least 2 acute and 2 preventative medications. Before permanent implantation, all participants underwent percutaneous trial stimulation. There was a 12-week blind period when patients were randomized to receive bilateral active stimulation or sham stimulation; after 12 weeks, all patients were converted to active stimulation. The primary end point of the study at 12 weeks was change from baseline in migraine days per month; there was no significant difference between groups. Following permanent implantation, however, patients with a positive percutaneous trial demonstrated a reduction of 8.8 migraine days per month compared with a reduction of only 0.7 migraine days for those patients for whom the trial failed to provide relief ($P<.001$). The most frequent adverse events were device infection, non–target area sensory phenomena, and pain at the implant site. These results were presented at the 14th Congress of the International Headache Society and the 51st Annual Scientific Meeting of the American Headache Society in September, 2009.

St. Jude Medical Trial

St. Jude Medical Neuromodulation sponsored a randomized, controlled, pivotal trial of ONS for CM; 150 patients from 15 centers were enrolled, with success defined as a 50% reduction in pain and no increase in headache frequency or duration. Patients were randomized to either a stimulation trial followed by device implantation and active stimulation for 12 weeks or a stimulation trial followed by device implantation but sham stimulation for 12 weeks. After 12 weeks, participants were unblinded but patients were followed for 1 year. Data collection from this study have been completed and publication is pending.

MECHANISM OF ACTION

The exact mechanism of peripheral neuromodulation for CM is unknown; however, there are 2 prevailing theories. The first proposed mechanism is similar to the pain gait theory implicated in the mechanism of action of spinal cord or peripheral nerve stimulation for somatic neuropathic pain.[31] The second theory, based on a PET imaging study, suggests that ONS results in retrograde modulation of the brainstem nuclei involved in the trigeminal-vascular system thus inhibiting or aborting migraine headaches.[32]

SUMMARY

Peripheral nerve stimulation, whether of the occipital nerve(s) alone or in combination with others, seems to be both safe and effective for the treatment of medically intractable migraine headaches. Further work is needed to optimize our knowledge regarding patient selection, stimulation targets and parameters, and device programing. At present, neurostimulation for migraine headache pain is performed in the United States on an off-label basis, but based on our experience and the increasing evidence in the medical literature, we can look forward to its approval by the FDA in the near future so that patients with severe, medically intractable headache pain may gain access to these potentially important therapies.

REFERENCES

1. Bigal ME, Serrano D, Reed M, et al. Chronic migraine in the population: burden, diagnosis, and satisfaction with treatment. Neurology 2008;71: 559–66.
2. Natoli JL, Manack A, Dean B, et al. Global prevalence of chronic migraine: a systematic review. Cephalalgia 2010;30:599–609.
3. Headache Classification Committee. The international classification of headache disorders: 2nd edition. Cephalalgia 2004;24(Suppl 1):1–160.
4. Pompili M, Di CD, Innamorati M, et al. Psychiatric comorbidity in patients with chronic daily headache and migraine: a selective overview including personality traits and suicide risk. J Headache Pain 2009;10:283–90.
5. Breslau N, Merikangas K, Bowden CL. Comorbidity of migraine and major affective disorders. Neurology 1994;44(Suppl 7):17–22.

6. Breslau N, Davis GC, Andreski P. Migraine, psychiatric disorders and suicide attempts: an epidemiological study of young adults. Psychiatry Res 1991; 37:11–23.
7. Bigal ME, Rapoport AM, Lipton RB, et al. Assessment of migraine disability using the migraine disability assessment (MIDAS) questionnaire: a comparison of chronic migraine with episodic migraine. Headache 2003;43:336–42.
8. Meletiche DM, Lofland JH, Young WB. Quality of life differences between patients with episodic and transformed migraine. Headache 2001;41: 573–8.
9. Munakata J, Hazard E, Serrano D, et al. Economic burden of transformed migraine: results from the American Migraine Prevalence and Prevention (AMPP) study. Headache 2009;49:498–508.
10. Blumenfeld AM, Varon SF, Wilcox TK, et al. Disability, HRQoL and resource use among chronic and episodic migraineurs: results from the International Burden of Migraine Study (IBMS). Cephalalgia 2011;31:301–15.
11. Lozano AM, Vanderlindon G, Bachou R, et al. Microsurgical C-2 ganglionectomy for chronic intractable occipital pain. J Neurosurg 1998;89(3):359–65.
12. Dubuisson D. Treatment of occipital neuralgia by partial posterior rhizotomy at C1-3. J Neurosurg 1995;82(4):581–6.
13. Bovim G, Fredriksen TA, Stolt-Nielsen A, et al. Neurolysis of the greater occipital nerve in cervicogenic headache. A follow up study. Headache 1992;32(4): 175–9.
14. Joseph B, Kumar B. Gallie's fusion for atlantoaxial arthrosis with occipital neuralgia. Spine (Phila Pa 1976) 1994;19(4):454–5.
15. Picaza JA, Hunter SE, Cannon BW, et al. Pain suppression by peripheral nerve stimulation. Chronic effects of implanted devices. Appl Neurophysiol 1977; 40(2–4):223–34.
16. Waisbrod H, Panhans C, Hansen D, et al. Direct nerve stimulation for painful peripheral neuropathies. J Bone Joint Surg Br 1985;67(3):470–2.
17. Matharu MS, Bartsch T, Ward N, et al. Central neuromodulation in chronic migraine patients with suboccipital stimulators: a PET study. Brain 2004;127(Pt 1): 220–30.
18. Schwedt TJ, Dodick DW, Trentman TL, et al. Occipital nerve stimulation for chronic cluster headache and hemicrania continua: pain relief and persistence of autonomic features. Cephalalgia 2006;26:1025–7.
19. Schwedt TJ, Dodick DW, Hentz J, et al. Occipital nerve stimulation for chronic headache–long-term safety and efficacy. Cephalalgia 2007;27:153–7.
20. Saper JR, Dodick DW, Silberstein SD, et al. Occipital nerve stimulation for the treatment of intractable chronic migraine headache: ONSTIM feasibility study. Cephalalgia 2011;31:271–85.
21. Burns B, Watkins L, Goadsby PJ. Treatment of medically intractable cluster headache by occipital nerve stimulation: long-term follow-up of eight patients. Lancet 2007;369:1099–106.
22. Magis D, Allena M, Bolla M, et al. Occipital nerve stimulation for drug-resistant chronic cluster headache: a prospective pilot study. Lancet Neurol 2007;6:314–21.
23. Reed KL, Black SB, Banta CJ, et al. Combined occipital and supraorbital neurostimulation for the treatment of chronic migraine headaches: initial experience. Cephalalgia 2010;30:260–71.
24. Mueller OM, Gaul C, Katsarava Z, et al. Occipital nerve stimulation for the treatment of chronic cluster headache - lessons learned from 18 months experience. Cent Eur Neurosurg 2011;72:84–9.
25. Popeney CA, Alo KM. Peripheral neurostimulation for the treatment of chronic, disabling transformed migraine. Headache 2003;43:369–75.
26. Weiner RL, Reed KL. Peripheral neurostimulation for the control of intractable occipital neuralgia. Neuromodulation 1999;2:369–75.
27. Oh MY, Ortega J, Bellotte JB, et al. Peripheral nerve stimulation for the treatment of occipital neuralgia and transformed migraine using a C1-2-3 subcutaneous paddle style electrode: a technical report. Neuromodulation 2004;7(2):103–12.
28. Slavin KV, Nersesyan H, Wess C, et al. Peripheral neurostimulation for treatment of intractable occipital neuralgia. Neurosurgery 2006;58(1):112–9 [discussion: 112–9].
29. Levy RM. Northwestern study of peripheral neurostimulation for HA. 2009.
30. Silberstein SD, Dodick DW, Saper J, et al. Safety and efficacy of peripheral nerve stimulation of the occipital nerves for the management of chronic migraine: results from a randomized, multicenter, double-blinded, controlled study. Cephalalgia 2012;32(16): 1165–79.
31. Melzack R, Wall PD. Pain mechanisms: a new theory. Science 1965;150(3699):971–9.
32. Delphine M, Allena M, Bolla M, et al. Central modulation in cluster headache patients treated with occipital nerve stimulation: an FDG-PET study. BMC Neurol 2012;11:2–9.

Neuromodulation of the Lumbar Spinal Locomotor Circuit

Nicholas AuYong, MD, PhD, Daniel C. Lu, MD, PhD*

KEYWORDS

• Central pattern generator • Spinal cord injury • Epidural stimulation • Locomotion

KEY POINTS

- The spinal cord has a self-contain neuronal network capable of driving complex locomotor behaviors, which remains functional following a spinal cord injury (SCI) and can be reengaged with neuromodulatory interventions.
- Epidural spinal stimulation is emerging as a promising technique to facilitate locomotor behavior, likely through increasing the baseline activation of the central pattern generation (CPG).
- An activated CPG following SCI can perform postural and locomotor-like activity by reacting to real-time environmental and movement-related sensory cues.

INTRODUCTION

The mammalian lumbar spinal cord contains the necessary circuitry to drive a wide variety of locomotor behaviors. This spinal capacity for locomotion in the absence of supraspinal influence was well recognized by the early twentieth century.[1] In that period, Sherrington's[2] reflex chain mechanism was the prevailing theory whereby spinal locomotion is generated from serial triggering of reflex actions by peripheral afferent feedback as a consequence of limb movement. Contemporary studies by Thomas Graham Brown[3,4] found to the contrary that acutely spinalized cats following lumbosacral dorsal rhizotomy exhibited rhythmic stepping behavior. Brown, therefore proposed that the spinal cord is inherently capable of driving rhythmic locomotor behavior in the absence of supraspinal or sensory input. This fundamental concept of a self-contained spinal mechanism for locomotion gave rise to the modern conceptualization of the locomotor central pattern generation (CPG).[5] There is now a growing body of evidence for a locomotor CPG mechanism in the human lumbar spinal cord[6] that is amenable to rehabilitation following a spinal cord injury (SCI).[7] A primary goal of SCI therapeutic development is to identify strategies that maximize the retained locomotor potential of the spinal locomotor circuits following injury.

Current therapeutic strategies aim to (1) increase baseline excitability of spinal interneuronal circuits underlying CPG function and (2) optimize sensorimotor integration processes governing locomotor activity (**Fig. 1**). Several approaches have been explored both individually and in combination to accomplish this. The most widely studied approaches are based on repetitive task-specific training[8,9] and pharmacologic neuromodulatory agents.[10–12] Recently, epidural stimulation (EDS) was used in conjunction with locomotor training[7] on a patient classified as ASIA B (American Spinal Injury Association classification). This patient regained full weight-bearing standing and was able to execute voluntary controlled movement in his lower extremity with EDS. Similar findings of voluntary-controlled locomotion was seen in rats treated with a combination

Department of Neurosurgery, University of California, Los Angeles, 650 Charles E Young Drive South, CHS 74-129, Los Angeles, CA 90095, USA
* Corresponding author.
E-mail address: DCLu@mednet.ucla.edu

Neurosurg Clin N Am 25 (2014) 15–23
http://dx.doi.org/10.1016/j.nec.2013.08.007
1042-3680/14/$ – see front matter

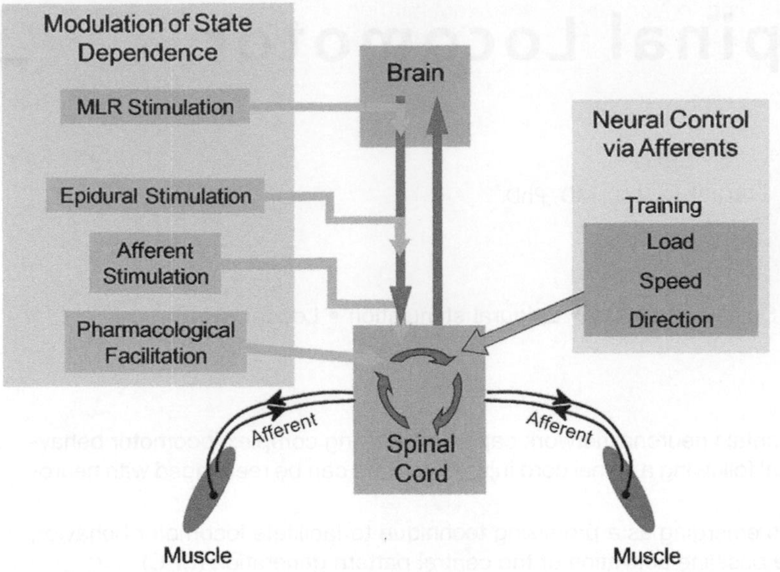

Fig. 1. This illustration provides a global perspective on the sources of neural control of posture and locomotion, which normally includes the exchange of information between the brain and the spinal cord and between the sensory receptors within the muscles, joints, and skin and the spinal cord. This article emphasizes the importance of the afferent information from the periphery as a source of control of posture or locomotor tasks, in conjunction with the spinal circuitry to which CPG is routinely attributed, when there can be no exchange of information between the brain and spinal cord (ie, following a complete SCI). Given that it is possible to generate locomotor movements with a tonic stimulation of the mesencephalic locomotor area, details of the control of posture and locomotion are not likely to be derived from a tonic signal from the brainstem. However, this tonic stimulation can be an important source of modulatory control of the spinal circuitry, as can be epidural stimulation, afferent stimulation, and pharmacologic modulation. Factors listed on the right side of the figure point out details of the physical environment that can be detected by the spinal cord and used to instruct the spinal circuitry to activate the appropriate motor pools at the appropriate time. The sensory perception of the factors listed in the box on the right side can play an important role in shaping the physiology of the spinal circuitry through repetitive activity (ie, training). Further evidence of the importance of the sensory information is demonstrated by the acute effects of unilateral deafferentation after which epidural stimulation will induce locomotor movements only on the intact side.

of EDS, locomotor training, and pharmacologic modulatory agents after a complete thoracic spinal transection[12,13] and after a double hemisection at different spinal levels.[14] Together, these studies suggest that EDS can effectively elevate the functional state of the spinal locomotor circuitry, thereby facilitating sensory-mediated locomotion and voluntary movements via spared supraspinal fibers. In this article, the physiologic basis of EDS and future directions of EDS-based spinal neuromodulation is discussed.

SPINAL SENSORIMOTOR CONTROL OF LOCOMOTOR BEHAVIOR

The spinal locomotor circuit normally operates under the direction of supraspinal input and sensory cues. Supraspinal areas, including the motor cortex, red nucleus, vestibular nuclei, reticular nuclei, and the mesencephalic locomotor area (MLR), are known to modulate spinal locomotor circuits.[15–17] In concert, spinal locomotor circuits are receiving a constant inflow of information from sensory receptors that gauge the environment and proprioceptive receptors that transduce both the limb configuration and movement state.[18,19] One fundamental concept is that even in a normal spinal cord, rhythmic locomotor behaviors, although initiated by supraspinal input, are largely a product of spinal interneuronal circuits (ie, CPG) but shaped by sensory information (see **Fig. 1**).

The underlying sensorimotor integration processes governing spinal locomotor behavior are highly sophisticated. This sophistication is demonstrated by the wide varieties of locomotor behaviors, such as trotting, galloping, backwards and sideways walking, and obstacle avoidance, that can be executed by spinal animals with sensory cues alone. The constant influx of sensory information must be interpreted and responded to in a contextually appropriate manner. For example, studies on stumbling responses in chronic spinal cats demonstrate that electrical stimulation of cutaneous receptors of the dorsum paw surface during the flexion phase enhanced ongoing flexion, a response that is appropriate of obstacle avoidance.[20,21] If this same stimulus elicits a flexion response when the paw is bearing weight, it would result in a fall. If the paw was in the stance phase and bearing weight, that same stimuli that enhanced flexion during the swing phase will instead enhance the ongoing extension. The mechanism underlying this locomotor phase-dependent selection of motor responses has been partly examined through intracellular recordings, demonstrating phasic modulation of cutaneous input postsynaptic potential in acute spinal cats,[22–24] chronic spinal cats,[22] and in decerebrate preparations.[25,26] Results from these studies suggest that the transmission of cutaneous information through oligosynaptic pathways strongly influences the spinal locomotor circuitry.[27–29]

Therefore, the CPG's responses to sensory information are not mere fixed reactions. They are highly contingent on the behavioral state (ie, rest vs walking), the task being performed (eg, stand vs walking), and the phase of the task being executed (eg, extension vs flexion phase of walking).[29] These characteristics argue that the spinal locomotor circuits operate with similarities to engineered intelligent control systems. In fact, even simple reflex responses in spinalized animals are modifiable through an instrumental learning paradigm.[30–33] Furthermore, noncontingent stimuli can actually block future attempts at instrumental learning through a central sensitization mechanism.[34] Therapeutic development for SCI should, therefore, take advantage of these features to promote functional recovery.

REHABILITATING THE INJURED SPINAL CORD

Two general strategies, based on leveraging the retained spinal locomotor ability following SCI, have been widely studied. These strategies are repetitive task-specific training[35] and pharmacologic modulation.[10,12] The basis of repetitive task-specific therapy is to optimize spinal locomotor performance through use-dependent plasticity.[35] Initial studies showed that with repetitive task-based training alone, spinal cats can regain weight-bearing stepping[36–38] or standing ability[38] comparable with normal cats.[39] Although there is a decline in locomotor performance following training cessation, repeated training leads to faster gains than with initial training, suggesting a use-dependent plasticity process.[9] This process is likely mediated by axonal sprouting, alterations in the strength of afferent pathways, and changes in the level of expression of neurotrophic factors and receptors brought on by locomotor training.[40,41] Functional improvements are largely limited to the task practiced in training. For example, stand training in spinal cats results in the recovery of weight-bearing standing ability; however, this does not translate into improvement of weight bearing during stepping.[38] In fact, stand-trained spinal cats step more poorly, suggesting that task-specific training can negatively affect the acquisition of other behaviors. Task-specific locomotor training in the form of overground and partial bodyweight support locomotor training have been studied in human patients with SCI.[42] Although human patients with SCI gain improvement in walking speed and maximal walking distance with training, their recovery does not match the results seen in spinal cats. Further, improvement in locomotor function in response to locomotor training is well documented in individuals that have had an incomplete spinal injury for more than 1 year, but full weight-bearing locomotion has not yet been achieved with training after a clinically complete injury.[42]

A variety of pharmacologic agents have been investigated for the purpose of promoting or enhancing locomotor activity.[10] These agents include drugs that target catecholamine receptors (eg, L-dopa, dopamine, and clonidine) and serotonin receptors (eg, quipazine).[10] Some agents, such as L-dopa[43] and clonidine,[44] can illicit locomotor activity from a nonlocomotor state, whereas agents affecting the serotonergic system result in the enhancement of muscle activation during locomotion.[45] These agents may partially mimic the cellular actions of supraspinal tracts on spinal locomotor circuits[10] and can modulate different aspects of locomotor activity following spinal transection in animal studies.[12] The differential enhancement in the features of spinal locomotion of agents acting on the serotonergic, dopaminergic, or noradrenergic pathways were found to be additive in combination therapy.[12] A potential clinical implication is that pharmacologic treatments may be tailored to the specific locomotor deficits in patients. To date, studies on drug therapy alone in human patients with SCI found only slight improvement in locomotor performance, less than the functional gains made with locomotor training alone.[11] It remains to be determined if further systematic evaluation of combination pharmacologic therapy alone will demonstrate greater improvements in human patients with SCI.

ELECTRICAL STIMULATION OF SPINAL LOCOMOTOR CIRCUITS

Spinal cord stimulation aims to activate and recruit intrinsic spinal mechanisms driving multi-joint motor actions.[46] Two main approaches have been used to deliver electrical stimulation directly to the spinal cord for this purpose, (1) intraspinal electrodes and (2) epidural grid-electrode arrays. Microstimulation of the spinal cord gray matter via intraspinal electrodes is an attractive means to precisely stimulate a small volume of neural tissue. The function of local spinal circuits in movement generation can be closely examined using this method. This strategy was initially applied in frogs,[47] rats,[48] and feline[49,50] models. A common finding from these studies is that intraspinal stimulation, only at distinct sites, resulted in a small set of unique force patterns. When simultaneous intraspinal stimulation was carried out at 2 separate sites, the resulting force patterns corresponded to the simple summation of force patterns generated if each site was stimulated independently. One hypothesis is that spinal circuits generate complex movement behaviors by superimposing basic movement building blocks.[51,52] A theoretical approach for the neuromodulation of spinal behavior, based on this hypothesis, is to drive behavior through intraspinal stimulation at multiple sites.[46] Only a small number of studies have shown that intraspinal stimulation can evoke locomotor activity[50,53]; however, this required multiple electrodes over multiple levels[50] or site-specific single-electrode stimulation following the administration of clonidine.[53] It remains to be determined if the modularity observed in spinal behavior is a result of modularity in the underlying spinal circuits or a consequence of the complex bidirectional interaction between spinal circuits, musculoskeletal system, and the environment.[54] Nevertheless, spinal neuromodulation via intraspinal stimulation is likely challenging to translate due to the technical issues of placing and securing multiple intraspinal electrodes without significant tissue damage.

Another means to deliver electrical stimuli directly to the spinal cord is with an epidural electrode-grid array. Epidural stimulation has been used for some time for the management of intractable pain.[55] Percutaneous and laminectomy-based placements of epidural electrodes are well established and common practice in neurosurgery. EDS was found to elicit locomotor-like activity in humans[56–58] and rats[13] with complete spinal cord injuries. Initial studies on epidural stimulation in human patients with SCI aimed to identify the optimal electrode placement site and stimulation parameters to promote locomotor activity.[56] Stimulation was delivered via quadripolar electrodes (Medtronic, Minneapolis, MN) percutaneously placed at the L1-2 level in patients with an ASIA A SCI, more than 1 year from injury.[6,56] The level of injury ranged from C5 to T8. Patients were examined in a supine position, and the responses to the stimulation of the ventral and dorsal surface were studied. The ventral spinal cord was targeted because projections from the MLR course ventrally. Because stimulation of the MLR in cats can dependably promote locomotor activity,[59] stimulation of the ventral cord may activate areas targeted by MLR projection fibers. However, ventral cord stimulation elicited only tonic muscle contraction in all 8 patients tested, with background rhythmic hip movements in 4 of 8 patients for the entirety of stimulation.[56] The tonic response was likely caused by activation of the anterior-horn motoneuronal pools.

In contrast, dorsal cord stimulation at L2 resulted in rhythmic, step-like electromyogram (EMG) activity associated with leg flexion and extension (nonpatterned 5–9 V, 25–50 Hz). When the electrode was located rostral or caudal from L2, only tonic or irregular rhythmic EMG activity was elicited, but there was no locomotor-like activity. With increasing amplitude of stimulus intensity at L2, EMG progressed from tonic to rhythmic activity, ultimately converting to organized rhythmic locomotor-like movements in both limbs (at 5.5 V, 30 Hz). This progression of activity was highly reproducible among the patients tested. Stimulation frequencies of 20 to 70 Hz were most effective for producing oscillatory movements of the legs. Bilateral locomotor-like activity was produced only with the electrode placed in the midline, whereas unilateral locomotor-like activity was observed when the electrode was offset from the midline. Similar findings were made with epidural stimulation in T10 spinal cats, with stimulation at the L5 level being most effective for producing step-like activity.[56] (Nota Bene The cat has 7 lumbar segments.) These studies demonstrate that EDS is able to invoke locomotor-like activity following complete SCI, further supporting the presence of a locomotor CPG in the human spinal cord. Additionally, activity is highly dependent on the site of stimulation, frequency of stimulation, and intensity of stimulation.

PHYSIOLOGIC BASIS OF EPIDURAL STIMULATION–INDUCED STEPPING

The biophysical effects of EDS were previously examined with finite-element, 3-dimensional, volume-conductor models[60,61] to examine the spatial current density and field potential distribution. These models accounted for the surrounding anatomic structures, including vertebral column, cerebrospinal fluid (CSF), dura matter, and, in some cases, spinal musculature. The thickness of the CSF layer between the dura and dorsal column were found to have a strong effect on the distribution of field potentials. Spatial geometry of the anode in relation to the cathode was also an important factor in the current spread. According to these models, the large proprioceptive dorsal root fibers were most likely to be stimulated at the dorsal root entry zone, with transverse fibers more easily stimulated than longitudinally oriented fibers.

The importance of dorsal roots in EDS-mediated locomotion was reaffirmed in experiments on spinal cats following unilateral dorsal roots section.[56] Epidural stimulation at the site of sectioning resulted in locomotor-like activity only on the contralateral side with intact dorsal roots. However, stimulation below the site of lesion elicited bilateral locomotor-like activity. Similar findings were reported in studies on T8 spinal rats following T12 to S2 unilateral deafferentation.[62] There was a progressive improvement in stepping limited to the non-deafferented side when EDS was applied at 3 to 7 weeks from injury. When the 5-hydroxytryptamine agonist quipazine was given at 7 weeks to facilitate stepping, only limited stepping was observed on the deafferented side while the non-deafferented side was stepping robustly on a treadmill. These findings demonstrate that the excitation of the locomotor CPG with EDS is mediated by sensory fibers in the dorsal roots. Epidural stimulation may produce an antidromic stimulation of Ia and propriospinal fibers that terminate in the dorsal horn and intermediate zone. Lumbar intermediate zone interneurons have been identified by immunohistochemistry to be activated during locomotion and likely operate as part of the CPG.[63–65]

Additional insight into the physiologic action of EDS is inferred from characteristic EMG responses to stimulation, seen in both animal models and human subjects. Examination of the motor responses evoked by epidural stimulation at L2 or S1 in normal[66] and T8 spinal rats[62] demonstrated 3 distinct components, an early response (ER) from direct muscle stimulation, a middle response (MR) with features consistent with a monosynaptic pathway, and a late response (LR) attributed to a polysynaptic pathway. MR and LR were evoked by low to medium intensity ($\leq$6 V) stimulation with a latency range of 4.5 to 7.0 milliseconds and 9 to 11 milliseconds, respectively. At high stimulation intensities (>6 V), MR and, in some cases, ER was evoked with a latency of and 2.5 to 3.0 milliseconds. Both MR and LR are modulated in a phase-dependent manner similar to sensory pathways. For example, MR evoked by L2 stimulation in the sartorius and medial gastrocnemius was facilitated during the swing phase and attenuated or suppressed during stance. In the vastus lateralis and medial gastrocnemius, LR evoked by S1 stimulation was facilitated during the stance phase. Phase-dependent modulation of ER, MR, and LR was also observed during stepping in T8 spinal rats.[62] A 40-Hz stimulation was able to elicit all 3 responses similar to a single pulse; however, LR responses during stepping on a treadmill were composed of a complex response rather than a single response.

The recovery of locomotor activity was related to the presence of the LR. Immediately following T8 transection in rats, LR was abolished, whereas MR in distal muscles was facilitated greater than 2-fold at 1 week and 3- to 4-fold 6 weeks after the injury with S1 stimulation.[67] The return of locomotor activity coincided with the return of LR 3 to 5 weeks following the injury with 40-Hz S1 stimulation. The amplitude of LR was 30% to 60 % of the preinjury levels at 6 weeks, never fully recovering. The optimal stimulation frequency was suggested to have an interstimulation period that allows for complete expression of LR.[62] Higher frequencies would interrupt LR with an elicited MR, whereas lower frequencies did not generate sustained locomotor activity.

EDS AND LOCOMOTOR TRAINING IN HUMAN PATIENTS WITH INCOMPLETE SCI

EDS has recently been investigated as part of a multimodal therapeutic strategy in human patients with incomplete human SCI[7,68,69] with partial weight-body training (PWBT). In a previous study in T7–9 spinal rats, the locomotor activity was more robust when their hindlimbs were loaded with 5% to 20% of their body weight along with EDS (40–50 Hz) at the L2 segment.[13] The combination of PWBT and epidural stimulation was examined in a 43-year-old male patient classified as C5-C6 ASIA C 3.5 years from injury.[68,69] Non-patterned stimulation was delivered above the threshold for producing paresthesia but less than the levels causing contraction. Increased speed and sustained effort during overground ambulation was subjectively less effortful, and the energy cost was reduced by 20% to 30%.[69]

Harkema and colleagues[7] investigated the combination of EDS with locomotor training in a 23-year-old SCI male patient classified as ASIA B who underwent epidural electrode placement 3.4 years after a C7–T1 subluxation injury. The patient underwent 26 months of body-weight support and manual assisted locomotor training before implantation without improvement. EDS was delivered via a 16-electrode array (Specify 5-6-5, Medtronic, Minneapolis, MN) over spinal cord segments L1 to S1. EDS of caudal spinal segments (L5–S1) with loading of bilateral lower extremities was sufficient to promote standing with 65% bodyweight support initially, which improved to full weight bearing with continued training. Both EDS at 30 to 40 Hz with locomotor-related sensory cues alternating loading of the legs and changes in the flexion-extension position were required to drive locomotor-like activity. Voluntary movements were observed in both legs 7 months after implantation and training; however, it was only with EDS. The results of this study are encouraging and provide a proof of principle that EDS can be safely and effectively applied in patients with SCI.

CONCEPTUALIZING THE EFFECTS OF EDS ON THE LOCOMOTOR CPG

Although Brown[4] envisioned a half-center organizational CPG scheme whereby antagonistic (ie, flexion and extension) half-centers governing the alternating action in a limb are coupled through mutual inhibition to half-centers governing the contralateral limb, it does not fully account for all the aspects of locomotion generation. Multilayer CPG models have been recently proposed with separate layers/modules for rhythm generation (RG) and motor pattern shaping.[70–74] In this theoretical framework, EDS may serve to elevate the activity of the RG layer, making it more responsive to sensory cues or spared supraspinal fibers crossing the lesion site.

Increased efficacy of EDS at rostral spinal levels bear similarities to previous studies on rostral lumbar spinal networks in the spinal cord of chick embryos,[75] neonatal rodents,[76–78] and cats.[44,79,80] Disruption of segments L3 to L5 pharmacologically or through mechanical sectioning abolishes locomotion generation in both acute and chronic spinal cats.[44,80] Disruption of lumbar segments rostral to L3 or caudal to L5 degrades locomotion quality or impairs spontaneous locomotor ability but does not abolish locomotor production completely. The differential regional contributions to locomotion expression indicate that the spinal network may consist of segmental interacting network modules, acting together to drive locomotor activity,[81,82] and may be coordinated through propriospinal connection.[75] This distributed network seems to be highly influenced by the rostral lumbar activity and corresponds to the known modulatory effects of hip afferents on locomotor activity.[83]

THE FUTURE OF SPINAL CORD NEUROMODULATION FOR LOCOMOTION

The concept that the injured spinal cord is amenable to rehabilitation is now firmly established in animal studies; however, clinical translation has proven challenging. Although repetitive task-specific training in spinal cats can lead to significant recovery following injury, similar functional gains in humans have been difficult to achieve. An effective pharmacologic approach for human patients also remains to be defined. In light of the recent findings, EDS seems to be a promising technique for reengaging the human locomotor CPG following SCI. Combination strategies including EDS are underway with promising initial results. A recent animal study by van den Brand and colleagues[14] investigated L2 and S1 EDS, a pharmacologic cocktail of serotonergic receptor agonists and dopamine agonist, and activity-based training in a staggered bilateral hemisection adult rat model. This combination approach was able to promote recovery of bipedal walking with the suggestion of voluntary motor control below the lesion site. In comparison with previous available techniques, EDS offers a new direction for further research.[7,84,85] Existing clinical practice in EDS electrode and generator placement for pain may bolster clinical translation of EDS in locomotor recovery.

REFERENCES

1. Clarac F. Some historical reflections on the neural control of locomotion. Brain Res Rev 2008; 57:13–21.
2. Sherrington CS. Further observations on the production of reflex stepping by combination of reflex excitation with reflex inhibition. J Physiol 1913;47: 196–214.
3. Brown TG. The intrinsic factors in the act of progression in the mammal. Proc R Soc Lond B Biol Sci 1911;84:308–19.
4. Brown TG. On the nature of the fundamental activity of the nervous centers; together with an analysis of the conditioning of rhythmic activity in progression, and a theory of the evolution of function in the nervous system. J Physiol 1914; 48:18–46.
5. Grillner S, Wallen P. Central pattern generators for locomotion, with special reference to vertebrates. Annu Rev Neurosci 1985;8:233–61.
6. Dimitrijevic MR, Gerasimenko Y, Pinter MM. Evidence for a spinal central pattern generator in humans. Ann N Y Acad Sci 1998;860:360–76.
7. Harkema S, Gerasimenko Y, Hodes J, et al. Effect of epidural stimulation of the lumbosacral spinal cord on voluntary movement, standing, and assisted stepping after motor complete paraplegia: a case study. Lancet 2011;377:1938–47.
8. Edgerton VR, Courtine G, Gerasimenko YP, et al. Training locomotor networks. Brain Res Rev 2008; 57:241–54.

9. de Leon RD, Hodgson JA, Roy RR, et al. Retention of hindlimb stepping ability in adult spinal cats after the cessation of step training. J Neurophysiol 1999; 81:85–94.
10. Rossignol S, Giroux N, Chau C, et al. Pharmacological aids to locomotor training after spinal injury in the cat. J Physiol 2001;533:65–74.
11. Domingo A, Al-Yahya AA, Asiri Y, et al. A systematic review of the effects of pharmacological agents on walking function in people with spinal cord injury. J Neurotrauma 2012;29:865–79.
12. Musienko P, van den Brand R, Märzendorfer O, et al. Controlling specific locomotor behaviors through multidimensional monoaminergic modulation of spinal circuitries. J Neurosci 2011;31: 9264–78.
13. Ichiyama RM, Gerasimenko YP, Zhong H, et al. Hindlimb stepping movements in complete spinal rats induced by epidural spinal cord stimulation. Neurosci Lett 2005;383:339–44.
14. van den Brand R, Heutschi J, Barraud Q, et al. Restoring voluntary control of locomotion after paralyzing spinal cord injury. Science 2012;336: 1182–5.
15. Armstrong DM. Supraspinal contributions to the initiation and control of locomotion in the cat. Prog Neurobiol 1986;26:273–361.
16. McCrea DA. Supraspinal and segmental interactions. Can J Physiol Pharmacol 1996;74:513–7.
17. Jahn K, Deutschländer A, Stephan T, et al. Supraspinal locomotor control in quadrupeds and humans. Prog Brain Res 2008;171:353–62.
18. Pearson KG. Proprioceptive regulation of locomotion. Curr Opin Neurobiol 1995;5:786–91.
19. Prochazka A. Proprioceptive feedback and movement regulation. Compr Physiol 1996. http://dx.doi.org/10.1002/cphy.cp120103. Published Online First.
20. Forssberg H, Grillner S, Rossignol S. Phase dependent reflex reversal during walking in chronic spinal cats. Brain Res 1975;85:103–7.
21. Forssberg H, Grillner S, Rossignol S. Phasic gain control of reflexes from the dorsum of the paw during spinal locomotion. Brain Res 1977;132: 121–39.
22. Andersson O, Grillner S, Lindquist M, et al. Peripheral control of the spinal pattern generators for locomotion in cat. Brain Res 1978;150:625–30.
23. Schomburg ED, Behrends HB. The possibility of phase-dependent monosynaptic and polysynaptic is excitation to homonymous motoneurons during fictive locomotion. Brain Res 1978;143:533–7.
24. Schmidt BJ, Meyers DE, Fleshman JW, et al. Phasic modulation of short latency cutaneous excitation in flexor digitorum longus motoneurons during fictive locomotion. Exp Brain Res 1988;71: 568–78.
25. Fleshman JW, Lev-Tov A, Burke RE. Peripheral and central control of flexor digitorum longus and flexor hallucis longus motoneurons: the synaptic basis of functional diversity. Exp Brain Res 1984;54:133–49.
26. Degtyarenko AM, Simon ES, Burke RE. Differential modulation of disynaptic cutaneous inhibition and excitation in ankle flexor motoneurons during fictive locomotion. J Neurophysiol 1996;76: 2972–85.
27. Schmidt BJ, Meyers DE, Tokuriki M, et al. Modulation of short latency cutaneous excitation in flexor and extensor motoneurons during fictive locomotion in the cat. Exp Brain Res 1989;77:57–68.
28. Burke RE. The use of state-dependent modulation of spinal reflexes as a tool to investigate the organization of spinal interneurons. Exp Brain Res 1999;128:263–77.
29. Rossignol S, Dubuc RJ, Gossard JP. Dynamic sensorimotor interactions in locomotion. Physiol Rev 2006;86:89–154.
30. Grau JW, Barstow DG, Joynes RL. Instrumental learning within the spinal cord: I. Behavioral properties. Behav Neurosci 1998;112:1366–86.
31. Grau JW, Joynes RL. Pavlovian and instrumental conditioning within the spinal cord: methodological issues. In: Michael MP, James WG, editors. Spinal cord plasticity: alterations in reflex function. New York: Springer; 2001. p. 13–53.
32. Crown ED, Grau JW. Preserving and restoring behavioral potential within the spinal cord using an instrumental training paradigm. J Neurophysiol 2001;86:845–55.
33. Liu GT, Ferguson AR, Crown ED, et al. Instrumental learning within the rat spinal cord: localization of the essential neural circuit. Behav Neurosci 2005; 119:538–47.
34. Ferguson AR, Crown ED, Grau JW. Nociceptive plasticity inhibits adaptive learning in the spinal cord. Neuroscience 2006;141:421–31.
35. Edgerton VR, de Leon RD, Harkema SJ, et al. Retraining the injured spinal cord. J Physiol 2001; 533:15–22.
36. Lovely RG, Gregor RJ, Roy RR, et al. Effects of training on the recovery of full-weight-bearing stepping in the adult spinal cat. Exp Neurol 1986;92: 421–35.
37. Barbeau H, Rossignol S. Recovery of locomotion after chronic spinalization in the adult cat. Brain Res 1987;412:84–95.
38. de Leon RD, Hodgson JA, Roy RR, et al. Full weight-bearing hindlimb standing following stand training in the adult spinal cat. J Neurophysiol 1998;80:83–91.
39. Belanger M, Drew T, Provencher J, et al. A comparison of treadmill locomotion in adult cats before and after spinal transection. J Neurophysiol 1996;76:471–91.

40. Edgerton VR, Tillakaratne NJ, Bigbee AJ, et al. Plasticity of the spinal neural circuitry after injury. Annu Rev Neurosci 2004;27:145–67.
41. Dunlop SA. Activity-dependent plasticity: implications for recovery after spinal cord injury. Trends Neurosci 2008;31:410–8.
42. Harkema SJ, Hillyer JJ, Schmidt-Read MM, et al. Locomotor training: as a treatment of spinal cord injury and in the progression of neurologic rehabilitation. Arch Phys Med Rehabil 2012;93:1588–97.
43. Grillner S, Zangger P. On the central generation of locomotion in the low spinal cat. Exp Brain Res 1979;34:241–61.
44. Marcoux J, Rossignol S. Initiating or blocking locomotion in spinal cats by applying noradrenergic drugs to restricted lumbar spinal segments. J Neurosci 2000;20:8577–85.
45. Barbeau H, Rossignol S. Initiation and modulation of the locomotor pattern in the adult chronic spinal cat by noradrenergic, serotonergic and dopaminergic drugs. Brain Res 1991;546:250–60.
46. Grill WM. Electrical activation of spinal neural circuits: application to motor-system neural prostheses. Neuromodulation 2000;3:97–106.
47. Giszter SF, Mussa-Ivaldi FA, Bizzi E. Convergent force fields organized in the frog's spinal cord. J Neurosci 1993;13:467–91.
48. Tresch MC, Kiehn O. Coding of locomotor phase in populations of neurons in rostral and caudal segments of the neonatal rat lumbar spinal cord. J Neurophysiol 1999;82:3563–74.
49. Lemay MA, Grill WM. Modularity of motor output evoked by intraspinal microstimulation in cats. J Neurophysiol 2004;91:502–14.
50. Mushahwar VK, Collins DF, Prochazka A. Spinal cord microstimulation generates functional limb movements in chronically implanted cats. Exp Neurol 2000;163:422–9.
51. Bizzi E, Cheung VCK, d'Avella A, et al. Combining modules for movement. Brain Res Rev 2008;57:125–33.
52. Giszter SF, Hart CB. Motor primitives and synergies in the spinal cord and after injury—the current state of play. Ann N Y Acad Sci 2013;1279:114–26.
53. Barthelemy D, Leblond H, Provencher J, et al. Nonlocomotor and locomotor hindlimb responses evoked by electrical microstimulation of the lumbar cord in spinalized cats. J Neurophysiol 2006;96:3273–92.
54. Tresch MC, Jarc A. The case for and against muscle synergies. Curr Opin Neurobiol 2009;19:601–7.
55. North RB, Kidd DH, Olin JC, et al. Spinal cord stimulation electrode design: prospective, randomized, controlled trial comparing percutaneous and laminectomy electrodes - part I: technical outcomes. Neurosurgery 2002;51:381–9.
56. Gerasimenko YP, Makarovskii AN, Nikitin OA. Control of locomotor activity in humans and animals in the absence of supraspinal influences. Neurosci Behav Physiol 2002;32:417–23.
57. Jilge B, Minassian K, Rattay F, et al. Initiating extension of the lower limbs in subjects with complete spinal cord injury by epidural lumbar cord stimulation. Exp Brain Res 2004;154:308–26.
58. Minassian K, Jilge B, Rattay F, et al. Stepping-like movements in humans with complete spinal cord injury induced by epidural stimulation of the lumbar cord: electromyographic study of compound muscle action potentials. Spinal Cord 2004;42:401–16.
59. Orlovskii GN, Severin FV, Shik ML. Locomotion induced by stimulation of the mesencephalon. Dokl Akad Nauk SSSR 1966;169:1223–6 [in Russian].
60. Coburn B. A theoretical study of epidural electrical stimulation of the spinal cord–part II: effects on long myelinated fibers. IEEE Trans Biomed Eng 1985;32:978–86.
61. Holsheimer J. Computer modelling of spinal cord stimulation and its contribution to therapeutic efficacy. Spinal Cord 1998;36:531–40.
62. Lavrov I, Dy CJ, Fong AJ, et al. Epidural stimulation induced modulation of spinal locomotor networks in adult spinal rats. J Neurosci 2008;28:6022–9.
63. Harrison PJ, Hultborn H, Jankowska E, et al. Labelling of interneurones by retrograde transsynaptic transport of horseradish peroxidase from motoneurones in rats and cats. Neurosci Lett 1984;45:15–9.
64. Kjaerulff O, Barajon I, Kiehn O. Sulphorhodamine-labelled cells in the neonatal rat spinal cord following chemically induced locomotor activity in vitro. J Physiol 1994;478(Pt 2):265–73.
65. Dai X, Noga BR, Douglas JR, et al. Localization of spinal neurons activated during locomotion using the c-fos immunohistochemical method. J Neurophysiol 2005;93:3442–52.
66. Gerasimenko YP, Lavrov IA, Courtine G, et al. Spinal cord reflexes induced by epidural spinal cord stimulation in normal awake rats. J Neurosci Methods 2006;157:253–63.
67. Lavrov I, Gerasimenko YP, Ichiyama RM, et al. Plasticity of spinal cord reflexes after a complete transection in adult rats: relationship to stepping ability. J Neurophysiol 2006;96:1699–710.
68. Carhart MR, He JP, Herman R, et al. Epidural spinal-cord stimulation facilitates recovery of functional walking following incomplete spinal-cord injury. IEEE Trans Neural Syst Rehabil Eng 2004;12:32–42.
69. Herman R, He J, D'Luzansky S, et al. Spinal cord stimulation facilitates functional walking in a chronic, incomplete spinal cord injured. Spinal Cord 2002;40:65–8.

70. Perret C, Gabelguen JM, Orsal D. Analysis of the pattern of activity in "knee flexor" motoneurons during locomotion in the cat. In: Stance and motion: facts and concepts. New York: Plenum Press; 1988. p. 133–41.
71. Koshland GF, Smith JL. Mutable and immutable features of paw-shake responses after hindlimb deafferentation in the cat. J Neurophysiol 1989; 62:162–73.
72. Kriellaars DJ, Brownstone RM, Noga BR, et al. Mechanical entrainment of fictive locomotion in the decerebrate cat. J Neurophysiol 1994;71:2074–86.
73. Burke RE, Degtyarenko AM, Simon ES. Patterns of locomotor drive to motoneurons and last-order interneurons: clues to the structure of the CPG. J Neurophysiol 2001;86:447–62.
74. McCrea DA, Rybak IA. Organization of mammalian locomotor rhythm and pattern generation. Brain Res Rev 2008;57:134–46.
75. Ho S, O'Donovan MJ. Regionalization and intersegmental coordination of rhythm-generating networks in the spinal cord of the chick embryo. J Neurosci 1993;13:1354–71.
76. Kjaerulff O, Kiehn O. Distribution of networks generating and coordinating locomotor activity in the neonatal rat spinal cord in vitro: a lesion study. J Neurosci 1996;16:5777–94.
77. Cowley KC, Schmidt BJ. Regional distribution of the locomotor pattern-generating network in the neonatal rat spinal cord. J Neurophysiol 1997;77: 247–59.
78. Kremer E, LevTov A. Localization of the spinal network associated with generation of hindlimb locomotion in the neonatal rat and organization of its transverse coupling system. J Neurophysiol 1997;77:1155–70.
79. Deliagina TG, Orlovsky GN, Pavlova GA. The capacity for generation of rhythmic oscillations is distributed in the lumbosacral spinal cord of the cat. Exp Brain Res 1983;53:81–90.
80. Langlet C, Leblond H, Rossignol S. Mid-lumbar segments are needed for the expression of locomotion in chronic spinal cats. J Neurophysiol 2005;93:2474–88.
81. Buschges A. Sensory control and organization of neural networks mediating coordination of multisegmental organs for locomotion. J Neurophysiol 2005;93:1127–35.
82. Grillner S, Markram H, De Schutter E, et al. Microcircuits in action - from CPGs to neocortex. Trends Neurosci 2005;28:525–33.
83. Dietz V, Harkema SJ. Locomotor activity in spinal cord-injured persons. J Appl Physiol 2004;96: 1954–60.
84. Minassian K, Hofstoetter U, Tansey K, et al. Neuromodulation of lower limb motor control in restorative neurology. Clin Neurol Neurosurg 2012;114: 489–97.
85. Musienko P, Heutschi J, Friedli L, et al. Multi-system neurorehabilitative strategies to restore motor functions following severe spinal cord injury. Exp Neurol 2012;235:100–9.

Spinal Cord Stimulation for the Treatment of Vascular Pathology

Milind Deogaonkar, MD[a], Zion Zibly, MD[a], Konstantin V. Slavin, MD, FAANS[b,*]

KEYWORDS

- Spinal neuromodulation • Spinal cord stimulation • Peripheral vascular disease
- Critical limb ischemia • Peripheral arterial disease

KEY POINTS

- Spinal cord stimulation (SCS) in peripheral vascular disease (PVD) treatment can result in significant decrease in pain and improvements in limb salvage.
- Key patient selection criteria have been defined for SCS for PVD.
- Mechanisms of action are unknown but likely relate to direct modulation of factors that regulate vascular tone, including nitric oxide and prostaglandin production and sympathetic neuromodulation.
- Surgical techniques for SCS for PCD do not significantly differ from SCS techniques for pain.

INTRODUCTION

Peripheral vascular disease (PVD) is a common disease mostly involving arteries of the extremities. It usually results from progressive narrowing of arteries in the lower extremities, caused by atherosclerosis.[1] PVD prevalence in the United States has ranged as high as 30% in adult populations and is closely associated with elevated risk of cardiovascular disease morbidity and mortality.[2,3] It is estimated that by 2020, 7 million people aged older than 40 years will suffer from PVD. Severe limb pain, claudication, ulcerations, and limb amputation are common complications of PVD, especially among patients with kidney disease and diabetes.[4,5] The universal treatment approach for PVD includes risk-factor modification, pharmacologic therapy, and revascularization.[6]

Early in the 1980s, individuals with refractory ischemic pain attributed to PVD were treated with spinal cord stimulation (SCS).[7] Since then, multiple studies have shown proved efficacy of SCS in PVD. Other studies inquired into the pathophysiology and mechanism of action; the changes in tissue oxygenation and blood flow were considered as markers for response. It was also consistently shown that SCS significantly improved multiple outcomes, such as exercise tolerance, limb salvage, and pain level in patients presenting with critical leg ischemia.[8]

This article describes the role of SCS in the treatment of PVD, the patient selection criteria along with the outcomes, and mechanism by which SCS works in PVD.

REVIEW OF PUBLISHED LITERATURE

Electrical stimulation of the posterior column (SCS) was first introduced in the late 1960s. It is thought to be based on the "gate-control" theory of pain described in 1965 by Melzack and Wall.[9] It is generally used for the treatment of pain and is currently an established treatment of neurogenic pain. It was not until 1976 when Cook and

[a] Department of Neurosurgery, Ohio State University, 480 Medical Center Drive, Columbus, OH 43210, USA;
[b] Department of Neurosurgery, University of Illinois, 912 South Wood Street, M/C 799, Chicago, IL 60612, USA
* Corresponding author.
E-mail address: kslavin@uic.edu

Neurosurg Clin N Am 25 (2014) 25–31
http://dx.doi.org/10.1016/j.nec.2013.08.013
1042-3680/14/$ – see front matter

colleagues[10,11] introduced SCS as a therapeutic option for vascular disease of the limbs. Since then, multiple studies were done to prove and assess the efficacy of SCS for the treatment of PVD (**Table 1**).

One of the large prospective, controlled studies was the Spinal Cord Stimulation European Peripheral Vascular Disease Outcome Study. The aim of the study was to evaluate the outcome of SCS on limb survival in individuals with critical leg ischemia. It concluded that SCS provided a significantly better limb survival rate than conservative treatment. In this study, the transcutaneous oxygen pressure (TcPO2), which is associated with high amputation rate, was assessed in 71 patients with PVD. Based on this prospective controlled study, the authors concluded that SCS provided a significantly better limb survival rate than conservative treatment. After a 12-month follow-up, limb survival was 33% higher in the patients treated with SCS. It was also shown that pain was significantly reduced in the SCS-treated group.[8]

Jivegard and colleagues[12] studied 51 patients presenting with atherosclerotic and diabetic limb ischemia. In this prospective, randomized, controlled study that followed patients for 18 months, there was no difference in microcirculation between the SCS and control groups. Nevertheless, the group of patients treated with SCS had better pain relief and significantly higher rate of limb salvage. In the same study, it was also noted that the most significant benefit from SCS was among those with inoperable limb ischemia and those presenting with arterial hypertension.

Tallis and colleagues[13] reported a case series of 10 patients presenting with severe, intractable symptoms of arteriographically proved arteriosclerosis and vascular ischemia. Some of the patients also demonstrated nonhealing ulcers and claudication. The authors measured cutaneous blood flow and muscle blood flow (by measuring Xenon 133 clearance). All patients had SCS trial before implantation of a permanent epidural SCS device. In this study all 10 patients showed improvement in mean claudication distance and improvement in the bicycle ergometer tolerance exercise. Most of the patients showed improvement in ischemic limb pain and ulcer healing. After SCS, there was a remarkable increase in the cutaneous blood flow and in the measured muscle blood flow within the group of patients that had positive clinical response to the SCS.

Reig and Abejon[14] reported their 20 years of experience with 98 SCS implants in patients

Table 1
Summary of SCS studies for the treatment of PVD

Author, Year	Patient (N)	SCS Trial	Results
Amann et al,[8] 2003	71	Yes	significant improvement in limb survival rate, significant reduction of pain
Reig & Abejon,[14] 2009	98	N/A	Significant reduction of pain, improvement in ischemic symptoms
Jivegard et al,[12] 1995	51	N/A	significant improvement in limb survival rate, significant reduction of pain
Brummer et al,[15] 2006	8	N/A	significant improvement in limb survival rate, significant reduction of pain
Ubbink et al,[16] 1999	120	Yes	significant improvement in limb survival rate in a specific group of patients
Claeys and Horsch,[31] 1996	86	No	Major improvement in stage IV Fontaine
Ubbink & Vermeulen,[19] 2013[a]	450	N/A	significant improvement in limb survival rate, significant reduction of pain
Tallis et al,[13] 1983	10	Yes	Significant reduction of pain, significant improvement of claudication and muscle blood flow
Petrakis and Sciacca,[32] 1999	150	Yes	Significant reduction of pain, improvement in ischemic symptoms and skin blood flow
Horsch et al,[18] 2004	258	N/A	Significant increase in limb survival
kumar et al,[17] 1997	39	Yes	Significant reduction of pain, improvement in ischemic symptoms and blood flow

[a] Review.

presenting with PVD. The authors measured clinical response, relief of pain, and ulcer healing. Almost 88% of the patients showed good clinical response with SCS. In this big retrospective cohort study, the authors concluded that SCS should be a therapeutic approach in treating PVD. Good pain relief was reported in more than 85% of the patients and most patients also reported improvement of their ischemic symptoms.

An important study was done among a group of patients with end-stage renal disease by Brummer and colleagues.[15] The importance of the study was defined by the fact that these patients were not candidates for limb-preservation surgeries and not considered to benefit from any revascularization procedures. Intensity of ischemic pain, quality of life, use of analgesic medications, limb survival, and outcome of skin ischemic lesions were evaluated before implantation of an SCS and at 6 and 12 months of follow-up. Of the eight patients that were studied, all showed significant improvement in pain, quality of life, limb survival, and absence of new skin ulcer development. This dynamic was most prominent in patients assessed at Fontaine stage III and IV.

The Dutch multicenter randomized controlled study followed 120 patients presenting with critical leg ischemia. In this study, Ubbink and colleagues[16] investigated the cutaneous microcirculation by means of capillary microscopy, laser Doppler perfusion, and transcutaneous oxygen measurements in the foot. The minimum follow-up period was 18 months. The authors reported that amputation frequency was higher in those patients with poor microcirculation and lower in those with good skin perfusion. In this important study, it was shown that in the group of patients with intermediate microcirculation SCS provided better chance for limb survival.

Kumar and colleagues[17] prospectively studied 39 patients with nonreconstructable ischemic vascular lower extremity disease. All patients had a successful SCS trial. The average follow-up was 21 months, and the analyzed parameters included pain control, microcirculatory changes measured by means of TcPO2, blood flow velocities, and pulse volumes. They concluded that SCS provides benefits as measured by TcPO2, blood flow velocities, and pulse volumes and improves microcirculation and macrocirculation.

In their retrospective study of 258 patients treated with SCS, Horsch and colleagues[18] followed the patients for a period of 18 months. All patients had to meet the following criteria: baseline TcPO2 less than 20 mm Hg, noncandidates for reconstructive surgery, and not treated with any medications for the PVD. The authors concluded that among the group of patients presenting with a low baseline TcPO2 (<10 mm Hg), limb survival was significantly improved. They also showed that patients treated with SCS had ischemic pain relief and improvement in microcirculation. This study led to a conclusion that baseline TcPO2 could serve as a predictor for SCS treatment outcome.

In their critical review of the literature, Ubbink and Vermeulen[19] summarized reports of nearly 450 patients in six studies. Based on this, they concluded that limb salvage after 12 months follow-up period was higher within the group of patients that were treated with SCS. Pain relief was also higher in the SCS patient group, and the need for analgesics and other pain relief medications was significantly lower. However, there was no significant statistical difference in ulcer healing.

PROPOSED MECHANISMS OF ACTION

The exact mechanism by which SCS acts in the treatment of PVD is not completely understood and several theories have been suggested. Because the SCS is implanted along the posterior epidural space, it stimulates mainly the dorsal columns of the spinal cord. Thus, SCS should stimulate sensory unmyelinated C fibers and myelinated A delta fibers that originate in the dorsal root ganglia.[20–26] This, in turn, activates cell signaling cascade that leads to release and activation of different molecules. The end point of this cascade is the release of nitric oxide, which causes vasodilatation, decrease in vascular resistance, and relaxation of the vascular wall (smooth muscles) (**Fig. 1**). Suppression or modulation of the sympathetic nervous system is also achieved by inhibition of the nicotine transmission at the ganglion and postganglionic junction.[21,27,28] In addition, reduction of pain is achieved by release of endogenous opioid-like peptides.[29] The exact nature of neurohumoral effects mediated by dorsal root small-diameter afferents or the sympathetic fibers remains unclear. Prostaglandin-mediated vasodilatation caused by antidromic stimulation of dorsal root afferents has been suggested. It has also been suggested that pain relief in itself might relieve vasoconstriction. Speculation has also centered on the release of vasoactive substances with local and possibly systemic effects, including vasoactive intestinal peptide, substance P, and calcitonin gene-related peptide.[17] It may be possible that several mechanisms are active simultaneously, with inhibition of autonomically mediated vasoconstriction and activation of vasoactive substances participating in the efficacy of SCS.[17,26]

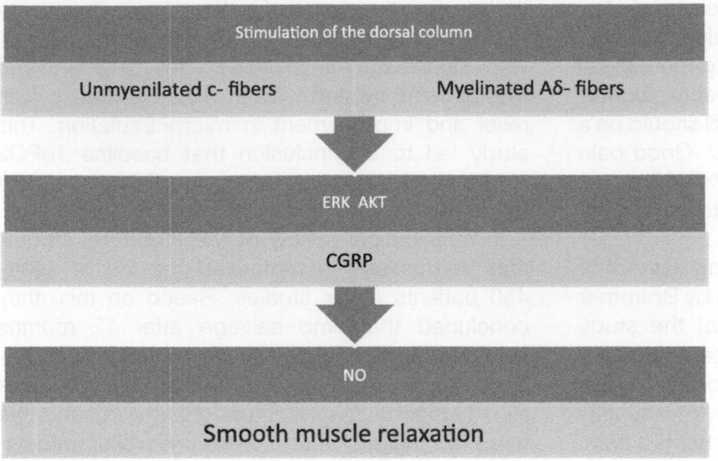

Fig. 1. SCS proposed mechanism of action. AKT, protein kinase B; CGRP, calcitonin gene related protein; ERK, extracellular regulated kinase; NO, nitric oxide.

PATIENT SELECTION

The selection of the right candidate for SCS among patients with PVD is based on certain basic criteria succinctly outlined by Kumar and colleagues[17] in their study. They are as follows:

1. End-stage lower limb PVD with pain unresponsive to medical therapy.
2. Severe, nonreconstructable arterial obstruction. This is demonstrated by an ankle/brachial index that is less than 0.4 (unless arteries were incompressible, as with diabetes), or by a great toe pressure less than 30 mm Hg.
3. Foot ulcers, if present, must be less than 2 cm in diameter and may not extend deep into the dermis.
4. Gangrene, if present, must be dry and must satisfy the ulcer conditions stated previously.
5. Patients with significant heart failure, pulmonary or renal insufficiency, or unstable angina are excluded.
6. A demonstrable pathology accounted for the pain.
7. Conservative therapies have failed or are contraindicated.
8. Untreated drug addiction problems do not exist.
9. Psychological assessment does not identify major barriers to treatment success.
10. Patients are motivated sufficiently to understand and cooperate with instructions on the use of the device and its adjustment, and are able to return for regular follow-up visits.
11. Patients are able to detect paresthesia in the painful area during the trial implantation screening period.
12. Patients report substantial pain relief after trial stimulation.
13. Patients have a life expectancy greater than 6 months.
14. Patients are able to give informed consent to the treatment.[17]

Some authors advocate not to perform an SCS trial because of a lack of objective response measures and also to reduce the risk of infection.[12,30]

Currently, it is considered a standard to treat patients with PVD with SCS based on their microcirculatory parameters. This has been shown to help with pain reduction, halt ulcer progression, and improve the chances of limb salvage. At present, patients are considered to be candidates for SCS if they are unable to have open or endovascular surgical procedures. Thus, this group includes patients with isolated resting limb pain (Fontaine stage III), and those with resting limb pain together with ulcers that are less than 3 cm in diameter (Fontaine IV). In addition, among the SCS candidates are those patients who had an unsuccessful revascularization and continue to present with limb pain or ischemia. The Dutch multicenter randomized controlled study, for example, showed that only patients who present with critical leg ischemia and intermediate cutaneous microcirculation could benefit from SCS treatment.[16]

Claeys and Horsch[31] carried out a randomized controlled study where 81 Fontaine stage IV patients with end-stage PVD treated with prostaglandins were treated with SCS. After a 12-month follow-up the authors concluded that SCS provides a significant benefit for Fontaine stage IV patients especially if the initial TcPO2 is higher than

10 mm Hg, making a case for this value to be considered as a parameter for patient selection.

To decide whether the TcPO2 could serve as a prognostic parameter for SCS permanent implantation, Petrakis and Sciacca[32] studied 150 patients with Fontaine stages III and IV. After a mean follow-up period of 71 months, SCS proved to improve skin blood flow and significantly reduce pain. They also concluded that TcPO2 increase after a 2-week SCS trial period is a good predictive index for subsequent successful treatment with permanent SCS.

Kumar and coworkers[17] suggested that trial stimulation parameters of excellent pain relief combined with an increase in TcPO2 of 10 mm Hg or greater, and an increase in peak flow velocity of 10 mm/s or more, give significant predilection for long-term success of SCS in the treatment of critical limb ischemia.

SURGICAL TECHNIQUE

Standard surgical technique of SCS for chronic pain is described in various published articles. The same technique is used while implanting SCS for PVD. There are, however, some differences in SCS for PVD compared with SCS for chronic pain.

1. Need of trial: Some studies have done a preimplant trial[17] but most studies do not comment on a preimplant trial. Rationale for skipping the trial is likely an inability to see clinical improvement in PVD during a short trial period.
2. Type of electrodes: Although very few studies comment on type of electrodes used for SCS, those who commented have used paddle lead implants more often. Nevertheless, the experience of the authors and personal communication with implanters worldwide suggest that percutaneous electrodes dominate in this surgical indication.
3. Placement of electrodes: All the SCS electrodes were placed in the dorsal epidural space with very few studies mentioning the exact location of the electrode contacts along the craniocaudal axis.

COMPLICATIONS

The estimated overall complication rate is 17% and includes hardware failure (lead migration, generator failure) and infection at the epidural lead site or generator site.[19] Based on meta-analysis of six studies comprising 450 patients that were treated with SCS for PVD, Ubbink and Vermeulen[19] reported that the risk of infection of the lead or generator pocket is less than 3%. The biggest study that examined the occurrence of SCS complications for all indications was done by Babu and colleagues.[33] In their comparative analysis of 13,774 patients who were implanted with either percutaneous or paddle lead SCS the authors reported that SCS paddle leads had higher chance of complication than percutaneous leads at 90 days after surgery, but after 2 years the percutaneous group had a higher rate of reoperations.[33,34] Kinfe and colleagues[35] reported in their series of 81 patients with SCS implantation for the treatment of pain a 2.5% risk of lead migration, which clearly represents another kind of a surgical complication. Other complications that are possible with SCS are cerebrospinal fluid leak and hypotensive headache, and spinal cord injury. The assumed risk of all these complications is below 3%, and depends on surgeon experience.

SUMMARY

Although there have been no masked studies to evaluate the benefit of SCS in the treatment of critical limb ischemia and end-stage PVD, there is plenty of evidence that supports its efficacy. It is clear that SCS, when done by an experienced functional neurosurgeon, is safe and effective. It is important to have clear criteria for patient selection and to understand that all patients should be therapeutically refractory (medication and revascularization) to qualify for SCS.

It is safe to conclude that SCS improves limb survival in patients with critical limb ischemia, gives significant pain control, improves blood circulation, and improves patients' quality of life by improving claudication.

REFERENCES

1. Selvin E, Erlinger TP. Prevalence of and risk factors for peripheral arterial disease in the United States: results from the National Health and Nutrition Examination Survey, 1999-2000. Circulation 2004;110: 738–43.
2. Newman AB, Shemanski L, Manolio TA, et al. Ankle-arm index as a predictor of cardiovascular disease and mortality in the Cardiovascular Health Study. The Cardiovascular Health Study Group. Arterioscler Thromb Vasc Biol 1999;19:538–45.
3. Murabito JM, Evans JC, Nieto K, et al. Prevalence and clinical correlates of peripheral arterial disease in the Framingham Offspring Study. Am Heart J 2002;143:961–5.
4. Creager MA, Luscher TF, Cosentino F, et al. Diabetes and vascular disease: pathophysiology,

clinical consequences, and medical therapy: part I. Circulation 2003;108:1527–32.
5. Luscher TF, Creager MA, Beckman JA, et al. Diabetes and vascular disease: pathophysiology, clinical consequences, and medical therapy: part II. Circulation 2003;108:1655–61.
6. White C. Clinical practice. Intermittent claudication. N Engl J Med 2007;356:1241–50.
7. De Vries J, De Jongste MJ, Spincemaille G, et al. Spinal cord stimulation for ischemic heart disease and peripheral vascular disease. Adv Tech Stand Neurosurg 2007;32:63–89.
8. Amann W, Berg P, Gersbach P, et al. Spinal cord stimulation in the treatment of non-reconstructable stable critical leg ischaemia: results of the European Peripheral Vascular Disease Outcome Study (SCS-EPOS). Eur J Vasc Endovasc Surg 2003;26: 280–6.
9. Melzack R, Wall PD. Pain mechanisms: a new theory. Science 1965;150:971–9.
10. Cook AW. Epidural stimulation for vascular disease of extremities. J Neurosurg 1981;55:664.
11. Cook AW, Oygar A, Baggenstos P, et al. Vascular disease of extremities. Electric stimulation of spinal cord and posterior roots. N Y State J Med 1976;76: 366–8.
12. Jivegard LE, Augustinsson LE, Holm J, et al. Effects of spinal cord stimulation (SCS) in patients with inoperable severe lower limb ischaemia: a prospective randomised controlled study. Eur J Vasc Endovasc Surg 1995;9:421–5.
13. Tallis RC, Illis LS, Sedgwick EM, et al. Spinal cord stimulation in peripheral vascular disease. J Neurol Neurosurg Psychiatry 1983;46:478–84.
14. Reig E, Abejon D. Spinal cord stimulation: a 20-year retrospective analysis in 260 patients. Neuromodulation 2009;12:232–9.
15. Brummer U, Condini V, Cappelli P, et al. Spinal cord stimulation in hemodialysis patients with critical lower-limb ischemia. Am J Kidney Dis 2006;47: 842–7.
16. Ubbink DT, Spincemaille GH, Prins MH, et al. Microcirculatory investigations to determine the effect of spinal cord stimulation for critical leg ischemia: the Dutch multicenter randomized controlled trial. J Vasc Surg 1999;30:236–44.
17. Kumar K, Toth C, Nath RK, et al. Improvement of limb circulation in peripheral vascular disease using epidural spinal cord stimulation: a prospective study. J Neurosurg 1997;86:662–9.
18. Horsch S, Schulte S, Hess S. Spinal cord stimulation in the treatment of peripheral vascular disease: results of a single-center study of 258 patients. Angiology 2004;55:111–8.
19. Ubbink DT, Vermeulen H. Spinal cord stimulation for non-reconstructable chronic critical leg ischaemia. Cochrane Database Syst Rev 2013;(2):CD004001.
20. Naoum JJ, Arbid EJ. Spinal cord stimulation for chronic limb ischemia. Methodist Debakey Cardiovasc J 2013;9:99–102.
21. Pedrini L, Magnoni F. Spinal cord stimulation for lower limb ischemic pain treatment. Interact Cardiovasc Thorac Surg 2007;6:495–500.
22. Tanaka S, Komori N, Barron KW, et al. Mechanisms of sustained cutaneous vasodilation induced by spinal cord stimulation. Auton Neurosci 2004;114:55–60.
23. Tanaka S, Barron KW, Chandler MJ, et al. Local cooling alters neural mechanisms producing changes in peripheral blood flow by spinal cord stimulation. Auton Neurosci 2003;104:117–27.
24. Tanaka S, Barron KW, Chandler MJ, et al. Role of primary afferents in spinal cord stimulation-induced vasodilation: characterization of fiber types. Brain Res 2003;959:191–8.
25. Provenzano DA, Nicholson L, Jarzabek G, et al. Spinal cord stimulation utilization to treat the microcirculatory vascular insufficiency and ulcers associated with scleroderma: a case report and review of the literature. Pain Med 2011;12:1331–5.
26. Provenzano DA, Jarzabek G, Georgevich P. The utilization of transcutaneous oxygen pressures to guide decision-making for spinal cord stimulation implantation for inoperable peripheral vascular disease: a report of two cases. Pain Physician 2008; 11:909–16.
27. Deer TR, Raso LJ. Spinal cord stimulation for refractory angina pectoris and peripheral vascular disease. Pain Physician 2006;9:347–52.
28. Reig E, Abejon D, del Pozo C, et al. Spinal cord stimulation in peripheral vascular disease: a retrospective analysis of 95 cases. Pain Pract 2001;1:324–31.
29. Wu M, Linderoth B, Foreman RD. Putative mechanisms behind effects of spinal cord stimulation on vascular diseases: a review of experimental studies. Auton Neurosci 2008;138:9–23.
30. Klomp HM, Spincemaille GH, Steyerberg EW, et al. Spinal-cord stimulation in critical limb ischaemia: a randomised trial. ESES Study Group. Lancet 1999; 353:1040–4.
31. Claeys LG, Horsch S. Transcutaneous oxygen pressure as predictive parameter for ulcer healing in endstage vascular patients treated with spinal cord stimulation. Int Angiol 1996;15:344–9.
32. Petrakis E, Sciacca V. Prospective study of transcutaneous oxygen tension (TcPO2) measurement in the testing period of spinal cord stimulation in diabetic patients with critical lower limb ischaemia. Int Angiol 2000;19:18–25.
33. Babu R, Hazzard MA, Huang KT, et al. Outcomes of percutaneous and paddle lead implantation for spinal cord stimulation: a comparative analysis of complications, reoperation rates, and health-care costs. Neuromodulation 2013. http://dx.doi.org/10.1111/ner.12065.

34. Huang KT, Hazzard MA, Babu R, et al. Insurance disparities in the outcomes of spinal cord stimulation surgery. Neuromodulation 2013. http://dx.doi.org/10.1111/ner.12059.

35. Kinfe TM, Schu S, Quack FJ, et al. Percutaneous implanted paddle lead for spinal cord stimulation: technical considerations and long-term follow-up. Neuromodulation 2012;15:402–7.

Sacral Neuromodulation for Refractory Overactive Bladder, Interstitial Cystitis, and Painful Bladder Syndrome

Aaron Laviana, MD, Forrest Jellison, MD, Ja-Hong Kim, MD*

KEYWORDS

• Sacral neuromodulation • Overactive bladder • Interstitial cystitis • Painful bladder syndrome • Urinary urge incontinence • Pelvic floor disorders • Chronic pelvic pain

KEY POINTS

- Sacral neuromodulation is a treatment option approved by the Food and Drug Administration for refractory overactive bladder syndrome, which consists of urinary frequency, urgency, nocturia, and urge incontinence.
- There is a growing body of evidence supporting off-label use of sacral neuromodulation for the treatment of interstitial cystitis, painful bladder syndrome, and chronic pelvic pain.

INTRODUCTION

Sacral neuromodulation (SNM) is a minimally invasive treatment modality for patients who fail conservative therapy, avoiding the morbidity of extensive surgery for many pelvic floor disorders. Since its approval by the Food and Drug Administration (FDA) in 1997 for urinary conditions related to overactive bladder (OAB) symptoms, the indications for use of SNM continue to expand; they now include nonobstructive urinary retention (1999) and, more recently, fecal incontinence (2011).

There are reports of the off-label use of SNM for other urinary conditions and pelvic floor disorders, such as neurogenic bladder and interstitial cystitis/painful bladder syndrome (IC/PBS).[1–5] Although it is considered off-label for IC/PBS, the American Urological Association (AUA) includes SNM in its treatment guideline algorithm (**Fig. 1**). Furthermore, SNM has demonstrated efficacy in treating chronic pelvic pain, which some experts consider a variant of complex visceral pain syndrome.[6,7]

This article focuses on the use of SNM for the treatment of OAB symptoms and IC/PBS, with detailed discussion on its mechanism of action, pertinent technical aspects, and relevant clinical conditions.

BACKGROUND

Mechanism of Action

The clinical benefits of SNM therapy are well established for the treatment of OAB and the urinary symptoms of IC/PBS.[4,8,9] Although the precise mechanism is not entirely understood, SNM treats a wide array of urinary conditions of the pelvic floor. Understanding the effects of SNM on voiding function involves knowing the micturition reflex and anatomy of the lower urinary tract. SNM stimulates the sympathetic, parasympathetic, and somatic fibers of the sacral nerves through a tined

Disclosures: The authors have no disclosures.
Division of Pelvic Medicine and Reconstructive Surgery, Department of Urology, UCLA School of Medicine, 200 Medical Plaza, Suite 140, Los Angeles, CA 90095, USA
* Corresponding author.
E-mail address: jhkim@mednet.ucla.edu

Neurosurg Clin N Am 25 (2014) 33–46
http://dx.doi.org/10.1016/j.nec.2013.08.001
1042-3680/14/$ – see front matter

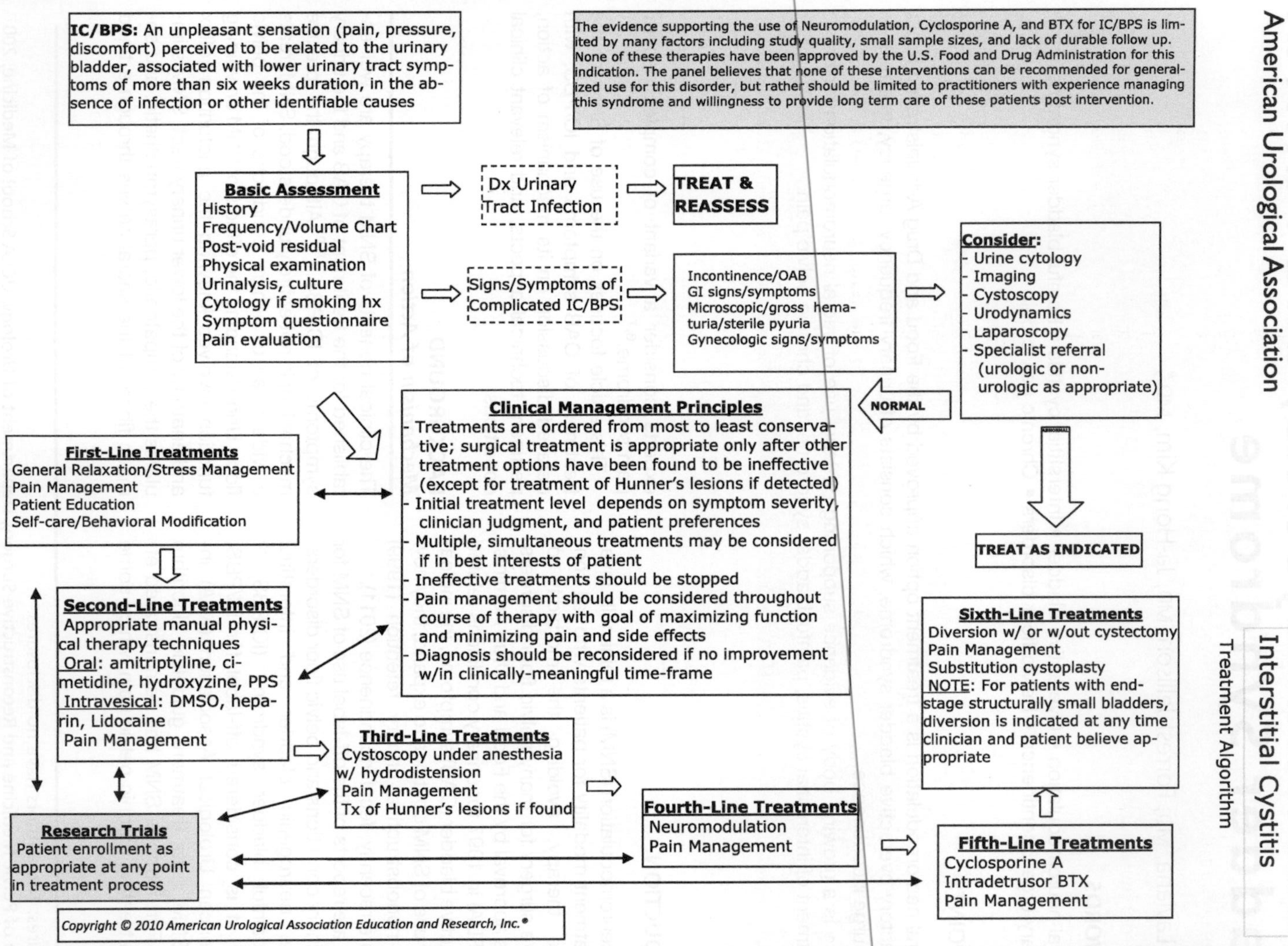

Fig. 1. The American Urological Association treatment algorithm for interstitial cystitis/painful bladder syndrome includes sacral neuromodulation for refractory cases (for complete guidelines see www.auanet.org/guidelines). (Hanno PM, Burks DA, Clemens JQ, et al. Guideline on the Diagnosis and Treatment of Interstitial Cystitis/Bladder Pain Syndrome (2011). American Urological Association Education and Research, Inc., ©2011; with permission. Available at: http://www.auanet.org/education/guidelines/ic-bladder-pain-syndrome.cfm.)

electrode placed through the S3 foramen.[10,11] It likely modulates this nerve at the sacral and suprasacral levels. The S3 nerves carry efferent autonomic, somatic, and afferent sensory fibers that innervate the bladder, urethral sphincter, and musculature of the pelvic floor. The parasympathetic efferent nerves activate the bladder and inhibit the urethral smooth muscle through the pelvic nerve. The sympathetic efferent nerves activate the bladder neck via the hypogastric nerve. Somatic nerves signal arrival from the Onuf nucleus and travel through the pudendal nerve to the external urinary sphincter. Finally, the sensory information of the bladder travels through the sympathetic and somatic pathways (**Fig. 2**).

The bladder functions differently from other visceral organs by being in the storage phase most of them time and activating only during the micturition stage in an "all-or-none" event.[11] OAB symptoms and IC/PBS involve disproportionately more excitatory signals to the bladder than inhibitory signals. SNM exerts its therapeutic effect by coordinating the bladder signals between storage and emptying phases, and mediating afferent feedback through the sympathetic and somatic pathways. SNM stimulation modulates voiding reflexes by decreasing sympathetic afferent signaling from C fibers that are normally inactive. SNM may therefore block increased sympathetic activity associated with IC/PBS. The somatic afferent pathways, when stimulated by SNM impulses, travel through the pudendal nerve and activate efferent preganglionic neurons of the bladder. Current studies suggest that SNM also changes activity in the brain. On positron emission tomography, the supraspinal effect of SNM stimulation modulates activity in the cingulate gyrus, midbrain, and pons.[12] The brains of patients with OAB show similar areas of changes on functional magnetic resonance imaging (MRI).[13] This exciting area of research has increasing potential for future applications in the treatment of OAB and IC/PBS.

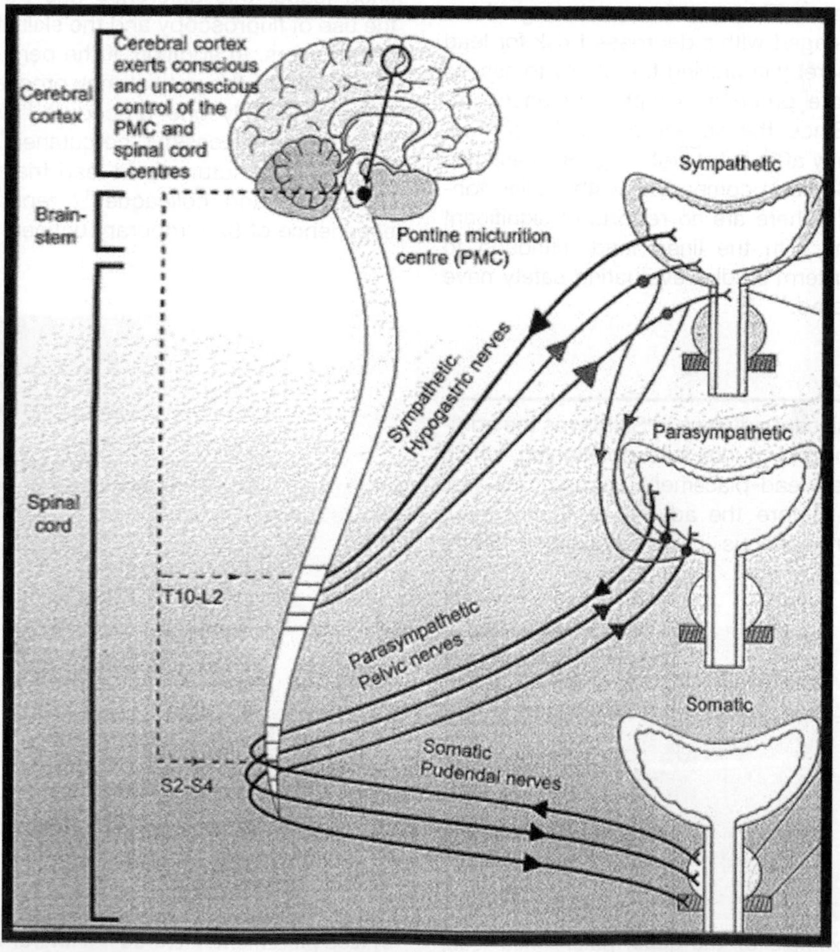

Fig. 2. Sacral neuromodulation. Although the precise mechanism is unknown, sacral neuromodulation stimulates sympathetic, parasympathetic, and somatic fibers of the sacral nerves at the S3 foramen.

TECHNICAL ASPECTS OF SNM

Tined Leads

Since FDA approval of SNM in 1997, in particular InterStim therapy (Medtronic, Minneapolis, MN, USA), numerous advances continue to be made. The first novel advance was the tined lead, approved by the FDA in 2002. Previously, nontined leads resulted in leads anchored to bone or fascia. Bone-anchored leads required general anesthesia, preventing the intraoperative elicitation of any sensory feedback. Although fascia-anchored leads allowed conscious sedations without general anesthesia, they required deep incisions, increasing the anesthetic requirement and minimizing sensory information. By contrast, percutaneous, self-anchoring, tined leads required only mild conscious sedation, allowing sensory and motor responses to augment fluoroscopic confirmation. The most current lead is the quadripolar tined lead, which is made of 4 sets of tines proximal to the electrodes (**Fig. 3**). These leads anchor to the subcutaneous tissue and muscle to prevent lead migration.[14] This modified anchoring allows SNM to be staged with a decreased risk for lead migration, thereby improving the ability to assess efficacy before proceeding with permanent implantation. Since the advent of the tined lead, loss of efficacy after initial first stage success has decreased 3-fold in comparison with earlier nontined leads.[15] There are no reports of significant complications with the tined lead, although to date no long-term studies evaluating safety have been conducted.[16]

Fluoroscopy

Another significant advance in SNM was the addition of fluoroscopy during lead positioning, which has enhanced lead placement accuracy as well as efficacy. Before the advent of fluoroscopy, bilateral percutaneous nerve evaluation (PNE) was the initial screening test used to determine placement of the leads. PNE consisted of passing a temporary electrode "blindly" through the S3 foramen, relying on motor responses and anatomic landmarks to guide placement. After placement, a nontined wire was percutaneously placed and secured to the skin with adhesive tape. Not surprisingly, these leads often became dislodged, and the number of patients proceeding to permanent implantation was significantly lower.[14,17] Anterior-posterior and lateral fluoroscopy now allows for much improved accuracy of lead placement into the proper foramen (**Fig. 4**).

With fluoroscopy becoming more common in clinical settings there has been a revival of PNE, because it allows initial testing to take place in an office setting under local anesthesia. The physician places the temporary leads bilaterally to maximize possible therapeutic benefit, and subsequently removes them at the end of the trial. Although PNE may not have as high a success rate as the intraoperative staged procedure with tined leads, this difference has decreased with the use of fluoroscopy and the skill of very experienced users. In addition, if the percutaneous trial is successful, the patient may proceed to implantation with only one procedure.[16] At the same time, an unsuccessful percutaneous trial does not prohibit a future tined-lead trial. By contrast, Sutherland and colleagues[15] reported on their experience of 82 temporary untined leads placed

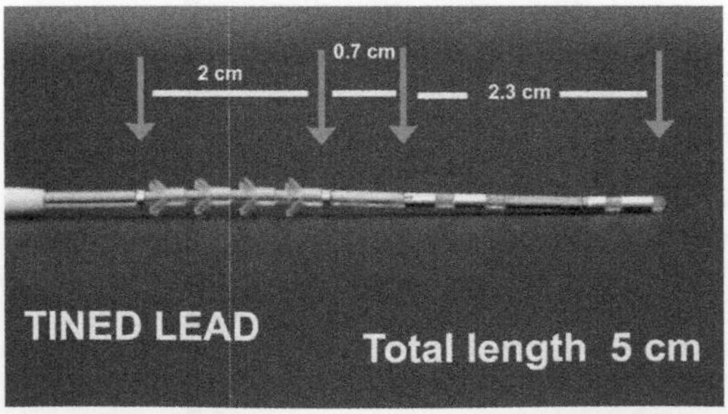

Fig. 3. An example of the quadripolar tined lead, which consists of 4 sets of tines proximal to the 4 electrodes.

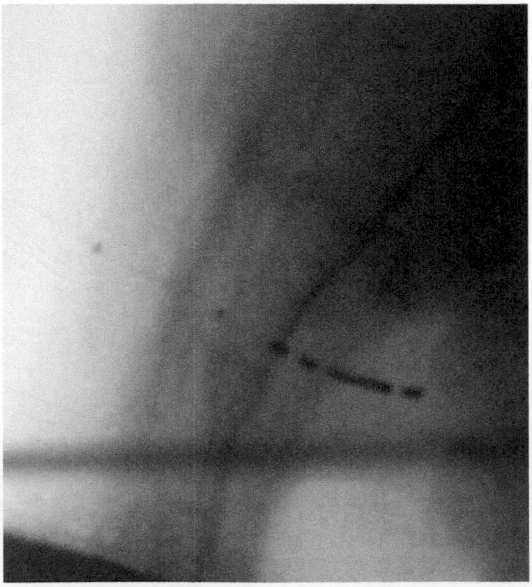

Fig. 4. Fluoroscopy now allows for improved accuracy of lead placement. Pictured is a lateral view of a tined lead in the S3 foramen. (*Courtesy of* Ja-Hong Kim, Los Angeles, CA.)

after a PNE trial and 73 quadripolar tined leads implanted as part of a staged procedure. 17 of 28 patients, who failed the first trial and underwent a successful second trial, initially received PNE. In addition, 4 of 5 patients requiring a third trial found success with a tined staged implant, and all 5 patients requiring a fourth trial found success with a tined staged implant.[15] It appears that performing staged trials with quadripolar tined leads may have higher implantation rates, although this may change over time as percutaneous techniques evolve.

Unilateral Versus Bilateral Test Phase

There is ongoing debate regarding unilateral versus bilateral neuromodulation of S3 for the treatment of OAB and urinary incontinence. Baxter and Kim[18] extensively reviewed the literature and found a paucity of data on this topic. Kessler and colleagues[19] noted the only 2 long-term failures among 16 permanent placements occurred in patients who underwent unilateral first-stage stimulation. Scheepens and colleagues,[20] by contrast, found no statistically significant difference in long-term outcome or progression to second stage between unilateral and bilateral temporary leads. This study, however, had 2 major weaknesses: it used a heterogeneous group of patients with pelvic floor disorders, and it was underpowered to reach significance. Pham and colleagues[21] performed a retrospective comparison of 55 patients undergoing unilateral test stimulation and 69 patients undergoing bilateral test stimulation for refractory voiding dysfunction. This group found that 76% progressed to permanent implantation in the bilateral group, compared with 58% in the unilateral group. Marcelissen and colleagues[22] found that in 12 patients with refractory OAB who had failed unilateral stimulation, 33% had improvement with bilateral stimulation during the first stage. Despite few studies comparing the unilateral to bilateral techniques, it appears that bilateral lead placement may allow more programming flexibility, in turn improving efficacy in the treatment of refractory OAB.

Evolution of Pulse Generator

Since the introduction of the InterStim II device in 2006, the size of the implantable pulse generator has decreased significantly. It is now 50% lighter and smaller, allowing for a smaller incision, less patient discomfort, and higher patient tolerability.[14] The main drawback with the reduced size of the internal pulse generator is shorter battery life. The smaller battery lasts 3 to 5 years, compared with 7 to 10 years for the original device. In more experienced users, however, improved lead placement parallel and in close proximity to the nerve minimizes stimulation thresholds needed for efficacy, thus optimizing battery life.[23] Finally, the Interstim II has more programming capabilities; whether this increases patient satisfaction remains to be determined.

Direct Pudendal Nerve Stimulation

The conventional approach to SNM was lead placement into the S3 foramen. More recently, there has been increasing interest in targeting the pudendal nerve as it originates from the S2, S3, and S4 nerve roots.[14] Pudendal nerve stimulation (PNS) provides broader sacral nerve root stimulation compared to targeting the S3 nerve root alone, and inhibits the micturition reflex, increases bladder capacity, and minimizes uninhibited detrusor contractions. Peters and colleagues[24] performed a prospective, single-blinded, randomized crossover trial comparing traditional SNM with PNS for voiding dysfunction. Thirty patients underwent placement of a sacral tined lead, with a second pudendal tined lead placed on the same side. There were no statistically significant voiding differences between the groups, but 79% of the patients found greater subjective improvement and comfort with the pudendal lead. Both groups experienced significant improvements in urinary urgency, frequency, bowel function, and pelvic pain.

Future Developments

In the near future, screening tools will enable clinicians to better understand which patients are ideal candidates for SNM. Technology will continue to enhance optimal lead placement. Rechargeable batteries with longer battery life are also likely, as are MRI-compatible devices. Finally, the development of novel stimulation targets, such as the dorsal genital nerve, for alternative clinical purposes may occur.

OVERACTIVE BLADDER SYNDROME

Background

OAB syndrome is a combination of urinary symptoms that are defined by the International Continence Society as urinary urgency (compelling desire to void) with or without urinary urge incontinence (UI) (loss of urine preceded by urgency) as well as frequency (>8 episodes daily) and nocturia (>1 episode nightly).[25] OAB has increased excitatory to inhibitory impulses during the filling phase of the bladder that can lead to urinary UI, urgency, frequency, or nocturia. The etiology is not fully understood, and is likely to affect a heterogeneous population of patients who have changes to their central and peripheral nervous systems.[26,27] OAB occurs in the absence of other conditions that present with similar symptoms, such as neurogenic bladder, bladder malignancies, radiation cystitis, bladder obstruction, and high-grade pelvic organ prolapse. It is important to evaluate patients who are refractory to behavioral and medical treatment before proceeding to SNM.

OAB negatively affects the health-related quality of life (HRQOL) of many patients, and poses a significant economic burden.[27–31] The estimated prevalence of OAB in the United States is 12% to 17%, of which one-third of patients primarily have UI.[30,32,33] It is equally prevalent in both genders, and increases with advancing age.[30,32,33] Patients may adapt by developing coping mechanisms, which include being near a toilet at all times or confining themselves to their homes to avoid incontinence accidents. Urgency and UI may cause social anxiety, which limits social interaction and sexual function.[34] Patients with OAB also report lower physical and mental health scores on HRQOL questionnaires.[35] Furthermore, many elderly patients with OAB have higher risk of traumatic falls and fractures because of their frequent rushed visits to the toilet, particularly during the night. This serious comorbidity of OAB, along with increased episodes of urinary tract infection, has led to increasing numbers of office visits in this patient population.[36,37]

The first line of treatment for OAB is behavioral modification and pelvic floor muscle therapy (AUA guideline). Routinely, physicians combine first-line therapy and a second-line treatment of anticholinergic medications. However, the lack of efficacy of these medications, and their side effects, often lead the patient to discontinue their use. Nearly 50% to 75% of patients fail medical therapy and conservative management, leading many to proceed to third-line treatments for refractory OAB. At present, this includes SNM, percutaneous tibial nerve stimulation (PTNS), and intradetrusor botulinum injections (BTX).[38]

Treatment Options for Refractory OAB: SNM, PTNS, and BTX

SNM, PTNS, and BTX all have their own unique considerations. SNM involves placement of a tined lead into the S3 sacral foramen to stimulate the corresponding sacral nerve. The mechanism of action of SNM is discussed in an earlier section. PTNS involves the percutaneous placement of a 25-gauge needle into the posterior tibial nerve, which modulates through the S3 dermatome by a mechanism similar to that of SNM. PTNS entails weekly treatments for 6 to 12 weeks followed by monthly treatments thereafter. The mechanism of action of BTX results in the chemical denervation of the bladder with decreased detrusor contractibility and afferent signaling of the bladder. Botulinum toxin A (BTX-A) temporarily blocks the release of presynaptic acetylcholine through cleavage of the synaptosomal-associated protein 25 (SNAP-25) and binding of synaptic vesicle protein 2.[39] In addition, it affects the afferent transmission by inhibiting the release of substance P, adenosine triphosphate, and downregulating P2×3 and TPRV1 receptors in the urothelium.[40]

SNM for Refractory OAB

Although the precise mechanism is not fully understood, SNM is the most clinically efficacious and utilized modality for the treatment of refractory OAB. Improvement in urinary symptoms from SNM reported in case series and randomized trials ranges from 64% to 88%.[9] Three randomized control trials reveal that SNM was successful in treating refractory OAB, as defined by a 50% improvement in urinary symptoms.[41–43] Weil and colleagues[42] conducted a randomized crossover study in which 21 patients in the treatment arm had immediate SNM implantation and 23 patients in the control arm had delayed SNM implantation for 6 months while receiving conservative treatment with medication and pelvic floor therapy. Seventy-five percent of study patients in the treatment arm showed improvement in the number of episodes of UI, with 56% reporting being completely dry. In a randomized controlled trial reported by Hassouna and colleagues,[41] patients treated with SNM had an 88% improvement in urinary urgency/frequency with a 46% decrease in the frequency of episodes at 12 months follow-up. In a study by Schmidt and colleagues,[43] 99 patients were randomized to immediate placement of SNM versus standardized medical therapy for 6 months. At 6 months follow-up, the number of daily incontinence episodes, severity of episodes, and numbers of absorbent pads or diapers replaced daily were significantly reduced in the immediate stimulation arm ($P<.001$). The cure or dry rate was 47%. In a systematic review that compiled 120 patients from randomized controlled trials and case series, 80% of patients with urinary UI were dry or completely cured after SNM.[44]

A 5-year longitudinal prospective study of a cohort of patients with SNM implants has supported the durability of SNM for treating refractory OAB. At 1-year follow-up, 84% of patients with

UI and 71% with urgency/frequency had improvement, which persisted at 5 years (68% and 56%, respectively).[45] Overall, studies have shown overall improvement for UI at 5 years ranging from 56% to 68%.[8,45] This long-term improvement is similar to those reported in several case series.[15,46,47] In a case series of a 104 patients with a follow-up of 22 months, there was improvement in each urinary symptom (frequency, urgency, UI, nocturia) associated with OAB symptoms (P<.01).[15] These findings were further supported by Foster and colleagues,[47] who reported that 79% of patients, with a mean follow-up of 27 months, were satisfied after implantation.

The majority of these studies occurred before the advent of recent SNM advances. SNM can treat a less severe degree of refractory OAB than was commonly encountered in these previous studies. The recently completed multicenter InSite study prospectively evaluated patients with less severe baseline UI (3.1 episodes daily) who had failed one but not all anticholinergic medications. At baseline and at 12 months, 272 patients completed a validated quality-of-life questionnaire. On each measure of the International Consultation on Incontinence Module Questionnaire (ICIQ), there was an improvement in Overactive Bladder Symptoms Quality of Life (OABqol), with an 80% decrease of urinary symptoms at 12 months.[48] The degree of pelvic pain and depression among study participants also improved, as did overall improvement.

Patients with OAB symptoms often have concomitant pelvic floor disorders that affect their quality of life.[15,49,50] Several studies report SNM improves symptoms of pelvic pain, bowel function, and sexual function.[48,50–53] Using a 0- to 10-point visual analog scale, the InSite study found that patients had improvement in their urinary symptoms and pelvic pain with SNM.[48] Jadav and colleagues[50] analyzed 43 women with urinary symptoms and fecal incontinence, and reported 53% had improvements in overall sexual function after SNM. The study also showed improvements in fecal incontinence, quality of life related to bowel function, and OAB symptoms (P<.05). A prospective pilot study of 8 patients with OAB or fecal incontinence found a trend toward improved sexual function, but this was underpowered to show significance.[54] In a prospective case series from the Cleveland Clinic, 24 patients with refractory OAB showed improved urinary and bowel symptom scores with overall quality of life improving for urinary function but not bowel function.[49]

Although there are 3 treatment modalities for refractory OAB, no treatment algorithm or level I evidence exists to guide the physician regarding which treatment to offer. Using the current literature, the physician is left to decide how to treat refractory OAB guided by clinical experience, expertise, patients' characteristics (age, activity level, ability to use a controller), concomitant symptoms (bowel, retention, pain), and potential side effects of treatment. Each treatment has unique advantages and side effects that require discussion with the patient. For example, PTNS requires weekly visits and monthly maintenance therapy, which may act as a barrier, preventing patients from choosing this method of treatment. Even though BTX and SNM are more established treatments, there is no evidence supporting the efficacy of one treatment over another. Both have been shown to improve OAB symptoms and urinary quality-of-life measures.[15,46,55–59] However, both have potentially serious side effects. For example, BTX may result in urinary retention with need for daily self-catheterizations, or urinary tract infections (UTI). In addition, it often requires repeat procedures. Although treatment with SNM has a very low risk of urinary retention and UTIs, it requires staged procedures and may result in pain, infection, or battery explants. At present, the ROSETTA randomized trial is accruing participants to compare the long-term efficacy of BTX and SNM in the management of refractory OAB syndrome.[60]

Complications of SNM

SNM is a minimally invasive surgical procedure. Most adverse events are minor and include pain, infection, and device explantation. Device removal is typically attributable to pain, infection, lack of clinical response, need for MRI, or loss of battery function. Infection rates range from 0% to 11%, pain ranges from 3% to 42%, and lead migration ranges from 1% to 21%.[41–45] The new advancement of tined leads has dramatically decreased complication rates, from 73% to 28% in one study.[15,61] Management of most SNM complications occurs without surgical intervention, and device explantation rates range from 3% to 11%.[8,62–66] Overall, SNM complication rates range from 11% to 20% when using the updated technology.[48,61,63–66]

INTERSTITIAL CYSTITIS/PAINFUL BLADDER SYNDROME

Background

As discussed earlier, SNM received FDA approval in 1997 as a treatment alternative for UI and in 1999 for nonobstructive urinary retention and urgency/frequency. Off-label use of SNM is increasingly garnering popularity following its successful use in patients with voiding disorders of neurologic origin. An increasing proportion of off-label use involves individuals with IC/PBS.[2]

IC/PBS is a chronic condition of pelvic pain and voiding dysfunction that is neither well defined nor understood, resulting in discord with regard to its diagnosis and treatment. While the theories on the pathophysiology of IC/PBS continue to evolve, known components include epithelial dysfunction, chronic inflammation, and peripheral and central nerve dysfunction.[67] The International Continence Society defines IC/PBS as "the complaint of suprapubic pain related to bladder filling, accompanied by other symptoms such as increased daytime and nighttime frequency, in the absence of proven urinary infection of other obvious pathology." The diagnosis of IC, specifically, is reserved for patients with "typical cystoscopic and histologic features," without further describing these features.[68] In 2007, the European Society for the Study of Bladder Pain Syndrome (ESSIC) recommended that the term "bladder pain syndrome" (BPS) be used with or instead of IC, and defined this syndrome as "chronic pain lasting greater than 6 months with pressure or discomfort perceived to be related to the bladder and accompanied by at least one other urinary symptom."[69] The Society for Urodynamics and Female Urology amended this definition and defined IC/PBS as "an unpleasant sensation (pain, pressure, discomfort) perceived to be related to the urinary bladder, associated with lower urinary tract symptoms of more than 6 weeks duration, in the absence of infection of other identifiable causes."[70] This change in definition allows treatment after a relatively short symptomatic period, preventing the delay in treatment that may occur with the 6-month definition.

Current literature suggests that IC/PBS is significantly burdensome and diagnosed with increasing frequency. Data from the RAND Interstitial Cystitis Epidemiologic (RICE) Study estimated that 2.7% to 6.5% of women in the United States have urinary symptoms consistent with a diagnosis of IC/PBS.[71] These women are often affected by urinary urgency and frequency, nocturia, pelvic pain, dyspareunia, and other overlapping urogynecologic conditions.[6,72] Konkle and colleagues[73] compared the RICE population cohort with a clinically based IC/BPS cohort, and found remarkable similarity with respect to demographics, symptoms, and quality of life. Given this similarity, they concluded that IC/BPS is likely underdiagnosed and undertreated in the United States.

Pathophysiology of IC/PBS

Understanding IC/PBS involves understanding the origins of the reproductive and urinary tract, which both stem from the embryologic mesoderm. In females, the urogenital sinus transforms into the urethra, bladder, vagina, vestibule, and vestibular glands. The endoderm that eventually forms the urothelium of the bladder, trigone, and urethra also forms the lower third of the vagina and vestibule. Similarly, there is shared innervation and muscular support of the bladder, urethra, and pelvis, creating overlapping symptoms. As a result, IC/PBS is frequently associated with pelvic floor dysfunction, vaginitis, and provoked vestibulodynia.[7,74]

Several studies suggest a defect in the urothelial lining, more specifically the glycosaminoglycan layer, as the primary cause of IC/PBS.[75–77] The chain of urothelial cell dysfunction, central and peripheral neural upregulation, a resultant inflammatory response, and mast-cell activation is believed to be responsible for the chronic sequelae related to IC/PBS.[76,78] When noxious stimuli irritate the urothelium, mast-cell activation within the bladder wall causes an inflow of K^+ ions to upregulate afferent nerves; this activates additional mast cells, exacerbating the cycle of "neuroupregulation and inflammation."[6,77,78] Sensory nerve upregulation then results in visceral allodynia and hyperalgesia in the bladder and surrounding pelvic organs.[78] Because of the intertwining neurologic, immunologic, and inflammatory response cycles, some investigators refer to IC/PBS as a component of "complex visceral pain syndrome."[6] Both conditions involve chronic neurogenic inflammation, primary afferent overactivity, and central sensitization that interact to perpetuate pain. These pain impulses emitted by the bladder can then manifest in any or all surrounding organs, causing dyspareunia, pelvic floor dysfunction, and irritable bowel syndrome. The ambiguity in the true origin of pain makes the diagnosis of true IC/PBS difficult, favoring the broader definition of complex visceral pain syndrome by some experts.[6,7]

SNM for IC/PBS

Similarly to IC/PBS, the exact understanding of how SNM alters bladder function is not entirely understood. One theory is that SNM restores balance between excitatory and inhibitory impulses to and from the pelvic organs at the sacral and suprasacral levels. An alternative theory is that SNM modulates the afferent and efferent pathways to improve bladder function. These pathways, in turn, affect urinary function as well as pain.[67,79]

Although not approved by the FDA for pain, multiple articles have demonstrated efficacy of SNM in patients with IC/PBS. Whitmore and colleagues[80] performed a multicenter, prospective, observational study assessing 33 patients with intractable IC who failed alternative therapies. Analysis of voiding diaries showed statistically significant decreases in urinary frequency, bladder pain, average volume voided, and maximum volume voided ($P<.05$) after SNM. There were no significant changes in nocturia. Maher and colleagues[81] analyzed 15 women with refractory IC/PBS. Eleven of 15 patients (73%) reported improvement in pelvic pain, daytime frequency, nocturia, and urgency after percutaneous sacral nerve root stimulation for 7 to 10 days. This same number proceeded to implantation of the sacral neuromodulator. Eighty-seven percent reported a 50% decrease in bladder pain and 47% experienced a 50% decrease in 24-hour voiding frequency. Quality-of-life parameters, including social functioning, bodily pain, and general health as measured by the Short Urinary Distress Inventory and SF-36 Health Survey, also significantly improved.

Comiter[2] prospectively evaluated 25 patients with refractory IC/PBS and treated 17 with sacral nerve stimulation for a mean of 14 months. At follow-up, urinary daytime and nighttime frequency significantly decreased ($P<.01$), mean voided volume increased from 111 to 264 mL ($P<.01$), and pain decreased from 5.8 to 1.6 on a 0- to 10-point visual analog pain scale ($P<.01$). Ninety-four percent of patients with a permanent stimulator demonstrated sustained improvement in bladder capacity, voided volumes, nocturia, pain, and Interstitial Cystitis Symptoms Index (ICSI)/Interstitial Cystitis Problem Index (ICPI) scores at their last postoperative visit.

Peters and Konstandt[82] assessed the efficacy of long-term SNM by retrospectively reviewing 21 patients who had failed a mean of 6 previous treatments for IC/PBS and subsequently underwent implantation of a permanent InterStim device. Patients reported a 36% decrease in narcotic requirements from 81.6 to 52.0 mg/d of morphine dose equivalents, and 4 of 18 patients taking narcotics preoperatively stopped all narcotics after implantation. Overall, 20 of 21 patients reported moderate or marked improvement in pain.

Several studies have assessed the long-term efficacy of SNM for IC/PBS. Rackley and colleagues[83] followed 27 patients with refractory IC/PBS, of whom 22 underwent implantation of SNM. Over a 2-year period, 5 devices were explanted (2 devices were removed because of infection, and 3 because of failure to maintain efficacy). Among those remaining with the device, 13 expressed continued benefit and 4 complained of loss of efficacy. The overall success rate at 2 years was 48% (13 of 27), suggesting that the device may lose some degree of success over time. Other studies have shown variable success rates in long-term efficacy with SNM for IC/PBS. Marinkovic and colleagues[84] reported a 64% reduction in pain at an average of 86 months follow-up in 30 patients who underwent SNM. Powell and Krader[85] presented their long-term experience with SNM in patients with PBS and found that at 59.9 months, 7 of 9 (77.8%) patients who proceeded to permanent generator implantation experienced success with the device, suggesting long-term durability. Gajewksi and Al-Zahrani[86] performed a retrospective review, reporting the long-term results of 78 patients with IC/BPS. Forty-six (59%) demonstrated a positive response to PNE and thus underwent implantation. These patients were then followed for an average of 62 months, and 13 of the 46 (28%) underwent removal, most commonly for poor outcome or painful stimulation. For the remaining patients, the improvement in Global Response Assessment was greater than 75% in 70% of patients, and between 50% and 75% in the other 30% of those retaining the device.[86]

Although the aforementioned studies demonstrate the benefit of treating refractory IC/PBS with SNM, there remains only Grade C evidence, as there are no prospective, multicenter, randomized controlled trials demonstrating its efficacy. In those IC/PBS patients who benefit from SNM, responses tend to occur almost immediately after implantation, which implies that earlier use may decrease patient dissatisfaction with alternative therapies. Further research is needed, however, to delineate who is an optimal candidate. Education is also crucial is managing patient expectations, as most do not experience a complete eradication of symptoms. Rather, the goal should be a significant improvement in quality of life, as SNM is considered an invasive treatment after other conservative modalities have failed.

As alluded to previously, there are many causes of chronic pelvic pain, only one of which is IC/PBS. Irritable bowel syndrome, endometriosis, constipation, and urinary retention are all known risk factors. An additional risk factor is pelvic floor muscle hypertonia. The pudendal nerve provides innervation to the pelvic floor, consisting of the levator ani muscles and the coccygeus. Dysfunction occurs when these muscles contract asynchronously with the bladder or one another.[7] Similar to the improvement shown with IC/PBS, SNM has been also proved to attenuate pelvic pain in this subset of patients.[87] The goal is to reduce pelvic floor hypertonicity, which helps with pelvic pain as well as daytime frequency and nocturia. SNM likely mitigates afferent sacral nerve root stimulation and inhibits the motor fibers innervating the pelvic floor musculature. Subsequently this reduces hypertonicity, which is believed to exist in approximately 85% of patients with IC/PBS.[88,89] Everaert and colleagues[90] performed one of the initial studies suggesting improvement in pelvic pain with SNM. After conservative treatment failed, S3 stimulation was effective in 16 of 26 patients, 11 of whom underwent implantation. At a mean of 36 months' follow-up, all had improvement in pain (visual analog score <3/10, >50% pain relief).

Siegel and colleagues[87] used SNM in 10 patients with chronic intractable pelvic pain, inserting the leads into the S3 and S4 foramen in 8 and 2 cases, respectively. After a follow-up of 19 months, the number of hours of pain decreased from 13.1 to 6.9, with 9 of 10 patients experiencing a decrease in pain. The severity of pain decreased from 9.7 to 4.4 on the 0- to 10-point visual acuity pain scale.

Chai and colleagues[91] assessed 6 consecutive patients with symptoms and cystoscopic findings compatible with IC. These patients underwent continuous bilateral S3 stimulation with PNE for 5 days. In addition to monitoring pain and voiding diaries, urine samples were taken before and after measuring for heparin-binding epidermal growth factor and antiproliferative factor. After stimulation, pelvic pain scores decreased from 7.0 to 2.3 on a visual acuity pain scale. Furthermore, urinary antiproliferative factor activity decreased from −76.1% to −4.5%, suggesting significantly decreased inflammatory activity.

Not all studies have suggested uniform improvement, however. In one of the largest literature reviews to date, Marcelissen and colleagues[92] concluded that there is still insufficient evidence to determine the role of SNM in the treatment of chronic pelvic pain. Additional studies are still needed.

Because bladder and pelvic pain often involve more than one sacral root, either unilaterally or bilaterally, the stimulation of only one nerve root may not be sufficient in controlling pain. As of yet no trial has compared unilateral with bilateral tined-lead placement, although several studies suggest efficacy of the bilateral approach. Steinberg and colleagues[1] retrospectively reviewed 15 patients who underwent bilateral S3 stimulators for refractory IC/PBS. At a mean follow-up of 14.1 months, the mean decrease in frequency and nocturia was 10.4 voids ($P<.001$) and 2.6 voids ($P<.001$), respectively. Patient satisfaction improved as measured by the Urinary Distress Inventory short form ($P<.001$) and four patients were noted to have an improvement in fecal incontinence with 2.75 fewer episodes per day ($P<.01$).

In a similar study, Zabihi and colleagues[3] reported their experience with bilateral S2-S4 caudal epidural SNM using 2 parallel tined leads in 30 consecutive patients with severe refractory IC and/or chronic pelvic pain. Seventy-seven percent had a successful trial stimulation leading to permanent implantation. In these patients, pain improved by 40% ($P = .04$), and their ICSI and ICPI scores improved by 35% ($P = .005$) and 38% ($P = .007$), respectively. Unique to this study was that it utilized a caudal approach for lead placement, allowing stimulation of the S2 to S5 nerves, rather than only the S3 nerve. Though these are all small studies, they suggest SNM may play a role in alleviating symptoms of chronic pelvic pain.

Explant Rate of Pulse Generator in IC/PBS Patients

At present, the manufacturer of SNM lists the battery life for the original model as 7 years and the newer, smaller model as 4.4 years.[93] Although these statistics have held up in small trials assessing battery longevity,[85] these devices are occasionally removed prematurely because of infection, device damage, lack of response, site-specific pain, or need for MRI.[15,46,62] There is some speculation that certain urologic disease states, such as IC/PBS, increase the risk of device explantation by 50%.[85] However, other studies that assessed only IC/PBS patients reported no explantations.[2] Recently, Cameron and colleagues[94] analyzed a 5% sample of Medicare beneficiaries from 1997 to 2007 to determine the greatest risk factors for device explantation. Mean follow-up was 60.5 months. In this data series, 558 batteries were implanted and 63 (11.3%) explanted. Of the 19 individuals who were diagnosed with interstitial cystitis, 11 (57.9%) had the pulse generator removed. In this multivariate analysis, the diagnosis of IC was the only risk factor that predicted early removal, with an odds ratio of 10.5 (95% confidence interval 3.9–28.4). It should be noted that Medicare patients tend to be more elderly, which may preclude the generalization of these data to the rest of the population. In addition, with no clinical information about bladder symptoms, there is no way to know how many batteries were still functional at the time of explantation. Nevertheless, IC/PBS patients may suffer from higher levels of pain than other patients with similar demographics undergoing SNM and may not be as able to tolerate this procedure. Further studies are needed to better support this hypothesis.

SUMMARY

Sacral neuromodulation is a minimally invasive procedure that has revolutionized the treatment of various pelvic floor conditions such as refractory OAB, UI, and IC/PBS. Although its exact mechanism of action remains to be fully understood, there is a growing body of evidence demonstrating its durable efficacy in the management of bothersome urinary and pelvic pain related symptoms. Future research will aim at evaluating novel stimulation targets using pudendal and caudal approaches, minimizing explant rates resulting from infection and battery life, and developing MRI-compatible protocols. Large clinical trials are needed to clearly identify the patients most likely to benefit from SNM, thus maximizing successful outcomes and minimizing costs.

REFERENCES

1. Steinberg AC, Oyama IA, Whitmore KE. Bilateral S3 stimulator in patients with interstitial cystitis. J Urol 2007;69(3):441–3.
2. Comiter CV. Sacral neuromodulation for the symptomatic treatment of refractory interstitial cystitis: a prospective study. J Urol 2003;169(4):1369–73.
3. Zabihi N, Mourtzinos A, Maher MG, et al. Short-term results of bilateral S2-S4 sacral neuromodulation for the treatment of refractory interstitial cystitis, painful bladder syndrome, and chronic pelvic pain. Int Urogynecol J Pelvic Floor Dysfunct 2008;19(4):553–7.
4. Bosch JL. An update on sacral neuromodulation: where do we stand with this in the management of lower urinary tract dysfunction in 2010? BJU Int 2010;106(10):1432–42.
5. Lay AH, Das AK. The role of neuromodulation in patients with neurogenic overactive bladder. Curr Urol Rep 2012;13(5):343–7.
6. Wesselmann U. Interstitial cystitis: a chronic visceral pain syndrome. J Urol 2001;57(6 Suppl 1):32–9.
7. Fariello JY, Whitmore K. Sacral neuromodulation stimulation for IC/PBS, chronic pelvic pain, and sexual dysfunction. Int Urogynecol J 2010;21(12):1553–8.
8. Siddiqui NY, Wu JM, Amudsen CL. Efficacy and adverse events of sacral nerve stimulation for overactive bladder: a systemic review. Neurourol Urodyn 2010;29(1):S18–23.
9. Banakhar MA, Al-Shaiji T, Hassouna M. Sacral neuromodulation and refractory overactive bladder: an emerging tool for an old problem. Ther Adv Urol 2012;4(4):179–85.
10. Elkelini MS, Abuzgaya A, Hassouna MM. Mechanism of action of sacral neuromodulation. Int Urogynecol J 2010;21(2):S439–46.
11. Leng WW, Chancellor MB. How sacral nerve stimulation neuromodulation works. Urol Clin North Am 2005;32:11–8.
12. Dasgupta R, Critchley HD, Dolan RJ, et al. Changes in brain activity following sacral neuromodulation for urinary retention. J Urol 2005;174(6):2268–72.
13. Tadic SD, Griffiths D, Schaefer W, et al. Brain activity underlying impaired continence control in older women with overactive bladder. Neurourol Urodyn 2012;31(5):652–8.
14. Spinelli M, Sievert KD. Latest technologic and surgical developments in using InterStim Therapy for sacral neuromodulation: impact on treatment success and safety. Eur Urol 2008;54(6):1287–96.
15. Sutherland SE, Layers A, Carlson A, et al. Sacral nerve stimulation for voiding dysfunction: one institution's 11-year experience. Neurourol Urodyn 2007;26(1):19–28.
16. Thompson JH, Sutherland SE, Siegel SW. Sacral neuromodulation: therapy evolution. Indian J Urol 2010;26(3):379–84.
17. Janknegt RA, Weil EH, Eerdmans PH. Improving neuromodulation technique for refractory voiding dysfunctions: two-stage implant. J Urol 1997;49(3):358–62.
18. Baxter C, Kim JH. Contrasting the percutaneous nerve evaluation versus staged implantation in sacral neuromodulation. Curr Urol Rep 2010;11(5):310–4.
19. Kessler TM, Madersbacher H, Kiss G. Prolonged sacral neuromodulation testing using permanent leads: a more reliable patient selection method? Eur Urol 2005;47(5):660–5.
20. Scheepens WA, de Bie RA, Weil EH, et al. Unilateral versus bilateral sacral neuromodulation in patients with chronic voiding dysfunction. J Urol 2002;168(5):2046–50.
21. Pham K, Guralnick ML, O'Connor RC. Unilateral versus bilateral stage 1 neuromodulator lead placement for the treatment of refractory voiding dysfunction. Neurourol Urodyn 2008;27(8):779–81.
22. Marcelissen TA, Leong RK, Serroyen J, et al. The use of bilateral sacral nerve stimulation in patients with loss of unilateral treatment efficacy. J Urol 2011;185(3):976–80.
23. Siegel SW, Moeller SE. Sacral neuromodulation for the treatment of overactive bladder (OAB). In: Raz S, Rodriquez L, editors. Female urology. 3rd edition. Philadelphia: WB Saunders Company; 2008. p. 266–76 Chapter 22.

24. Peters KM, Feber KM, Bennett RC. Sacral versus pudendal nerve stimulation for voiding dysfunction: a prospective, single-blinded, randomized, crossover trial. Neurourol Urodyn 2005;24(7):643–7.
25. Abrams P. Urgency: the key to defining overactive bladder. BJU Int 2005;96(Suppl 1):1–3.
26. Tadic S, Holstege G, Griffiths DJ. The CNS and bladder dysfunction. F1000 Med Rep 2012;4:20.
27. Coyne KS, Payne C, Bhattacharyya SK, et al. The impact of urinary urgency and frequency on health-related quality of life in overactive bladder: results from a national community survey. Value Health 2004;7(4):455–63.
28. Coyne KS, Sexton CC, Irwin DE, et al. The impact of overactive bladder, incontinence and other lower urinary tract symptoms on quality of life, work productivity, sexuality and emotional well-being in men and women: results from the EPIC study. BJU Int 2008;101(11):1388–95.
29. Liberman JN, Hunt TL, Stewart WF, et al. Health-related quality of life among adults with symptoms of overactive bladder: results from a community-based survey. Urology 2001;57(6):1044–50.
30. Stewart WF, Van Rooyen JB, Cundiff GW, et al. Prevalence and burden of overactive bladder in the United States. World J Urol 2003;20(6):327–36.
31. Irwin DE, Mungapen L, Milsom I. The economic impact of overactive bladder syndrome in six Western countries. BJU Int 2009;103(20):202–9.
32. Irwin DE, Milson I, Hunskaar S. Population-based survey of urinary incontinence, overactive bladder, and other lower urinary tract symptoms in five countries: results of the EPIC study. Eur Urol 2006;50(6):1306–14.
33. Milsom I, Abrams P, Cardoza L, et al. How widespread are the symptoms of overactive bladder and how are they managed? A population-based prevalence study. BJU Int 2001;87(9):760–6.
34. Abrams P, Kelleher CJ, Kerr LA, et al. Overactive bladder significantly affects quality of life. Am J Manag Care 2000;6(11):S580–90.
35. Kannan H, Radican L, Turpin RS, et al. Burden of illness associated with lower urinary tract symptoms including overactive bladder/urinary incontinence. J Urol 2009;74(1):34–8.
36. Brown JS, McGhan WF, Chokroverty S. Comorbidities associated with overactive bladder. Am J Manag Care 2000;6(11):S574–9.
37. Darkow T, Fontes CL, Williamson TE. Costs associated with the management of overactive bladder and related comorbidities. Pharmacotherapy 2005;25(4):511–9.
38. Sears CL, Lewis C, Noel K, et al. Overactive bladder medication adherence when medication is free to patients. J Urol 2010;183(3):1077–81.
39. Dong M, Yeh F, Tepp WH, et al. SV2 is the protein receptor for botulinum neurotoxin A. Science 2006;312(5773):592–6.
40. Apostolidis A, Popat R, Yiangou Y, et al. Decreased sensory receptors P2X3 and TRPV1 in suburothelial nerve fibers following intradetrusor injections of botulinum toxin for human detrusor overactivity. J Urol 2005;174(3):977–82; [discussion 982-3].
41. Hassouna MM, Siegel SW, Nyebolt AA, et al. Sacral neuromodulation in the treatment of urgency-frequency symptoms: a multicenter study on efficacy and safety. J Urol 2000;163(6):1849–54.
42. Weil EH, Ruiz-Cerda JL, Eerdmans PH, et al. Sacral root neuromodulation in the treatment of refractory urinary urge incontinence: a prospective randomized clinical trial. Eur Urol 2000;37(2):161–71.
43. Schmidt RA, Jonas U, Oleson KA, et al. Sacral nerve stimulation for treatment of refractory urinary urge incontinence. Sacral Nerve Stimulation Study Group. J Urol 1999;162(2):352–7.
44. Brazzelli M, Murray A, Fraser C. Efficacy and safety of sacral nerve stimulation for urinary urge incontinence: a systemic review. J Urol 2006;175(3 Pt 1):835–41.
45. van Kerrebroeck PE, van Voskuilen AC, Heesakkers JP, et al. Results of sacral neuromodulation therapy for urinary voiding dysfunction: outcomes of a prospective, worldwide clinical study. J Urol 2007;178(5):2029–34.
46. Sigel SW, Catanzaro F, Dijkema HE, et al. Long-term results of a multicenter study on sacral nerve stimulation for treatment of urinary urge incontinence, urgency-frequency, and retention. J Urol 2000;56(6 Suppl 1):87–91.
47. Foster RT Sr, Anoia EJ, Webster GD, et al. In patients undergoing neuromodulation for intractable urge incontinence a reduction in 24-hr pad weight after the initial test stimulation best predicts long-term patient satisfaction. Neurourol Urodyn 2007;26(2):213–7.
48. Comiter C, Bennett J, Pinson T, et al. Evaluation of quality of life improvements at twelve months in subjects with overactive bladder treated with sacral neuromodulation using the InterStim system. Urodynamics/Incontinence/Female Urology: incontinence, Evaluation & Therapy (II) Moderated Poster. AUA 2013 [abstract 1034].
49. Gill BC, Swartz MA, Rackley RR. Improvement of bowel dysfunction with sacral neuromodulation for refractory urge urinary incontinence. Int Urogynecol J 2012;23(6):735–41.
50. Jadav AM, Wadhawan H, Jones GL. Does sacral nerve stimulation improve global pelvic function in women? Colorectal Dis 2013;15(7):848–57.
51. El-Gazzaz G, Zutshi M, Salcedo L, et al. Sacral neuromodulation for the treatment of fecal incontinence and urinary incontinence in female

patients: long-term follow-up. Int J Colorectal Dis 2009;24(12):1377–81.
52. Kim DH, Faruqui N, Ghoniem GM. Sacral neuromodulation outcomes in patients with urge urinary incontinence and concomitant urge fecal incontinence. Female Pelvic Med Reconstr Surg 2010;16(3):171–8.
53. Killinger KA, Hangas JR, Wolfert C, et al. Secondary changes in bowel function after successful treatment of voiding symptoms with neuromodulation. Neurourol Urodyn 2011;30(1):133–7.
54. van Voskuilen AC, Oerlemans DJ, Gielen N, et al. Sexual response in patients in patients treated with sacral neuromodulation for lower urinary tract symptoms or fecal incontinence. Urol Int 2012;88(4):423–30.
55. Fowler CJ, Auerbach S, Ginsberg D, et al. OnabotulinumtoxinA improves health-related quality of life in patients with urinary retention due to idiopathic overactive bladder: a 36-week, double-blinded, placebo-controlled, randomized, dose-ranging trial. Eur Urol 2012;62(1):148–57.
56. Anger JT, Weinberg A, Suttorp MJ, et al. Outcomes of intravesical botulinum toxin for idiopathic overactive bladder symptoms: a systemic review of the literature. J Urol 2010;183(6):2258–64.
57. Nitti VW, Dmochowski R, Herschorn S, et al. OnabotulinumtoxinA for the treatment of patients with overactive bladder and urinary incontinence: results of a phase 3, randomized, placebo controlled trial. J Urol 2013;189(6):2186–93.
58. Chapple C, Sievert KD, Macdiamid S, et al. OnabotulinumtoxinA 100 U significantly improves all idiopathic overactive bladder symptoms and quality of life in patients with overactive bladder and urinary incontinence: a randomised, double-blind, placebo-controlled trial. Eur Urol 2013;64(2):249–56.
59. Dmochowski R, Chapple C, Nitti VW, et al. Efficacy and safety of onabotulinumtoxinA for idiopathic overactive bladder: a double-blind, placebo controlled, randomized, dose ranging trial. J Urol 2010;184(6):2416–22.
60. Meikle S, Amundsen C, Richter H, et al. Refractory overactive bladder: sacral neuromodulation v. BoTulinum Toxin Assessment (ROSETTA) Trial. NIH. Available at: Clinicaltrialsfeeds.org.
61. van Voskuilen AC, Oerlemans DJ, Weil EH, et al. Medium-term experience of sacral neuromodulation by tined lead implantation. BJU Int 2007;99(1):107–10.
62. van Voskuilen AC, Oerlemans DJ, Weil EH, et al. Long term results of neuromodulation by sacral nerve stimulation for lower urinary tract symptoms: a retrospective single center study. Eur Urol 2006;49(2):366–72.
63. Spinelli M, Weil E, Ostardo E. New tined lead electrode in sacral neuromodulation: experience from a multicenter European study. World J Urol 2005;23(3):225–9.
64. Aboseif SR, Kim DH, Rieder JM. Sacral neuromodulation: cost considerations and clinical benefits. J Urol 2007;70(6):1069–73.
65. Hijaz A, Vasavada S. Complications and troubleshooting of sacral neuromodulation therapy. Urol Clin North Am 2005;32(1):65–9.
66. Guralnick ML, Benouni S, O'Connor RC, et al. Characteristics of infections in patients undergoing staged implantation for sacral nerve stimulation. J Urol 2007;69(6):1073–6.
67. Moldwin RM, Evans RJ, Stanford EJ, et al. Rational approaches to the treatment of patients with interstitial cystitis. J Urol 2007;69(Suppl 4):73–81.
68. Abrams P, Cardozo L, Fall M, et al. The standardisation of terminology of lower urinary tract function: report from the Standardisation Subcommittee of the International Continence Society. Neurourol Urodyn 2002;21(2):167–78.
69. van de Merwe JP, Nordling J, Bouchelouche P, et al. Diagnostic criteria, classification, and nomenclature for painful bladder syndrome/interstitial cystitis: an ESSIC proposal. Eur Urol 2008;53(1):60–7.
70. Hanno P, Dmochowski P. Status of international consensus on interstitial cystitis/bladder pain syndrome/painful bladder syndrome: 2008 snapshot. Neurourol Urodyn 2009;28(4):274–86.
71. Berry S, Bogart L, Soto M, et al. Presented at the American Urological Association Annual Meeting. Chicago, April 25–29, 2009.
72. Butrick CW. Interstitial cystitis/bladder pain syndrome: management of the pain disorder: a urogynecology perspective. Urol Clin North Am 2012;39(3):377–87.
73. Konkle KS, Berry SH, Elliott MN, et al. Comparison of an interstitial cystitis/bladder pain syndrome clinical cohort with symptomatic community women from the RAND Interstitial Cystitis Epidemiology study. J Urol 2012;187(2):508–12.
74. Myers DL, Aguilar VC. Gynecologic manifestations of interstitial cystitis. Clin Obstet Gynecol 2002;45(1):233–41.
75. Parsons CL. The role of the urinary epithelium in the pathogenesis of interstitial cystitis/prostatitis/urethritis. J Urol 2007;69(Suppl 4):9–16.
76. Sant GR, Kempuraj D, Marchand JE, et al. The mast cell in interstitial cystitis: role in pathophysiology and pathogenesis. J Urol 2007;69(Suppl 4):34–40.
77. Whitmore K, Siegel JF, Kellogg-Spadt S. Interstitial cystitis/painful bladder syndrome as a cause of sexual pain in women: a diagnosis to consider. J Sex Med 2007;4(3):720–7.

78. Nazif O, Teichman JM, Gebhart GF. Neural upregulation in interstitial cystitis. J Urol 2007;69(Suppl 4): 24–33.
79. Peters KM, Carey JM, Konstandt DB. Sacral neuromodulation for the treatment of refractory interstitial cystitis: outcomes based on technique. Int Urogynecol J Pelvic Floor Dysfunct 2003;14(4): 223–8.
80. Whitmore KE, Payne CK, Diokno AC, et al. Sacral neuromodulation in patients with interstitial cystitis: a multicenter clinical trial. Int Urogynecol J Pelvic Floor Dysfunct 2003;14(5):305–8.
81. Maher CF, Carey MP, Dwyer PL, et al. Percutaneous sacral nerve root neuromodulation for intractable interstitial cystitis. J Urol 2001;165(3): 884–6.
82. Peters KM, Konstandt D. Sacral neuromodulation decreases narcotic requirements in refractory interstitial cystitis. BJU Int 2004;93(6):777–9.
83. Rackley R, Vasavada S, Daneshagani F, et al. Neuromodulation for interstitial cystitis 2005. Clev Clin Glickman Urol Inst. Available at: http://my.clevelandclinic.org/Documents/Urology/AUA%20Abstracts%202005.pdf.
84. Marinkovic SP, Gillen LM, Marinkovic CM. Minimum 6-year outcomes for interstitial cystitis treated with sacral neuromodulation. Int Urogynecol J 2011; 22(4):407–12.
85. Powell CR, Kreder KJ. Long-term outcomes of urgency-frequency syndrome due to painful bladder syndrome treated with sacral neuromodulation and analysis of failures. J Urol 2010;183(1): 173–6.
86. Gajewski JB, Al-Zahrani AA. The long-term efficacy of sacral neuromodulation in the management of intractable cases of bladder pain syndrome: 14 years of experience in one centre. BJU Int 2011; 107(8):1258–64.
87. Siegel S, Paszkiewicz E, Kirkpatrick C, et al. Sacral nerve stimulation in patients with chronic intractable pelvic pain. J Urol 2001;166(5):1742–5.
88. Peters KM, Carrico DJ, Kalinowski SE. Prevalence of pelvic floor dysfunction in patients with interstitial cystitis. J Urol 2007;70(1):16–8.
89. Finamore PS, Goldstein HB, Whitmore KE. Pelvic floor muscle dysfunction: a review. J Pelvic Med Surg 2008;14(6):417–22.
90. Everaert K, Plancke H, Lefevere F, et al. The urodynamic evaluation of neuromodulation in patients with voiding dysfunction. Br J Urol 1997;79(5):702–7.
91. Chai TC, Zhang C, Warren JW, et al. Percutaneous sacral third nerve root neurostimulation improves symptoms and normalizes urinary HB-EGF levels and antiproliferative activity in patients with interstitial cystitis. J Urol 2000;55(5):643–6.
92. Marcelissen T, Jacobs R, van Kerrebroeck P, et al. Sacral neuromodulation as a treatment for chronic pelvic pain. J Urol 2011;186(2): 387–93.
93. Sacral Nerve Stimulation. 2012. Available at: http://professional.medtronic.com/therapies/sacral-nerve-stimulation-interstim-therapy/index.htm.
94. Cameron AP, Anger JT, Madison R, et al. Battery explantation after sacral neuromodulation in the Medicare population. Neurourol Urodyn 2012; 32(3):238–41.

Neuromodulation for Movement Disorders

Rob Dallapiazza, MD, PhD[a], M. Sean McKisic, MD[a],
Binit Shah, MD[b], W. Jeff Elias, MD[a,*]

KEYWORDS

• Neuromodulation • DBS • Stereotactic surgery • Focused ultrasound • Essential tremor
• Parkinson's disease

KEY POINTS

- Since the advent of stereotactic neurosurgery, various neuromodulation modalities have been used to confirm target localization.
- Electrical stimulation is the most common form of neuromodulation and is highly effective in treating essential tremor and Parkinson disease.
- Further experimental refinement of chemical and ultrasound neuromodulation may lead to highly selective and minimally invasive treatments of movement disorders.
- Magnetic and ultrasound neuromodulation have the potential for neuromodulation without open cranial surgery.

INTRODUCTION

The treatment of movement disorders represents an ideal application for neuromodulation of the central nervous system. Essential tremor (ET) and Parkinson disease (PD) are the most common movement disorders that are treated surgically. Although there are no curative therapies, the symptoms of both diseases are managed initially and effectively with medicine, but severe and refractory impairments occur during disease progression, requiring surgery to maintain quality of life. Over the past 2 decades, surgical neuromodulation has seen a dramatic resurgence in the treatment of ET and PD with the popularization and refinement of high-frequency, deep brain stimulation (DBS).

The critical element for successful DBS, or any stereotactic intervention, is precise anatomic localization and method for physiologic verification. This has significantly improved with modern neuroimaging, stereotactic equipment, and electrophysiology. However, even during the pioneering days of stereotactic neurosurgery when pallidotomy and thalamotomy were common procedures for the treatment of involuntary movements, surgeons recognized the need for precise localization and reversible means to confirm their target. This ensured the best outcomes. Surgeons creatively modulated neural circuitry with a variety of methods, including chemical inhibition, thermoregulation, focused ultrasound, and electrical stimulation.

Modern movement disorder surgery uses neuromodulation in 2 ways. First, it is used intraoperatively to verify the stereotactic target in the thalamus or basal ganglia by measuring the clinical or electrophysiologic responses to electrical stimulation. Second, neuromodulation is used chronically with DBS for treatment (**Figs. 1** and **2**).

Chemical Neuromodulation

Chemical neuromodulation refers to injection or infusion of a pharmacologically active substance within the nervous system. This application has the theoretical benefit of targeting specific receptors with precise effects. While chemical

[a] Department of Neurosurgery, University of Virginia School of Medicine, Charlottesville, VA, USA; [b] Department of Neurology, University of Virginia School of Medicine, Charlottesville, VA, USA
* Corresponding author.
E-mail address: wje4r@virginia.edu

Neurosurg Clin N Am 25 (2014) 47–58
http://dx.doi.org/10.1016/j.nec.2013.08.002
1042-3680/14/$ – see front matter

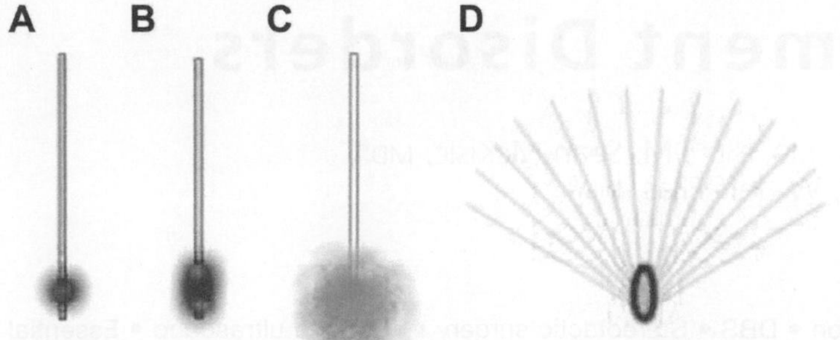

Fig. 1. Therapeutic zones by each neuromodulation modality. (*A*) Monopolar DBS electrodes produce a spherical zone of effect. (*B*) Bipolar DBS electrode configuration produces an elliptical-shaped zone. (*C*) Chemical infusions have a spherical zone of effect with a tail that tracts up the catheter. (*D*) Focused ultrasound lesions are elliptical or disc-shaped secondary to the configuration of the ultrasound transducers around the head during treatment.

neuromodulation is principally used in animal models for experimental purposes, there are several studies that have reported chemical neuromodulation in the human brain for movement disorders. In 1955, Cooper published a series of 5 patients in whom he injected procaine into the globus pallidus before creating a permanent lesion with ethanol for tremor in advanced PD.[1,2] He used

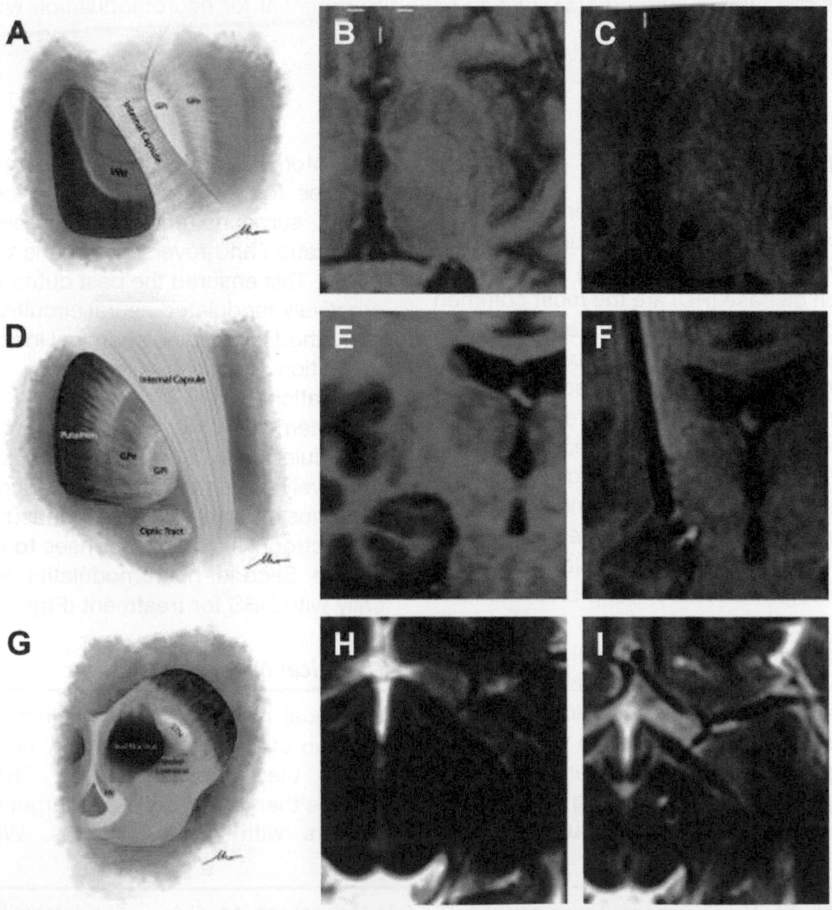

Fig. 2. Targets for DBS. (*A–C*) Targeting of the Vim nucleus is shown in the axial plane before (*B*) and after (*A*) DBS electrode implantation. (*D–F*) In the coronal plane, the GPi can be seen lateral to the internal capsule and medial to the putamen. (*E, F*) T1 MRI with an electrode targeting the GPi. (*G–I*) Axial T2 MRI showing the red nucleus and cerebral peduncle, often the STN can be seen. (*H, I*) Electrode targeting of the STN. Illustrations by M. Sean McKisic.

Central Neuromodulation

roentgenography for initial catheter placement with minor modifications of catheter position based on small volume tests of procaine until the "physiologic landmark" was identified by reduced tremor and rigidity in the contralateral limbs without evidence of motor weakness. He reported improved tremor and rigidity in 6 months of follow up for 3 of these patients. Similarly, Narabayashi and colleagues[3,4] used early stereotactic methods to inject procaine into the pallidum before permanent lesioning in patients with choreoathetosis. As with Cooper, small volumes of local anesthetic were used to determine whether the site of putative lesioning would be safe. In the series of 80 patients, improvement in athetosis was reported in approximately 60% of patients.

Infusion of local anesthetic was also applied to the thalamus during treatment of tremor. During radiofrequency thalamotomy, Parrent and colleagues[5] first infused 1 to 2 μL of lidocaine in 10 patients with tremor. They observed a transient suppression of tremor with a mean onset of 69 seconds and duration of 171 seconds. Interestingly, the lidocaine infusions correlated with microstimulation effects in 67% of cases.

As the understanding of neurotransmitter systems advanced with the use of selective antagonists and agonists, so did its application to movement disorders. In 1984, Penn and Kroin[6,7] used intrathecal baclofen, a GABA-B receptor agonist, to alleviate spasticity of spinal origin. Shortly thereafter, they targeted the globus pallidum with muscimol, a GABA-A receptor agonist, during pallidotomy surgery for a patient with PD. Within 20 minutes, bradykinetic movements increased and rigidity resolved, although tremor worsened.[8]

Intraoperative microinjections of muscimol into deep brain nuclei of patients with PD have been reported to transiently inhibit either the globus pallidus internus (GPi) or subthalamic nucleus (STN) neurons. The effect of muscimol infusion elicits a temporary clinical effect that is similar to stimulation or lesioning. Levy and colleagues[9] targeted the STN with muscimol in 7 patients with PD. Modern microelectrode recording techniques were used to confirm target location, and small doses of lidocaine and muscimol were injected into the STN with simultaneous microelectrode recording in 2 patients. Injection of lidocaine blocked nearby neural firing within minutes and improved contralateral limb rigidity with peak effect 10 to 20 minutes after injection. Dyskinesias were noted while blocking the STN with lidocaine. In 2 of 3 patients, these effects wore off during the procedure. Muscimol injection had a similar effect by decreasing tremor in the contralateral limb of both patients tested, and altered the spectrum of a single neuron oscillatory frequency. No adverse events were noted with injection of muscimol. The clinical improvements with muscimol infusion were correlated closely with successful final treatment effects.

Pahapill and colleagues[10] reported infusion of muscimol into the Vim nucleus of patients with ET. Similarly, microelectrode recordings were used to confirm tremor-synchronous neurons in the lateral thalamus, and microelectrode stimulation ceased tremor. Subsequent microinfusion of muscimol reliably reduced tremor with a latency of 7 minutes and for a mean duration of 9 minutes.

Although chemical neuromodulation is principally used in experimental models, these examples in humans are important advances in understanding the basic pathophysiology of movement disorders and its potential application as a therapeutic tool (**Table 1**).

Table 1
A summary of chemical infusions into the human thalamus and basal ganglia during movement disorder surgery

Study	n	Target	Drug	Concentration	Dose/Infusion
Cooper,[1] 1955	5	GPi	Procaine	NS	<250 μL
Narabayashi et al,[4] 1960	80	GPi	Procaine	NS	1–2 μL
Parrent et al,[5] 1993	10	Thalamus	Lidocaine	2%	1–2 μL
Penn et al,[8] 1998	1	GPi	Muscimol	8.8 mM	2.5 μL
Levy et al,[9] 2001	4	STN	Lidocaine	2%	3.5–23 μL
	2	STN	Muscimol	8.8 mM	5–10 μL
Pahapill et al,[10] 1999	6	Thalamus	Muscimol	8.8 mM	1–5 μL
	3	Thalamus	Saline		

Abbreviations: GPi, globus pallidus internus; STN, subthalamic nucleus.

Cryogenic Neuromodulation

During the 1950s, scientists and surgeons were examining the effects of cooling on nervous tissues and function. Results from these experiments showed that cooling various structures of the brain to 0 to 10°C produced a reversible inhibition of neural activity, and that cooling below −20° could create a permanent lesion. In 1961, Mark and colleagues[11] used a refrigeration probe to cool the region of the third nerve nucleus in cats and demonstrated reversible pupillary dilation. Rowbotham and colleagues[12] applied this concept to humans for the treatment of glioma. Cooper published a report of 100 cryothalamotomies for parkinsonism and concluded that the procedure was the ideal technique for movement disorder surgery, as it provides a reversible, physiologic test before the creation of a stable lesion.[13–15] Although the study does not specifically cite examples of neuromodulation during the course of the target localization, subsequent commentary notes, "I have had the pleasure of seeing Dr Cooper turn a Babinski on and off by adjustment of a valve. This is truly impressive (Cambell JB)."

Thermal Neuromodulation

During the same period as cryogenic thalamotomies, radiofrequency waves were also being used to produce thermal lesions within the brain. Experimental models demonstrated reversible inhibition of neural activity. Using a model similar to Mark and colleagues,[11] Brodkey and colleagues[16] used radiofrequency stimulation to heat the Edinger-Westphal (EW) nucleus in cats. They found that heating the EW nucleus to 44 to 49°C produced a reversible dilation of the pupil that returned to baseline size within 20 minutes of heating. The premise that low-temperature heating can produce reversible lesions in the brain is based on these studies. It is now recognized that low-temperature heating can cause thermal injury depending on the duration of exposure such that tissue ablation even occurs at approximately 43°C when exposed for a duration of 240 minutes.[17]

Ultrasound Neuromodulation

Interestingly, even before the publication of cryothalamotomy and radiofrequency lesioning in the basal ganglia, Fry and colleagues[18,19] reported the use of high-intensity ultrasound to create destructive lesions of the internal capsule in cats. The goal of their research was to provide neurosurgeons with a tool to perform functional neurosurgery in the treatment of movement disorders. They sonicated the feline lateral geniculate nucleus with lower doses of acoustic energy and temporarily suppressed visual evoked responses recorded at the cortex.[20] These experiments necessitated craniotomy because the skull reflected and absorbed the ultrasound waves. The recent decade has led to advances in ultrasound transducer design so that transcranial delivery of high-intensity ultrasound is possible and precise in humans.[21,22] Our group observed neuromodulation of the sensory, ventrolateral thalamus in 5 of 15 patients with ET undergoing focused ultrasound thalamotomy although likely from thermal mechanisms.[23] In the laboratory, ultrasound neuromodulation has been demonstrated in vivo in rodents with low-intensity, pulsed parameters and without heating.[24,25]

Magnetic Neuromodulation

Transcranial magnetic stimulation (TMS) is a noninvasive technique used for measuring and modulating cortical plasticity introduced by Barker and colleagues[26] in 1985. TMS is delivered via an electrical coil placed on the scalp, which generates a magnetic field that traverses the cranium and induces an electrical field in the cortex. This electrical field depolarizes neurons and has been used extensively to measure cortical plasticity in a variety of neurologic disorders. This contrasts with transcranial electrical stimulation where current flow is achieved directly through the skull via leads injected into the scalp. Repetitive pulsing of TMS, known as repetitive transcranial magnetic stimulation (rTMS), has been used in the past 2 decades to modulate cortical excitability in ways that treat neurologic and psychiatric disease. rTMS is currently approved for use in medication-refractory depression in the United States and Canada. It has been studied in neurologic diseases such as PD, tremor, dystonia, tics, spasticity, and epilepsy.[27] High-frequency rTMS (>1 Hz) increases cortical excitability[28] and low-frequency rTMS (<1 Hz) reduces cortical excitability.[29] Paradigms of stimulation based on these observations have driven the design of studies investigating rTMS in movement disorders.

rTMS has been studied extensively for PD motor features with the hypothesis that high-frequency, cortically excitatory stimulation can overcome decreased output from the basal ganglia via the thalamus. Elahi and colleagues[30] performed a meta-analysis of studies with high-frequency and low-frequency rTMS to the motor cortex on PD motor scores. All of the studies had sham-controlled arms and compared the sham group with active groups (either low-frequency or high-frequency rTMS). In the pooled effect, they found a significant reduction in the UPDRS part III (motor) of 6.68 points (95% confidence interval = −9.66 to −3.69) in the high-frequency studies and no significant change on UPDRS part III in the low-frequency studies. It should be noted that the power of the analysis in both paradigms was low. Recent studies have looked at intermittent bursts of very high frequency stimulation to the motor cortex,[31] stimulation of the supplementary motor area,[32] and of the cerebellum[33] and have shown promising results. This is tempered, however, by other studies showing no significant motor benefit of high-frequency stimulation of the motor cortex.[34,35] Further studies are needed to identify the paradigms and sites of stimulation that may be effective in treating motor features of PD.

Levodopa-induced dyskinesia is a common, disabling feature of PD characterized by excessive, often uncontrollable, movements in the medicated PD state. Use of low-frequency and high-frequency rTMS over the motor cortex, supplemental motor area, and cerebellum have demonstrated mixed results on dyskinesia and UPDRS motor scores.[36–39]

In essential tremor, the role of excitation of the motor cortex seems promising. Studies have shown that DBS to the Vim increases motor cortex excitability[40] and subdural motor cortex stimulation has shown benefit in ET.[40] Hellriegel and colleagues[41] investigated very high frequency rTMS (50 Hz) over the motor cortex in ET and found significant reduction in tremor as measured by accelerometry. However, this benefit was not appreciated by the study subjects and patient ratings of change were no different between active and sham stimulation. The role of the cerebellum as part of the cerebello-thalamo-cortical pathway in essential tremor has been explored via cerebellar rTMS. Popa and colleagues[42] used 1-Hz bilateral cerebellar stimulation and found significant improvement in tremor amplitude and functional disability due to tremor that was persistent for 3 weeks.

Electrical Neuromodulation: DBS

Shortly after the development of a stereotactic frame applicable to the human skull by Spiegel and Wycis[43–46] in 1947, many teams of neurosurgeons and neurophysiologists began electrical recordings and stimulation of subcortical structures in the human brain. The principal investigations in these studies were patients with psychiatric disease; however, they quickly moved to movement disorders. Spiegel and Wycis[43–46] published reports using stereotactic surgery to treat Huntington disease, choreoathetosis, and PD shortly after their description of the stereoencephatome. In these operations, electrical stimulation was used to ensure the electrode was not in an eloquent structure, such as the internal capsule. During these operations, the surgical conditions made it difficult to assess symptoms; however, subsequent surgeries used electrical stimulation of the target to monitor clinical symptoms. It was noted that electrical stimulation of the target could mimic the effects of a lesion. In 1961, Alberts and colleagues[47] found that stimulation of the ventrolateral thalamus or internal segment of the globus pallidus at 60 Hz could evoke or abate tremor. Chronic electrical stimulation of the thalamus and pallidum was also described to locate targets for subsequent lesioning. In 1965, Sem-Jacobsen[48] reported chronic stimulation of the thalamus with multiple implanted electrodes to determine the optimal target for lesioning. In his description, he noted that electrodes could be kept in place for months without complication. In 1972, Bechtereva and colleagues[49] reported chronic electrode placement in the ventrolateral thalamus with intermittent high-frequency stimulation, the results of which were used for later ablative procedures. These and many other studies set the stage for modern DBS. In 1987, Benabid and colleagues[50] published their results of unilateral Vim thalamotomy and unilateral continuous, high frequency Vim stimulation with an implanted electrode in patients with PD. The principal benefits of stimulation compared with lesion are well noted, but include the ability for neuromodulation. These studies demonstrated that tremor was optimally suppressed with higher frequency (>130 Hz) stimulation, and that this suppression could be maintained chronically with implanted neurostimulator devices.[50,51] This opened the door to electrical neuromodulation of several different subcortical structures previously targeted by lesioning for the treatment of movement disorders.

ACUTE ELECTRICAL NEUROMODULATION FOR STEREOTACTIC TARGET LOCALIZATION DURING SURGERY

Technique

Stereotactic technique is used for both ablative and DBS surgeries in the treatment of movement disorders. Modern frame-based, and more recently skull-mounted devices, are typically precise for electrode insertion to approximately 1 mm.[52–54] Almost all preoperative planning relies on magnetic resonance imaging (MRI) sequences uploaded to a computer-based neuronavigation platform so that coordinates can be determined by either direct visualization of the target structure or by indirect methods by using calculations from the midcommissural point. Anatomic software is available for most of these navigation programs so that stereotactic brain atlases can be overlain on the patient's MRI or computed tomography images.

Regardless of whether the surgical procedure involves lesioning or stimulation, it is imperative to localize and confirm the target before the therapeutic treatment. Microelectrode recordings through small, higher-impedance electrodes in the extracellular space can identify discharges from a single or small group of neurons along the planned trajectory. Neurons of the striatum, pallidum, and ventrolateral thalamus have characteristic firing patterns that can be recognized and used to determine electrode location. These microelectrodes with exposed tips of approximately 5 μm can also be used for microstimulation with amplitudes ranging from 0 to 100 μA although high-stimulation currents will subsequently affect the impedance of the electrode.[55]

Although the use of microelectrode recordings for target localization remains debated, electrical stimulation is always applied through a macroelectrode (typical diameter ≥1 mm) such as those used for lesioning or for DBS. Macrostimulation applies repetitive low-amplitude voltage or currents at the electrode tip to elicit a clinical response, thus mapping the region for efficacious treatment or the identification of critical surrounding structures that should be avoided. High-frequency (100+ Hz) stimulation is used to simulate the chronic therapy that is typically used in the outpatient clinic setting. Low frequencies (2–10 Hz) can be used to preferentially activate large, myelinated axons like those of the pyramidal tract encountered in the posterior limb of internal capsule. As a comparison, cortical stimulation during awake craniotomy surgery typically uses 50-Hz to 60-Hz stimulation, which is ideal for mapping cortex and subcortical tracts.

Vim Thalamus

The ventral intermediate nucleus of the thalamus is the preferred of target to treat tremors. This nucleus receives projections from the spinal cord and deep cerebellar nuclei and has reciprocal connections with the cerebral cortex. Anatomically, it is "intermediately" positioned between the motor (ventral oral) and sensory (ventral caudal) thalamus and medially adjacent to the posterior limb of the internal capsule. The Vim nucleus is not readily discernable from the adjacent thalamic nuclei by MRI likely due to its small size and relatively hypocellular composition,[56] and so electrophysiologic or clinical testing is even more important for target confirmation. Because stimulation of Vim thalamus suppresses tremor immediately, intraoperative localization ultimately relies on the demonstration of tremor suppression with high (>100 Hz) stimulation, typically through a macroelectrode in the awake patient. Capsular stimulation from a laterally positioned electrode will activate descending corticobulbar or corticospinal tracts, thus eliciting tonic motor contractions of the face or upper extremity. Electrodes positioned posterior of Vim will stimulate sensory thalamus leading to localized and persistent paresthesias of the face or upper or lower extremities. Medial or anteriorly placed electrodes will often be ineffective in relieving tremor. Microstimulation mapping is more precise than macrostimulation for identifying the exact border between Vim and Vc.[57] Either of these methods can be used to confirm target location before lesioning or final placement of chronic stimulating electrodes.

GPi, Internal Segment

The GPi is a common target for the surgical treatment of dystonias and the medication-refractory, motor symptoms of PD. This disc-shaped nucleus has a volume of approximately 500 mm^3, and represents the primary outflow of basal ganglia. In contrast to stimulation of the Vim nucleus, acute stimulation of the GPi through a macroelectrode requires several minutes before clinical improvement in parkinsonism can be observed. Therefore, macroelectrode stimulation during GPi targeting focuses on avoiding the critical surrounding structures, namely the internal capsule medially and optic tract inferiorly. Most commonly, the posterior ventrolateral portion of the nucleus, the somatosensory region, is targeted for therapy toward the junction of the optic tract and internal capsule. Low-frequency (2 Hz) stimulation of corticobulbar in the 2-V to 4-V range can aid in finding the appropriate distance of GPi from the internal capsule. In a dark room, phosphenes and other visual phenomena in the contralateral visual field can be elicited with optic tract stimulation at high (130+ Hz) stimulation.

STN

The STN is commonly targeted for the treatment of PD. As part of the intrinsic circuitry of the basal ganglia, it provides excitatory, glutamatergic output to the GPi. Macroelectrode stimulation is quite valuable in determining electrode placement in the STN and frequently results in transient paresthesias of the distal extremities. Stimulation of the STN will produce immediate tremor arrest and reduced rigidity that returns when stimulation is stopped. Bradykinesia can be more difficult to assess and is often susceptible to lesional effects from macroelectrode insertion and repetitive high-frequency stimulation testing. Placement of an electrode in the anterolateral direction will result in stimulation of the cerebral peduncle, resulting in contralateral facial or hand contractions. Posteriorly placed electrodes near the medial leminiscus result in persistent or hemibody paresthesias. Medially placed electrodes will stimulate the red nucleus or the oculomotor nerve, resulting in unilateral eye deviation and/or diplopia. Identification of symptoms related to these structures guide subsequent electrode placement. Stimulation-induced dyskinesia is perceived as a favorable prognosis for a favorable outcome.

CLINICAL OUTCOMES OF CHRONIC ELECTRICAL NEUROMODULATION FOR MOVEMENT DISORDERS

DBS for Essential Tremor

Numerous studies of Vim ablation and stimulation have demonstrated dramatic improvements of appendicular tremors in ET. In one of the first reports of thalamotomy for PD, Speakman[58] treated 73 patients with 4-year follow-up and found that 56 patients were improved. Akbostanci and colleagues[59] reported the results of 37 patients treated with Vim thalamotomy for ET. At follow-up, 60.5% of patients had no tremor and an additional 13.9% of patients had mild tremor that did not interfere with activities of daily living.

There are several studies that demonstrate the efficacy of Vim DBS for essential tremor.[60–64] A systematic review of the literature published in 2009 found 17 studies that evaluated patients treated with Vim DBS for essential tremor.[65] All studies were retrospective case series and provide class IV evidence showing a reduction in tremor scores compared before or after surgery or with DBS turned off or on. Collectively, these studies suggest that Vim DBS improves tremor by 70% to 90%.

The durability of thalamic ablation and stimulation on tremor has been reported in long-term retrospective series.[66,67] Improvements in tremor severity are significant for as long as 7 years. However, with radiofrequency-thalamotomy, up to 20% of patients experienced tremor recurrence. Similarly, with thalamic DBS, tolerance to stimulation develops in up to 30% of patients; however, this can be improved by adjusting DBS settings.[68]

DBS for PD

In 1994, DBS was applied to the pallidum for treatment of PD.[69] The efficacy of chronic bilateral pallidal DBS was observed as comparable to pallidal lesioning.[70,71] Most studies report 30% to 50% improvement in motor symptoms with bilateral pallidal stimulation. Tremor is reduced by approximately 80%, and rigidity and akinesia improves by approximately 60%. The effects were reversible when stimulation was stopped, and parameters could be titrated to maximize therapeutic effects while minimizing negative size effects with bilateral implants.[70,72]

Like the GPi, the STN was recognized in experimental models of PD to be hyperactive.[73,74] STN lesions in nonhuman 1-methyl-4-phenyl-1,2,3,6-tetrahydropyridine primates alleviated parkinsonian signs, thus paving the way to explore the subthalamus as a potential stereotactic target for PD.

Subthalamotomy has never been widely accepted because of concerns for hemiballismus, primarily due to observations in humans with stroke in the region of the subthalamus and by the confirmation in the 1940s by Whittier and Mettler,[75,76] who were able to experimentally reproduce this by subthalamic lesions in primates. Unilateral subthalamotomy for medication refractory PD has proven beneficial in the alleviation of contralateral off-medication motor symptoms in a large series of 21 patients[77] and another series of 89 patients followed for up to 36 months.[78] In the former study, significant improvements were noted on UPDRS ratings with bradykinesia, rigidity, and tremor. Improvements remained at 2 years and were most pronounced for tremor. With regard to the "on" state, contralateral dyskinesia was reduced during the 2-year study and the mean dose of levodopa was decreased by 34% to 47% while the total *on* time without dyskinesia increased fourfold. In the study by Alvarez and colleagues,[79] significant reductions in part 3 of the off-medication UPDRS were noted at 12 (50%), 24 (30%), and 36 months (18%) following unilateral subthalamotomy.

There are several reported case series and large, multicenter trials that demonstrate the efficacy of STN-DBS.[80–87] These studies uniformly demonstrate improvement (reduction) in the duration of "off" medication time and a 48% to 58% improvement in motor function in patients who underwent bilateral STN-DBS compared with preoperative baselines.

Two multicenter, prospective, randomized control trials compared STN-DBS to best medical therapy.[88,89] In these studies, the primary outcomes were quality of life and motor function. As in previous studies, participants were evaluated with the PDQ and UPDRS. At 6-month follow-up evaluation, patients treated with STN-DBS had significant improvements in motor function, while not taking medications in both studies compared with best medical treatment. Further, quality-of-life measurements based on the PDQ demonstrated improvement in several categories, including activities of daily living and mobility. These studies concluded that STN-DBS was more effective at controlling severe motor complications in PD than medical management.

Long-term data regarding the efficacy STN-DBS have now been published. Several case series demonstrate the long-term durability of the effects of STN-DBS with 5-year and 10-year follow-up.[90–92] These studies show continued improved function in motor scores and activities of daily living compared with baseline preoperative function. In general, PD medication dosages were decreased by approximately 50%, as were medication-related dyskinesias. However, some studies reported worsening of postural stability, gait, axial DOPA-unresponsive symptoms, and cognitive neurologic decline. From these studies, it is unclear whether the decline in some symptoms was a factor of untreated disease progression in these patients or whether STN-DBS was a contributing factor.

Rigorous trials of STN versus GPi DBS include 3 randomized, double-blind, controlled trials documenting similar motor improvements as tested using UPDRS in the nonmedicated state.[93–95] The only consistent difference between targeting the STN and GPi-DBS are that there are significant reductions in levodopa medications and more cognitive and psychological sequelae with STN-DBS.

COMPARING NEUROMODULATION MODALITIES

There is no perfect technique for neuromodulation. Ideally, a combination of neuromodulation techniques could be used for both stereotactic localization in surgery and therapeutic uses in a chronic setting. Each of the modalities has its merits and limitations.

Chemical infusions theoretically have the potential for neuromodulation in a very selective fashion such that nuclear groups as well as axonal tracts could be manipulated independently. Most importantly, various neurotransmitter systems could be targeted for investigation and treatment. Unfortunately, chemical neuromodulation is relegated as a research tool today. If it becomes further developed, chemical infusions would likely be delivered with convective properties and image guidance for monitoring with a surrogate imaging tracer. Modern implanted infusion pumps are quite precise and reliable, although expensive. A more temporary infusion system can be implemented in the operating room environment, but semichronic infusions require externalized pump systems that are cumbersome with the risk of infection.

Cryogenic neuromodulation has been minimally used since the 1950s. There are currently no commercial systems available to implement this in the operating room. Importantly, the safety of neuronal cooling is poorly understood, and requires further investigation.

There is a long tradition of using thermal neuromodulation at subthreshold temperatures before permanent therapeutic ablation. Thermal modulation can now be implemented without surgery with the advent of contemporary transcranial-focused ultrasound devices. Importantly, the concept of a reversible thermal lesion should be questioned, as thermal doco occurs on a continuum proportional to the risk of neuronal damage.

Safety considerations with rTMS include possible induction of seizures, particularly with high-frequency paradigms.[96,97] Caution must be exercised, particularly in patients with a history of seizures and those who may be on medications that can reduce seizure threshold. Other reported adverse effects include temporary hearing loss and tinnitus associated with sound emitted by the TMS coil, local pain and cephalgia, and syncope.[27]

Contemporary transcranial-focused ultrasound systems can deliver acoustic energy through the intact scalp and cranium. Additionally, these treatments can be monitored in real time with MRI and MR thermometry. Because the technique is independent of an implanted stereotactic device, adjustments can be made in any dimension without invasive intracerebral penetrations. On the other hand, current ultrasound neuromodulation in humans depends on high-intensity wave forms. These are the ultrasound perimeters used for tissue ablation, and so thermal mechanisms analogous to radiofrequency energy are responsible for neuronal manipulation. Future systems may use low-intensity pulsed ultrasound, which does not result in heating. Ultrasound neuromodulation can be used today only for acute intraprocedural localization of a stereotactic target, as there is no current device available for chronic use.

Electrical neuromodulation is time tested, as more than 100,000 patients have been treated with DBS. The major advantage of electrical neuromodulation relates to its safety and reversibility.

Electrode configurations and stimulation parameters can be altered such that the electrical field is adjustable as well. Obviously, electrical neuromodulation relies on a surgically implanted electrode with some small risk of a hemorrhagic complication. Chronic neurostimulation devices are expensive and associated with inherent hardware complications, such as lead fracture, lead migration, scalp erosion, and device infection. These systems are expensive to implant and maintain with battery replacements. There is some selectivity of electrical stimulation, although this remains unknown. The electrical field likely affects neurons of all types, as well as traversing axonal pathways.

SUMMARY

Neuromodulation has been used extensively in movement disorder surgery for ET and PD. Acute and chronic electrical neuromodulation are currently the only modalities that are commonly used clinically. Chemical neuromodulation has been used in the past and experimentally in movement disorder surgery. This modality is a promising experimental tool for understanding the subcortical circuitry that underlies movement disorders. Transcranial magnetic stimulation and focused ultrasound neuromodulation are emerging, noninvasive modalities that are likely to have a large impact on therapy for movement disorders.

REFERENCES

1. Cooper IS. Chemopallidectomy: an investigative technique in geriatric parkinsonians. Science 1955;121(3137):217–8.
2. Cooper IS, Poloukhine N. Chemopallidectomy: a neurosurgical technique useful in geriatric parkinsonians. J Am Geriatr Soc 1955;3(11):839–59.
3. Narabayashi H, Okuma T, Shikiba S. Procaine oil blocking of the globus pallidus. AMA Arch Neurol Psychiatry 1956;75(1):36–48.
4. Narabayashi H, Shimazu H, Fujita Y, et al. Procaine-oil-wax pallidotomy for double athetosis and spastic states in infantile cerebral palsy: report of 80 cases. Neurology 1960;10:61–9.
5. Parrent AG, Tasker RR, Dostrovsky JO. Tremor reduction by microinjection of lidocaine during stereotactic surgery. Acta Neurochir Suppl (Wien) 1993;58:45–7.
6. Penn RD, Kroin JS. Intrathecal baclofen alleviates spinal cord spasticity. Lancet 1984;1(8385):1078.
7. Penn RD, Kroin JS. Continuous intrathecal baclofen for severe spasticity. Lancet 1985;2(8447): 125–7.
8. Penn RD, Kroin JS, Reinkensmeyer A, et al. Injection of GABA-agonist into globus pallidus in patient with Parkinson's disease. Lancet 1998;351(9099): 340–1.
9. Levy R, Lang AE, Dostrovsky JO, et al. Lidocaine and muscimol microinjections in subthalamic nucleus reverse Parkinsonian symptoms. Brain 2001;124(Pt 10):2105–18.
10. Pahapill PA, Levy R, Dostrovsky JO, et al. Tremor arrest with thalamic microinjections of muscimol in patients with essential tremor. Ann Neurol 1999; 46(2):249–52.
11. Mark VH, Chato JC, Eastman FG, et al. Localized cooling in the brain. Science 1961;134(3489): 1520–1.
12. Rowbotham GF, Haigh AL, Leslie WG. Cooling cannula for use in the treatment of cerebral neoplasms. Lancet 1959;1(7062):12–5.
13. Cooper I. A cryogenic method for physiologic inhibition and production of lesions in the brain. J Neurosurg 1962;19:853–8.
14. Cooper IS, Lee AS. Cryostatic congelation: a system for producing a limited, controlled region of cooling or freezing of biologic tissues. J Nerv Ment Dis 1961;133:259–63.
15. Cooper IS. Cryogenic surgery of the basal ganglia. JAMA 1962;181:600–4.
16. Brodkey JS, Miyazaki Y, Ervin FR, et al. Reversible heat lesions with radiofrequency current. a method of stereotactic localization. J Neurosurg 1964;21: 49–53.
17. Sapareto SA, Dewey WC. Thermal dose determination in cancer therapy. Int J Radiat Oncol Biol Phys 1984;10(6):787–800.
18. Fry WJ, Barnard JW, Fry FJ, et al. Ultrasonically produced localized selective lesions in the central nervous system. Am J Phys Med 1955;34(3):413–23.
19. Fry WJ, Mosberg WH Jr, Barnard JW, et al. Production of focal destructive lesions in the central nervous system with ultrasound. J Neurosurg 1954; 11(5):471–8.
20. Fry FJ, Ades HW, Fry WJ. Production of reversible changes in the central nervous system by ultrasound. Science 1958;127(3289):83–4.
21. Arvanitis CD, Livingstone MS, McDannold N. Combined ultrasound and MR imaging to guide focused ultrasound therapies in the brain. Phys Med Biol 2013;58(14):4749–61.
22. Martin E, Jeanmonod D, Morel A, et al. High-intensity focused ultrasound for noninvasive functional neurosurgery. Ann Neurol 2009;66(6):858–61.
23. Elias WJ, Huss D, Voss T, et al. A pilot study of focused ultrasound thalamotomy for essential tremor. N Engl J Med 2013;369:640–8.
24. Yoo SS, Bystritsky A, Lee JH, et al. Focused ultrasound modulates region-specific brain activity. Neuroimage 2011;56(3):1267–75.

25. Tyler WJ, Tufail Y, Finsterwald M, et al. Remote excitation of neuronal circuits using low-intensity, low-frequency ultrasound. PloS One 2008;3(10): e3511.
26. Barker AT, Jalinous R, Freeston IL. Non-invasive magnetic stimulation of human motor cortex. Lancet 1985;1(8437):1106–7.
27. Rossi S, Hallett M, Rossini PM, et al. Safety, ethical considerations, and application guidelines for the use of transcranial magnetic stimulation in clinical practice and research. Clin Neurophysiol 2009; 120(12):2008–39.
28. Pascual-Leone A, Valls-Sole J, Wassermann EM, et al. Responses to rapid-rate transcranial magnetic stimulation of the human motor cortex. Brain 1994;117(Pt 4):847–58.
29. Chen WH, Mima T, Siebner HR, et al. Low-frequency rTMS over lateral premotor cortex induces lasting changes in regional activation and functional coupling of cortical motor areas. Clin Neurophysiol 2003;114(9):1628–37.
30. Elahi B, Elahi B, Chen R. Effect of transcranial magnetic stimulation on Parkinson motor function—systematic review of controlled clinical trials. Mov Disord 2009;24(3):357–63.
31. Degardin A, Devos D, Defebvre L, et al. Effect of intermittent theta-burst stimulation on akinesia and sensorimotor integration in patients with Parkinson's disease. Eur J Neurosci 2012;36(5): 2669–78.
32. Shirota Y, Ohtsu H, Hamada M, et al. Supplementary motor area stimulation for Parkinson disease: a randomized controlled study. Neurology 2013; 80(15):1400–5.
33. Minks E, Marecek R, Pavlik T, et al. Is the cerebellum a potential target for stimulation in Parkinson's disease? Results of 1-Hz rTMS on upper limb motor tasks. Cerebellum 2011; 10(4):804–11.
34. Benninger DH, Iseki K, Kranick S, et al. Controlled study of 50-Hz repetitive transcranial magnetic stimulation for the treatment of Parkinson disease. Neurorehabil Neural Repair 2012;26(9):1096–105.
35. Zamir O, Gunraj C, Ni Z, et al. Effects of theta burst stimulation on motor cortex excitability in Parkinson's disease. Clin Neurophysiol 2012;123(4): 815–21.
36. Filipovic SR, Rothwell JC, van de Warrenburg BP, et al. Repetitive transcranial magnetic stimulation for levodopa-induced dyskinesias in Parkinson's disease. Mov Disord 2009;24(2):246–53.
37. Koch G, Brusa L, Caltagirone C, et al. rTMS of supplementary motor area modulates therapy-induced dyskinesias in Parkinson disease. Neurology 2005; 65(4):623–5.
38. Koch G, Brusa L, Carrillo F, et al. Cerebellar magnetic stimulation decreases levodopa-induced dyskinesias in Parkinson disease. Neurology 2009;73(2):113–9.
39. Wagle-Shukla A, Angel MJ, Zadikoff C, et al. Low-frequency repetitive transcranial magnetic stimulation for treatment of levodopa-induced dyskinesias. Neurology 2007;68(9):704–5.
40. Molnar GF, Sailer A, Gunraj CA, et al. Changes in cortical excitability with thalamic deep brain stimulation. Neurology 2005;64(11):1913–9.
41. Hellriegel H, Schulz EM, Siebner HR, et al. Continuous theta-burst stimulation of the primary motor cortex in essential tremor. Clin Neurophysiol 2012; 123(5):1010–5.
42. Popa T, Russo M, Vidailhet M, et al. Cerebellar rTMS stimulation may induce prolonged clinical benefits in essential tremor, and subjacent changes in functional connectivity: an open label trial. Brain Stimul 2013;6(2):175–9.
43. Spiegel EA, Wycis HT. Effect of thalamic and pallidal lesions upon involuntary movements in choreoathetosis. Trans Am Neurol Assoc 1950;51: 234–7.
44. Spiegel EA, Wycis HT. Stereoencephalotomy in the treatment of parkinsonian tremor. J Am Geriatr Soc 1954;2(5):317–20.
45. Spiegel EA, Wycis HT. Stereoencephalotomy. Trans Am Neurol Assoc 1948;73(73 Annual Meet):160–3.
46. Spiegel EA, Wycis HT, Marks M, et al. Stereotaxic apparatus for operations on the human brain. Science 1947;106(2754):349–50.
47. Alberts WW, Wright EW Jr, Levin G, et al. Threshold stimulation of the lateral thalamus and globus pallidus in the waking human. Electroencephalogr Clin Neurophysiol 1961;13:68–74.
48. Sem-Jacobsen CW. Depth electrographic stimulation and treatment of patients with Parkinson's disease including neurosurgical technique. Acta Neurol Scand Suppl 1965;13(Pt 1):365–77.
49. Bechtereva NP, Bondartchuk AN, Gretchin VB, et al. Structural-functional organization of the human brain and the pathophysiology of the Parkinsonian type hyperkineses. Confin Neurol 1972; 34(2):14–7.
50. Benabid AL, Pollak P, Louveau A, et al. Combined (thalamotomy and stimulation) stereotactic surgery of the VIM thalamic nucleus for bilateral Parkinson disease. Appl Neurophysiol 1987; 50(1–6):344–6.
51. Benabid AL, Pollak P, Gervason C, et al. Long-term suppression of tremor by chronic stimulation of the ventral intermediate thalamic nucleus. Lancet 1991;337(8738):403–6.
52. Holloway KL, Gaede SE, Starr PA, et al. Frameless stereotaxy using bone fiducial markers for deep brain stimulation. J Neurosurg 2005;103(3):404–13.
53. Shamir RR, Joskowicz L, Spektor S, et al. Target and trajectory clinical application accuracy in

neuronavigation. Neurosurgery 2011;68(1 Suppl Operative):95–101 [discussion: 2].

54. Thani NB, Bala A, Lind CR. Accuracy of magnetic resonance imaging-directed frame-based stereotaxis. Neurosurgery 2012;70(1 Suppl Operative): 114–23 [discussion: 23–4].
55. Slavin KV, Holsapple J. Microelectrode techniques: equipment, components, and systems. In: Israel Z, Burchiel K, editors. Microelectrode recording in movement disorder surgery. New York: Thieme Medical Publishers; 2004. p. 14.
56. Hirai T, Ohye C, Nagaseki Y, et al. Cytometric analysis of the thalamic ventralis intermedius nucleus in humans. J Neurophysiol 1989;61(3):478–87.
57. Sierens DK, Bakay RA. Is MER necessary in movement disorder surgery?. In: Israel Z, Burchiel K, editors. The case in favor. Microelectrode recording in movement disorder surgery. New York: Thieme Medical Publishers; 2004. p. 186.
58. Speakman T. Results of thalamotomy for Parkinson's disease. Can Med Assoc J 1963;28(89): 652–6.
59. Akbostanci MC, Slavin KV, Burchiel KJ. Stereotactic ventral intermedial thalamotomy for the treatment of essential tremor: results of a series of 37 patients. Stereotact Funct Neurosurg 1999; 72(2–4):174–7.
60. Hariz GM, Blomstedt P, Koskinen LO. Long-term effect of deep brain stimulation for essential tremor on activities of daily living and health-related quality of life. Acta Neurol Scand 2008; 118(6):387–94.
61. Hubble JP, Busenbark KL, Wilkinson S, et al. Effects of thalamic deep brain stimulation based on tremor type and diagnosis. Mov Disord 1997; 12(3):337–41.
62. Koller W, Pahwa R, Busenbark K, et al. High-frequency unilateral thalamic stimulation in the treatment of essential and parkinsonian tremor. Ann Neurol 1997;42(3):292–9.
63. Lyons KE, Pahwa R, Busenbark KL, et al. Improvements in daily functioning after deep brain stimulation of the thalamus for intractable tremor. Mov Disord 1998;13(4):690–2.
64. Pahwa R, Lyons KL, Wilkinson SB, et al. Bilateral thalamic stimulation for the treatment of essential tremor. Neurology 1999;53(7):1447–50.
65. Flora ED, Perera CL, Cameron AL, et al. Deep brain stimulation for essential tremor: a systematic review. Mov Disord 2010;25(11):1550–9.
66. Zhang K, Bhatia S, Oh MY, et al. Long-term results of thalamic deep brain stimulation for essential tremor. J Neurosurg 2010;112(6):1271–6.
67. Blomstedt P, Hariz GM, Hariz MI, et al. Thalamic deep brain stimulation in the treatment of essential tremor: a long-term follow-up. Br J Neurosurg 2007;21(5):504–9.
68. Hariz MI, Shamsgovara P, Johansson F, et al. Tolerance and tremor rebound following long-term chronic thalamic stimulation for parkinsonian and essential tremor. Stereotact Funct Neurosurg 1999;72(2–4):208–18.
69. Siegfried J, Lippitz B. Bilateral chronic electrostimulation of ventroposterolateral pallidum: a new therapeutic approach for alleviating all parkinsonian symptoms. Neurosurgery 1994;35(6):1126–9 [discussion: 9–30].
70. Blomstedt P, Hariz GM, Hariz MI. Pallidotomy versus pallidal stimulation. Parkinsonism Relat Disord 2006;12(5):296–301.
71. Kumar R, Lozano AM, Montgomery E, et al. Pallidotomy and deep brain stimulation of the pallidum and subthalamic nucleus in advanced Parkinson's disease. Mov Disord 1998;13(Suppl 1):73–82.
72. Kumar R, Lang AE, Rodriguez-Oroz MC, et al. Deep brain stimulation of the globus pallidus pars interna in advanced Parkinson's disease. Neurology 2000;55(12 Suppl 6):S34–9.
73. DeLong MR. The neurophysiologic basis of abnormal movements in basal ganglia disorders. Neurobehav Toxicol Teratol 1983;5(6):611–6.
74. DeLong MR. Primate models of movement disorders of basal ganglia origin. Trends Neurosci 1990;13(7):281–5.
75. Whittier JR, Mettler FA. Subthalamic lesion in the primate. Fed Proc 1947;6(1 Pt 2):226.
76. Whittier JR, Mettler FA. Studies on the subthalamus of the rhesus monkey; hyperkinesia and other physiologic effects of subthalamic lesions; with special reference to the subthalamic nucleus of Luys. J Comp Neurol 1949;90(3):319–72.
77. Patel NK, Heywood P, O'Sullivan K, et al. Unilateral subthalamotomy in the treatment of Parkinson's disease. Brain 2003;126(Pt 5):1136–45.
78. Obeso JA, Jahanshahi M, Alvarez L, et al. What can man do without basal ganglia motor output? The effect of combined unilateral subthalamotomy and pallidotomy in a patient with Parkinson's disease. Exp Neurol 2009;220(2):283–92.
79. Alvarez L, Macias R, Lopez G, et al. Bilateral subthalamotomy in Parkinson's disease: initial and long-term response. Brain 2005;128(Pt 3): 570–83.
80. Benabid AL, Pollak P, Gross C, et al. Acute and long-term effects of subthalamic nucleus stimulation in Parkinson's disease. Stereotact Funct Neurosurg 1994;62(1–4):76–84.
81. Ford B, Winfield L, Pullman SL, et al. Subthalamic nucleus stimulation in advanced Parkinson's disease: blinded assessments at one year follow up. J Neurol Neurosurg Psychiatry 2004;75(9): 1255–9.
82. Herzog J, Volkmann J, Krack P, et al. Two-year follow-up of subthalamic deep brain stimulation in

Parkinson's disease. Mov Disord 2003;18(11): 1332–7.

83. Limousin P, Krack P, Pollak P, et al. Electrical stimulation of the subthalamic nucleus in advanced Parkinson's disease. N Engl J Med 1998;339(16): 1105–11.
84. Pahwa R, Wilkinson SB, Overman J, et al. Bilateral subthalamic stimulation in patients with Parkinson disease: long-term follow up. J Neurosurg 2003; 99(1):71–7.
85. Rodriguez-Oroz MC, Gorospe A, Guridi J, et al. Bilateral deep brain stimulation of the subthalamic nucleus in Parkinson's disease. Neurology 2000; 55(12 Suppl 6):S45–51.
86. Rodriguez-Oroz MC, Obeso JA, Lang AE, et al. Bilateral deep brain stimulation in Parkinson's disease: a multicentre study with 4 years follow-up. Brain 2005;128(Pt 10):2240–9.
87. Kumar R, Lozano AM, Kim YJ, et al. Double-blind evaluation of subthalamic nucleus deep brain stimulation in advanced Parkinson's disease. Neurology 1998;51(3):850–5.
88. Deuschl G, Schade-Brittinger C, Krack P, et al. A randomized trial of deep-brain stimulation for Parkinson's disease. N Engl J Med 2006;355(9): 896–908.
89. Weaver FM, Follett K, Stern M, et al. Bilateral deep brain stimulation vs best medical therapy for patients with advanced Parkinson disease: a randomized controlled trial. JAMA 2009;301(1):63–73.
90. Castrioto A, Lozano AM, Poon YY, et al. Ten-year outcome of subthalamic stimulation in Parkinson disease: a blinded evaluation. Arch Neurol 2011; 68(12):1550–6.
91. Gervais-Bernard H, Xie-Brustolin J, Mertens P, et al. Bilateral subthalamic nucleus stimulation in advanced Parkinson's disease: five year follow-up. J Neurol 2009;256(2):225–33.
92. Krack P, Batir A, Van Blercom N, et al. Five-year follow-up of bilateral stimulation of the subthalamic nucleus in advanced Parkinson's disease. N Engl J Med 2003;349(20):1925–34.
93. Moro E, Lozano AM, Pollak P, et al. Long-term results of a multicenter study on subthalamic and pallidal stimulation in Parkinson's disease. Mov Disord 2010;25(5):578–86.
94. Nakamura K, Christine CW, Starr PA, et al. Effects of unilateral subthalamic and pallidal deep brain stimulation on fine motor functions in Parkinson's disease. Mov Disord 2007;22(5):619–26.
95. Weaver FM, Follett KA, Stern M, et al. Randomized trial of deep brain stimulation for Parkinson disease: thirty-six-month outcomes. Neurology 2012; 79(1):55–65.
96. Chen R, Gerloff C, Classen J, et al. Safety of different inter-train intervals for repetitive transcranial magnetic stimulation and recommendations for safe ranges of stimulation parameters. Electroencephalogr Clin Neurophysiol 1997; 105(6):415–21.
97. Wassermann EM, Grafman J, Berry C, et al. Use and safety of a new repetitive transcranial magnetic stimulator. Electroencephalogr Clin Neurophysiol 1996;101(5):412–7.

Neuromodulation for Dystonia
Target and Patient Selection

Kelly A. Mills, MD[a], Philip A. Starr, MD, PhD[b,*], Jill L. Ostrem, MD[a]

KEYWORDS

- Deep brain stimulation • Globus pallidus • Subthalamic nucleus • Brain target • Outcomes
- Predictive factors

KEY POINTS

- Greater understanding of the influence of patients' baseline characteristics on therapeutic response to deep brain stimulation (DBS) helps to more accurately counsel patients on expected outcome.
- Primary generalized dystonia has good evidence for a robust improvement in movement and disability after globus pallidus internus (Gpi) DBS.
- Specific types of secondary dystonia (tardive, cerebral palsy, neurodegeneration with brain iron accumulation) have reasonable outcomes after GPi DBS, whereas other secondary dystonias deserve more study.
- GPi has the strongest evidence in primary and secondary dystonia, but alternative brain targets such as the subthalamic nucleus or thalamus are being explored.

INTRODUCTION

Dystonia is a clinical syndrome of sustained muscle contractions producing twisting and repetitive movements or abnormal postures, often resulting in simultaneous contraction of agonist and antagonist muscles.[1] Medical therapies with anticholinergic and GABAergic medications are helpful in some cases, but often limited by side effects. Pallidotomy and thalamotomy were used extensively for the treatment of dystonia after it was observed that pallidotomy for Parkinson disease (PD) improved PD-related dystonia. Deep brain stimulation (DBS) therapy has shown significant and sustained success in the treatment of dystonia (especially in primary dystonia) when medical therapy fails to improve symptoms and there is disability.[2]

Most patients with dystonia over the last decade have been treated with globus pallidus internus (GPi) DBS. In recent years, DBS has been applied to treat a broader range of patients with dystonia (focal and secondary) and new brain targets for stimulation have been explored. In this article, the current status of DBS for treating patients with various types of dystonia is reviewed. Predictors of outcome and alternative brain targets are also discussed to help guide patient selection and target choice.

Classification

Three parallel classification schemes are used to describe dystonia, including categorization by age at onset, distribution, and cause (**Table 1**).[1,3] Age at onset is divided into early and late onset and can be helpful in understanding the underlying cause and likelihood of spread (eg, early-onset primary dystonia is more likely to become generalized than late onset). Distribution refers to the extent to which the dystonia occurs across the body. Cause is an attempt to classify the dystonia

[a] UCSF Department of Neurology, PADRECC, San Francisco VA Medical Center, UCSF Box 1838, 1635 Divisadero Street, Suite 520, San Francisco, CA 94143-1838, USA; [b] UCSF Department of Neurosurgery, PADRECC, San Francisco VA Medical Center, UCSF Box 1838, 1635 Divisadero Street, Suite 520, San Francisco, CA 94143-1838, USA
* Corresponding author.
E-mail address: StarrP@neurosurg.ucsf.edu

Neurosurg Clin N Am 25 (2014) 59–75
http://dx.doi.org/10.1016/j.nec.2013.08.014
1042-3680/14/$ – see front matter

Table 1
Current classification of dystonia

Age at Onset (y)	Distribution	Cause
Early (≤26)	Focal	Primary
Late (>26)	Segmental Multifocal Generalized Hemidystonia	Dystonia-plus Secondary Heredodegenerative Feature of another disease (eg, tics, PD, corticobasal syndrome, progressive supranuclear palsy)

by underlying cause. Classification can provide prognostic information and is essential when predicting potential benefit from therapies such as DBS. When no cause (with the exception of known genetic mutations) can be determined, then the dystonia is considered primary, which also implies the absence of other neurologic symptoms (with the exception of tremor). Familial early-onset dystonia are often caused by mutations in TOR1A (DYT1)[4] or THAP1 (DYT6),[5] whereas late-onset sporadic and familial dystonia typically presenting with cranial or cervical dystonia (CD) have been associated with THAP1 (DYT6), CIZ1, and GNAL, although these are more commonly without a known mutation.

Dystonia-plus syndromes are nonneurodegenerative conditions associated with other neurologic features such as myoclonus, parkinsonism, or autonomic dysfunction and include dopa-responsive dystonia, myoclonus-dystonia, and rapid-onset dystonia-parkinsonism. Secondary dystonia is diagnosed when symptoms can be related to acquired insults such as central nervous system (CNS) structural lesions, hypoxic injury, metabolic disease, or medication exposure (tardive). Heredodegenerative dystonias have a neurodegenerative cause, follow a progressive course, and may include other findings on examination but have dystonia as a prominent feature. A separate category has also been considered to capture dystonia associated with other neurodegenerative diseases that may not always be a central symptom (eg, corticobasal syndrome [CBS], progressive supranuclear palsy [PSP], PD, paroxysmal dyskinesia).[3]

PATIENT SELECTION

Although each patient's surgical candidacy should be evaluated individually considering their level of disability from dystonia, inclusion and exclusion criteria are helpful in patient selection (**Table 2**). The degree of disability required to warrant DBS may be dependent on the patient's expected baseline level of function, caregiver burden, and the degree of potential improvement in the disabling symptom. There are also several prognostic indicators to consider when accurately describing the risk/benefit ratio in any given case (**Box 1**).

Influence of Dystonia Type on Outcome

The quality of information predicting response to DBS in a specific type of dystonia is variable, with class 1 data for primary generalized dystonia (PGD) to class IV data for several types of secondary and heredodegenerative dystonia. The expected surgical outcome is discussed based on evidence available for the various etiologic classifications.

Primary Generalized Dystonia

The most rigorously studied group of patients with dystonia receiving DBS are those with PGD (**Tables 3** and **4**) and includes many patients who have tested positive for the TOR1A (DTY1) mutation. Early work suggested a 59% to 86% improvement in the Burk-Fahn-Marsden Dystonia Rating Scale Movement Score (BFMDRS-m) in open-label trials of patients with PGD receiving bilateral GPi DBS,[6–12] although more moderate effects were also reported in several other studies.[13,14] In 2005, Vidailhet and colleagues[15] reported a randomized, prospective multicenter trial in patients with PGD in which patients underwent double-blind video assessment 3 months after surgery and showed a 29% improvement in the BFMDRS-m score with DBS on compared with DBS off. After 12 months, these patients showed a 51% reduction in BFMDRS-m and a 44% improvement in the disability score.

Table 2
Relative inclusion and exclusion criteria in DBS for dystonia

Inclusion Criteria	Exclusion Criteria
Unequivocal diagnosis of dystonia	Young age (generally <7 y)
Failure of previous medical treatment	Low weight
Disability to patient or caregivers sufficient to warrant surgery	High infection risk Inability to follow-up Actively suicidal Unrealistic expectations

Box 1
Patient/dystonia characteristics to consider during DBS evaluation

Dystonia classification
Prominent involuntary movement type
Prominent pain
Age at the time of surgery
Disease duration
Psychiatric disease/depression
Cognitive function
Fixed skeletal deformities

In 2006, Kupsch and colleagues[16] established class I evidence for the treatment of primary dystonia with GPi DBS using a double-blind, multicenter, randomized trial controlled with sham stimulation for the first 3 months. DBS improved the BFMDRS-m and disability (BFMDRS-d) scores by 39.9% and 38%, respectively, compared with baseline. The sham surgery group showed only 4.9% and 11% improvement in movement and disability scores. Follow-up at 6 months showed 45% and 41% improvement in the BFMDRS-m and BFMDRS-d scores when compared with baseline in the patients with PGD.

A third European, multicenter, prospective study was performed with blinded evaluations of BFMDRS-m score, with masking of the patient's head and body for video recordings at 6 and 12 months, and included both patients with PGD and patients with CD. Dystonia movement scores improved by 43.8% (blinded assessment), and quality of life improved by 53.9% on the health-related quality-of-life score.[17]

More recently, long-term follow-up from other PGD cohorts shows a sustained benefit at 3,[18] 7,[19] and 10[20] years (see **Table 4**). Long-term follow-up of the French patients showed a sustained benefit of 58% and 46% improvement from baseline after 3 years in BFMDRS-m and BFMDRS-d scores, respectively.[2] Five-year, intention-to-treat outcome data on 20 of the original 24 patients with generalized dystonia in the German study showed a 58.1% improvement in BFMDRS-m score compared with baseline,[21] although nonresponders existed.

Primary cervical and craniocervical dystonia

Primary CD is more likely to begin later in life and is less likely to spread to other body segments or have a known single allelic genetic mutation than PGD. These differences suggest that CD may respond differently from DBS.

There are now at least 8 series with more than 2 years of follow-up data using unblinded assessments (see **Table 3**)[22–29] and at least 4 long-term follow-up series of the same patients (see **Table 4**)[18,21,30,31] showing a wide range of improvement in patients with CD (28%–70.2% in Toronto-Western Spasmodic Torticollis Rating Scale [TWSTRS] severity, 52.1%–76.1% in TWSTRS disability, and 37.5%–87.1% in TWSTRS pain subscores). The first prospective study using blinded video assessments in 8 patients at a median of 30 months postoperatively showed a 70% improvement in total TWSTRS score.[29] A prospective series of 10 patients using blinded video ratings at an average of 7.7 years postoperatively showed 47.6% improvement in the TWSTRS severity score.[31] No further statistically significant improvement was found in any of the subscores after the first year of follow-up, although benefit was sustained up to 10 years in some patients. The study by Kupsch and colleagues[16] included 16 patients with CD and showed a 45% improvement in BFMDRS-m score at 3 months in a double-blind assessment and 58.1% improvement after 5 years (data combined with PGD). The patients with CD in the study by Kupsch and colleagues also had most of their improvement in the first 12 months compared with patients with generalized dystonia, who continued to improve over 3 years.

The effectiveness of bilateral GPi DBS has also been evaluated in patients with idiopathic craniocervical dystonia (ICCD or Meige syndrome).[32–36] Several studies have shown sustained benefit in ICCD, with an average of 53% to 85% improvement in BFMDRS-m score after 25% to 78 months of follow-up[37–40] and 1 case report of continued response after 10 years.[41]

Secondary dystonia

Although secondary dystonia is considered to show less improvement after GPi DBS than primary dystonia, overall outcomes vary depending on the cause. One group in which there is substantial evidence for a reasonable benefit from bilateral GPi DBS is those with tardive dystonia (**Table 5**), a chronic movement disorder caused by previous exposure to dopamine receptor blocking agents such as neuroleptics or antiemetics[42–47] (reviewed in Ref.[48]). In a prospective, multicenter, open-label study using double-blind stimulation on and off testing in 10 patients, a 50% improvement in the Extrapyramidal Symptoms Rating Scale was found after 6 months of bilateral GPi DBS.[43] A smaller open-label series with longer follow-up showed a 62% improvement in BFMDRS-m score at 12 months and 71% improvement at last

Table 3
GPi DBS for dystonia studies with more than 5 patients

Type of Dystonia	N	Scale (Subscale)	Baseline Score	Follow-Up Time (mo)	Follow-Up Score	Percent Improvement
Vercueil et al,[6] 2001						
PGD[a]	1	BFMDRS (m/d)	—	12	—	67/81
PGD[a]	1	BFMDRS (m/d)	—	6	—	70/50
PGD DYT1+	1	BFMDRS (m/d)	—	12	—	86/86
PGD DYT1−	1	BFMDRS (m/d)	—	24	—	41/43
Craniocervical	1	BFMDRS (m/d)	—	6	—	66/66
Krauss et al,[25] 2002						
Cervical	5	TWSTRS (s/d/p)	20.5/40.5/6	20	7.5/12.7/3	62/69/50
Yianni et al,[7] 2003						
PGD DYT1+	2	BFMDRS (m)	—	12	—	85[b]
PGD DYT1−	11	BFMDRS (m)	—	12	—	46[b]
Cervical	7	TWSTRS (s/d/p)	21.3/21.7/15.1	12	10/14/8.3	50/38/43
Cif et al,[8] 2003						
PGD DYT1+	15	BFMDRS (m/d)	60.8/16.7	24–36+	14.2/5.7	71/63
PGD DYT1−	17	BFMDRS (m/d)	56.5/16.4	24–36	15.1/9.5	74/49
Kupsch et al,[9] 2003						
PGD DYT1+	1	BFMDRS (m)	34.5	3–12	27	22
PGD DYT1−	3	BFMDRS (m)	40	3–13	20	50
Segmental	1	BFMDRS (m)	32	3–14	19	41
Katayama et al,[10] 2003						
PGD	5	BFMDRS (m)	18–62	6	4–23	51–92
Coubes et al,[11] 2004						
PGD DYT1+	17	BFMDRS (m)	62.5	24	12.4	83
PGD DYT1−	14	BFMDRS (m)	56.3	24	13.4	75
Eltahawy et al,[13] 2004						
PGD DYT1+	1	BFMDRS (m)	88	6	66	25
PGD DYT1−	1	BFMDRS (m)	48	6	16	21
Cervical	3	TWSTRS (t)	37.7	6	16	57
Krause et al,[14] 2004						
PGD DYT1+	4	BFMDRS (m)	72	12–66	34	53
PGD DYT1−	6	BFMDRS (m)	73.9	12–67	50	32
Cervical	1	BFMDRS (m)	6	12–68	6	0
Vidailhet et al,[15] 2005						
PGD DYT1+	**7**	**BFMDRS (m/d)**	**55.1/14.72**	**12**	**26.1/85**	**53/45.6**
PGD DYT1−	**15**	**BFMDRS (m/d)**	**41.96/10.2**	**12**	**18.7/5.5**	**55.4/45**
Bittar et al,[26] 2005						
PGD DYT1+	2	BFMDRS (t)	103.8[c]	24	55.8	46[c]
PGD DYT1−	4	BFMDRS (t)	—	24	—	—
Cervical	6	TWSTRS (t)	6	24	23.7	59
Zorzi et al,[50] 2005						
PGD DYT1+	1	BFMDRS (m/d)	47/11	4	14/6	70/45
PGD DYT1−	8	BFMDRS (m/d)	68.9/17.9	19.1	46.5/12.6	32/37

(continued on next page)

Table 3
(continued)

Type of Dystonia	N	Scale (Subscale)	Baseline Score	Follow-Up Time (mo)	Follow-Up Score	Percent Improvement
Diamond et al,[122] 2006						
PGD DYT1+	5	UDRS	44.6	27.5	4.8	89[c]
PGD DYT1−	5	—	—	—	—	—
Kupsch et al,[16] 2006						
PGD DYT1+	**6**	**BFMDRS (m/d)**	**36.4/10.0**	**6**	**20.2/5.9**	**45/41[d]**
PGD DYT1−	**4**	**BFMDRS (m/d)**	—	—	—	—
Primary[a]	**14**	**BFMDRS (m/d)**	—	—	—	—
Cervical	**16**	**BFMDRS (m/d)**	—	—	—	—
Starr et al,[27] 2006						
PGD DYT1+	6	BFMDRS (m)	59.6	13.2	24.2	59[c]
PGD DYT1−	1	BFMDRS (m)	94	—	—	—
Segmental	3	BFMDRS (m)	22.6	21.7	12	47
Craniocervical	1	BFMDRS (m)	30	9	3	90
Generalized[a]	2	BFMDRS (m)	83	10.5	72.8	12
Hung et al,[22] 2007						
Cervical	10	TWSTRS (s/d/p)	21.9/18/11.7	12–67	9.9/7.4/5.8	54.8/52.1/50.5
Alterman et al,[123] 2007						
PGD DYT1+	12	BFMDRS (m/d)	35/8	38.9/9.0	4/2	89/75[c]
PGD DYT1−	3	BFMDRS (m/d)	—	—	—	—
Tisch et al,[92] 2007						
PGD DYT1+	7	BFMDRS (m/d)	38.9/9.0	6	11.9/4.1	69.5/58[c]
PGD DYT1−	8	—	—	—	—	—
Ostrem et al,[36] 2007						
Craniocervical	6	BFMDRS (m/d)	22/6	6	6.1/3.7	72/38
	—	TSWSTRS (t)	39		17	54
Kiss et al,[79] 2007						
Cervical	**10**	**TWSTRS (s/d/p)**	**14.7/14.9/26.6**	**12**	**8.4/5.4/9.2**	**43/64/65**
Cersosimo et al,[124] 2008						
PGD bilateral DBS	3	BFMDRS (m/d)	42.8/12.6	33–84	23.7/8.7	44.7/31
PGD DBS + lesion	5	BFMDRS (m/d)	60.2/19	15–94	28.4/10.8	52.8/43.2
Isaias et al,[19] 2009						
PGD DYT1+	17	BFMDRS (m)	44	84	13.6	82[c]
PGD DYT1−	7	—	—	—	—	—
PGD DYT1+ FSD	3	BFMDRS (m)	10.6	84	5.6	62[c]
PGD DYT1− FSD	3	—	—	—	—	—
Valldeoriola et al,[17] 2010						
PGD DYT1+	**6**	**BFMDRS (m/d)**	**46.4/12.4**	6–12	**26.1/7.64**	**43/38[c,d]**
PGD DYT1−	**16**	**BFMDRS (m/d)**	—	6–13	—	—
Cervical	**2**	**BFMDRS (m/d)**	—	6–14	—	—
Cacciola et al,[28] 2010						
Cervical	10	TWSTRS (t)	55.7	37.6	17.6	68
Groen et al,[125] 2010						
PGD DYT6+	5	BFMDRS (m)	38.9	6	25.6	34

(*continued on next page*)

Table 3
(continued)

Type of Dystonia	N	Scale (Subscale)	Baseline Score	Follow-Up Time (mo)	Follow-Up Score	Percent Improvement
Yamada et al,[23] 2012						
Cervical	8	TWSTRS (s/d/p)	—	24–36	—	70.2/76.1/87.1
Borggraefe et al,[70] 2010						
PGD DYT1+	3	BFMDRS (m)	52	13	8.7	83
PGD DYT1−	3	BFMDRS (m)	51	16.7	19	63
Panov et al,[74] 2012						
PGD DYT6+	3	BFMDRS (m)	—	24	—	61
PGD DYT1+	23	—	—	24	—	87
Skogseid et al,[29] 2012						
Cervical	8	TWSTRS (s/d/p)	28/15/22	30	7/2/2002	73/92/91

Series in bold type have class I evidence.

Abbreviations: AIMS, Abnormal Involuntary Movement Scale; BFMDRS, Burke-Fahn-Marsden Dystonia Rating Scale (d, disability subscore; m, motor score); ESRS, Extrapyramidal Symptom Rating Scale; TWSTRS, Toronto-Western Spasmodic Torticollis Rating Scale (d, disability; p, pain; s, severity).

[a] Unknown subtype.
[b] Estimated averages.
[c] DYT1+ and DYT1− groups analyzed together.
[d] Generalized and segmental groups combined.

follow-up (mean of 34 months).[46] Both of these studies also reported a benefit in choreiform involuntary movements.

Cerebral palsy (CP) is a common cause of secondary dystonia in children and adults. Most reports of CP treated with DBS have consisted of small series or part of larger series combined with other types of dystonia,[8,27,49–51] but larger series also exist in both children[52] and adults[53] (**Table 6**). A series of cognitively intact adults with CP and normal brain magnetic resonance imaging assessed by blinded raters 1 year after bilateral GPi DBS showed 21% and 18% improvements in the BFMDRS-m and BFMDRS-d scores, respectively.[53] Several quality-of-life measures also improved, whereas psychiatric and cognitive function did not decline. In contrast, another group reported less substantial results in adults.[52] Gimeno and colleagues[54] reported no clear improvement in BFMDRS-m scores but did find significant improvement in perceived caregiver burden and goal attainment scaling after GPi DBS. A meta-analysis including 68 cases of CP treated with DBS (60 bilateral GPi, 3 unilateral GPi, 1 unilateral GPi contralateral subthalamic nucleus [STN], 1 ventralis oralis anterior) at a median of 12 months of follow-up showed 23.6% and 9.2% improvements in BFMDRS-m and BFMDRS-d scores, respectively.[55] Patients with CP with a BFMDRS-m score greater than 85 were more likely to be a nonresponder (<20% improvement), which suggested an inverse correlation between dystonia severity and likelihood of improvement.

Other types of secondary dystonia have also been treated with DBS, including Fahr disease,[56] multiple sclerosis, and poststroke dystonia,[57,58] although data remain at the level of case reports and small case series.

Heredodegenerative dystonia

Patient or caregiver quality of life may be improved by DBS in some heredodegenerative dystonia cases. Dystonia and some of the behavior symptoms associated with Lesch-Nyhan disease have been reported to improve after DBS[59] (Ostrem and Starr, personal communication, 2013). GM1 gangliosidosis[60] and X-linked (Lubag) dystonia-parkinsonism have also been treated with DBS with some success.[61–65]

Perhaps most studied is neurodegeneration with brain iron accumulation (NBIA) secondary to PANK2 mutations, with improvements in the BFMDRS-m score ranging from 20%[66] to 91%[67] after DBS. An open-label, multicenter series of 23 patients with NBIA showed a 28.5% improvement after 2 to 6 months and a 25.7% improvement at 9 to 15 months in the BFMDRS-m score.[68] These patients also showed a median of 83.3% improvement in global quality-of-life scores at 9 to 15 months of follow-up, despite the slight worsening of BFMDRS-m score.

Table 4
Long-term follow-up studies of GPi DBS for dystonia

Type of Dystonia	N	Scale (Subscale)	Baseline Score	Follow-Up Time (mo)	Follow-Up Score	Percent Improvement
Vidailhet et al,[2] 2007						
From Vidailhet et al,[15] 2005						
PGD DYT1+	7	BFMDRS (m/d)	46.3/11.6	36	19.3/6.3	58/46[a]
PGD DYT1−	15	—	—	—	—	—
Loher et al,[18] 2008						
From Krauss et al,[24,25,49] 1999, 2002, 2003						
Primary genetic	1	BFMDRS (m/d)	71/17	36	17/4	76/76
Primary[b]	1	BFMDRS (m/d)	91/20	36	39.5/11	56/45
Cervical	4	TWSTRS (s/d/p)	20.5/40.5/6	36	14.8/15.8/3.8	28/61/38
Moro et al,[30] 2009						
From Hung et al,[22] 2007						
Cervical	8	TWSTRS (t)	24	28.6	11.1	53.8
Cif et al,[20] 2010						
From Cif et al,[8] 2003						
PGD DYT1+	18	BFMDRS (m/d)	54.7/14.6	3–10	13.7/4.4	75/70
PGD DYT1+ second lead	8	BFMDRS (m/d)	63.9/15.9	3–10	25.5/8.28	60/48
Volkmann et al,[21] 2012						
From Kupsch et al,[16] 2006						
PGD	20	BFMDRS (m/d)	43.4/10	60	18.2/5.3	58/47[c]
Cervical	12	BFMDRS (m/d)	—	—	—	—
Walsh et al,[31] 2013						
From Hung et al,[22] 2007						
Cervical	10	TWSTRS (s/d/p)	21.5/12.6/20.3	7.7	10.6/7.7/7.5	51/39/63

Series in bold type have class I evidence.
Abbreviations: AIMS, Abnormal Involuntary Movement Scale; BFMDRS, Burke-Fahn-Marsden Dystonia Rating Scale (m, motor score; d, disability subscore); ESRS, Extrapyramidal Symptom Rating Scale; TWSTRS, Toronto-Western Spasmodic Torticollis Rating Scale (d, disability; p, pain; s, severity).
[a] DYT1+ and DYT1− groups analyzed together.
[b] Unknown subtype.
[c] Generalized and segmental groups combined.

Summary

The strongest evidence for a beneficial effect exists for PGD and segmental dystonia (class I), suggesting an expected 44% to 58% improvement in BFMDRS-m scores sustained up to 3 years (see **Tables 3** and **4**). Primary CD was also included in a class I study, with several class III studies showing improvements in movement, disability, and pain. Secondary dystonia has a variable response based on cause, but the strongest evidence exists from class IV trials, supporting improvement in tardive dystonia and dyskinetic CP (see **Tables 5** and **6**).

Influence of Genetic Status on Outcome

The question of a differential response in patients with PGD based on the presence of a TOR1A mutation (DYT1+) has been raised after small series showed better outcomes in patients with DYT1+ than patients with DYT1−,[6,7,69] whereas others did not.[8,11] The larger, prospective, multicenter trials mentioned earlier did not show a difference between patients with DYT1+ and DYT1− PGD.[2,15,16] However, more recent evidence in children and adolescents[70] and a retrospective metaregression[71] indicate DYT1+ status as an

Table 5
Studies of GPi DBS for tardive dystonia

Study	N	Scale (Subscale)	Baseline Score	Follow-Up Time (mo)	Follow-Up Score	Percent Improvement
Trottenberg et al,[42] 2005	5	BFMDRS (m/d)	32/8	6	—	87/96
Damier et al,[43] 2007	10	ESRS	73.1	6	27.8	62
	—	AIMS	25	—	11.3	55
Sako et al,[44] 2008	6	BFMDRS (m/d)	30.8/9.3	21	3.8/1.8	88/80
Gruber et al,[45] 2009	9	BFMDRS (m/d)	30.9/11.6	40.7	5.5/3.4	82/71
	—	AIMS	23.1	—	4.3	81
Chang et al,[46] 2010	4	BFMDRS (m)	49.7	34	14.5	71
	—	ESRS	10.5	—	2	81
Capelle et al,[47] 2010	4	BFMDRS (m/d)	43/6	27.3	7/2	84/67

Abbreviations: AIMS, Abnormal Involuntary Movement Scale; ESRS, Extrapyramidal Symptom Rating Scale.

independent predictor of good outcome. Also, a recent prospective, multicenter, blinded-rater trial[17] showed DYT1+ status as a positive predictor of good outcome in a multivariate analysis of variance.

Recent discovery of a THAP1 mutation (DYT6) has allowed retrospective outcome analysis of patients with dystonia who received DBS. Although a case of DBS for CD in a DYT6+ has been reported showing a robust response,[72] other series may suggest an early plateau or possible loss of benefit after 12 months.[73,74] These studies also may show less benefit in oromandibular and laryngeal dystonia, which are often early and prominent symptoms in DYT6+ dystonia. When compared retrospectively, patients with DYT6+ primary dystonia had a smaller degree of improvement postoperatively compared with patients with DYT1+ primary dystonia (61% vs 87% at 24 months).[74]

Summary

The impact of DYT1 status on motor outcome after DBS is still controversial, with mixed findings between short-term and long-term follow-up.[2,11,17,21] It is also possible that as we learn more about the genetics of patients with DYT1− PGD, such as the impact of DYT6 on surgical outcomes, we will be able to better answer this

Table 6
Studies of GPi DBS for CP

Study/Dystonia Type	N	Scale (Subscale)	Baseline Score	Follow-Up Time (mo)	Follow-Up Score	Percent Improvement
Vidailhet et al,[53] 2009						
Choreathetosis CP	13	BFMDRS (m/d)	44.2/12.6	12	34.7/10.3	21/18
Marks et al,[52] 2011						
Dystonic CP <16 y old	8	BFMDRS (m/d)	61.1/18.3	6	35/16	43/14
	—	Barry-Albright	21.1	6	16.9	20
Dystonic CP >16 y old	6	BFMDRS (m/d)	91.5/24.8	6	82.8/24	9/3
	—	Barry-Albright	25.5	6	24.8	3
Gimeno et al,[54] 2012						
Dystonic CP	5	BFMDRS (m/d)	—	12	—	5.9
Glutaric aciduria	1	—	—	—	—	1.5[(−)]
Koy et al,[55] 2013						
CP	68	BFMDRS (m/d)	64.9/18.54	12	50.5/16.8	23.6/16.8

question. In practice, the presence of a DYT1 mutation assures us that the patient has primary dystonia and that they are in a group that is highly likely to respond to DBS, which allows us to stop looking for other secondary causes of dystonia.

Influence of Dystonia Symptoms on Outcome

Phasic versus tonic movement

Some studies suggest that mobile dystonia responds better than tonic dystonia. Certainly, tonic dystonia that progresses to fixed contractures is associated with a worse outcome.[75-77] Electromyographic (EMG) data can be used to predict the timing and degree of motor improvement in dystonic movements after pallidal DBS.[78] Patients with a dominant frequency pattern of phasic activity on EMG experienced earlier improvements than those patients with baseline EMG hyperactivity without a clear burst frequency.

Patients with PGD with (n = 6) and without (n = 24) fixed skeletal deformities showed 82.7% and 69.8% improvement in the BFMDRS-m score at a range of 2.4 to 13.6 months of follow-up after treatment with GPi DBS.[76] Although patients with a fixed deformity at a given joint may not recover much mobility after DBS, pain can be significantly reduced through relaxation of the dystonic contractions.

Pain

Independent of motor scores, several studies have shown improvements in pain scores in both primary[17,79,80] and secondary[54] dystonia. Not all pain may be the result of dystonia. For example, patients with CD may also have coexisting cervical spine disease, which is not expected to improve if the pain is coming from degenerative spine changes.

Summary

Phasic movements or mobile dystonia are likely to improve sooner and to a greater degree than tonic movements and fixed skeletal deformities after GPi DBS. Pain is also significantly improved in both primary and secondary dystonia after GPi DBS, independent of motoric improvement. Especially in cases in which there is significant surgical risk (such as in young or cognitively impaired patients), close attention to the type of movement targeted and the presence and cause of pain can help to more accurately weigh risks and benefits.

Age at Surgery and Outcome

Age at the time of surgery and outcome after DBS for dystonia has been closely studied, and is addressed here separately from disease duration and age of dystonia onset. Concerns over increased infection and lead breakage rate have been raised in young children, whereas older individuals with poor mobility may be at increased risk for infection and skin breakdown over the hardware. It is also possible that age is an independently associated prognosticator, independent of infection or hardware complication risk.

In PGD and CD, some studies have suggested that younger age predicts a better response to DBS. Children with PGD ranging from 7.8 to 17.8 years in age showed 75% and 71% improvement in the BFMDRS-m and BFMDRS-d scales, respectively.[51] Another group showed that young age (<21 years old) may portend a better motor and disability response than older patients (>21 years old),[81] and this was replicated by another group even when disease duration was taken into account.[82] On the contrary, the prospective Spanish study discussed earlier showed a positive correlation between degree of motor improvement and age at the time of surgery,[17] and a meta-analysis of previously reported cases showed no correlation between outcome and age at the time of surgery.[83] Such correlations have not been examined specifically in CD, although long-term follow-up data suggest a good response despite the later age of surgery (33–67 years old).[31]

In our experience, motor and disability outcomes in secondary dystonia may be complicated by increased risk for hardware-related malfunction or infection. Of our 6 reported patients treated with GPi DBS for hyperkinetic CP, the improvement in motor and disability was modest (10% and 20%, respectively).[51] Overall, the infection rate was 57% in children younger than 10 years, but was 0% in those older than 10 years, and all infections occurred in patients with either secondary or heredodegenerative dystonia.[51] A meta-analysis of 68 patients in whom GPi DBS was performed for CP showed no correlation between age at the time surgery and motor outcome.[55] Conflicting data exist for the impact of age at surgery on motor outcomes in patients with secondary dystonia. Although younger patients have higher infection and device complication rates, older patients are more likely to have fixed skeletal deformities. This finding may suggest an optimum window of intervention in late childhood.

In PGD and CD, older age may be associated with more improvement in motor outcome but not disability. There is little evidence for efficacy in children younger than 7 years, but we recommend a case-by-case decision based on cognitive impairment, skin integrity/health, weight, and the likelihood of complications. No upper age limit has been established.

Disease Duration

Shorter disease duration in patients with DYT1+ PGD has been associated with improved surgical outcomes, especially in children older than 10 years without fixed deformities.[84] However, in a more heterogeneous sample of patients with DYT1+ and DYT1− PGD and cervical dystonia, there was no correlation found between disease duration and motor outcome,[17] and a study of patient predictors in 28 patients with CD treated with bilateral GPi DBS showed no correlation between disease duration and degree of improvement.[85]

A meta-analysis using 137 patients from 24 studies[83] showed mixed results when evaluating the impact of disease duration on motor outcome. A metaregression using 466 patients from 157 studies[71] showed that in primary dystonia, shorter disease duration was associated with a better motor outcome ($P = .008$).

In a retrospective series of 70 consecutive children treated with GPi DBS for primary or secondary dystonia,[86] there was a negative correlation between BFMDRS-m improvement and disease duration. These investigators also showed that this negative correlation exists between motoric improvement and the ratio of disease duration/age at surgery, establishing that disease duration is a factor independent of age at the time of surgery. This study also showed that there was no reduction in efficacy in those with musculoskeletal deformities. Most data suggest that increasing disease duration is associated with worsening motor outcomes, although minimal data on correlation with change in quality of life are available.

Psychiatric Disease/Depression

The potential impact of bilateral DBS on premorbid psychiatric illness in PD has raised concern about its use in patients with dystonia. Depression is common in dystonia (≤30% in some studies[87]) and there are reports of suicide in depressed patients undergoing DBS for dystonia.[88,89]

When the impact of depression after DBS for dystonia has been studied in outcome studies, most have reported no change or improvement in depression. In the study by Vidailhet and colleagues,[2] the Beck Depression Inventory (BDI) was stable at 3 years, and an improvement in the BDI was seen at 6 months after surgery in the German study.[16] These 2 studies did exclude patients with severe depression. The Spanish DBS study[17] included patients with a mean preoperative BDI of 34.87 (moderately depressed), but the BDI improved to 27.12 ($P<.01$) at 12 months after surgery, with no suicides. The European Quality of Life 5D questionnaire anxiety/depression score also improved. Patients treated with GPi DBS for tardive dystonia, many of whom suffer from psychotic diseases or mood disorders requiring antipsychotic use, did not show worsening of psychiatric illness after DBS.[45,47]

It is still important to be aggressive in treating depression through comanagement with a mental health professional before surgery to ensure that patients are psychiatrically stable before having neurosurgical intervention.

Cognitive Function

There is no clear evidence from the largest trials of GPi DBS for dystonia[2] that there is a significant impact on cognition, although these contain mostly patients with primary dystonia.[90,91] Small, open-label trials in patients with tardive dystonia[45] and patients with CP without baseline cognitive impairment[53] do not show worsened cognition postoperatively. No cognitive outcome data are available for heredodegenerative dystonia.

TARGET SELECTION

Although most trials evaluating the efficacy of DBS for dystonia have used the GPi as the brain target, some consideration has been given to other brain targets to minimize potential side effects of GPi stimulation, to treat specific features of certain dystonic syndromes (like tremor), which may not respond entirely to GPi DBS, or for patients who are considered nonresponders to GPi DBS.

GPi

The benefits of GPi DBS in dystonia are discussed earlier and are described in **Tables 3–6**. In long-term follow-up of the largest prospective trials, blinded video assessment trials show sustained improvements to 3[2] and 5 years.[21] Significant long-term benefits in disability and quality-of-life measures have also been established in prospective trials using this target, with improvements in the BFMDRS-d score ranging from 41% to 75%.[2,18,20,21]

Potential limitations

Stimulation-induced side effects It has recently been recognized that patients who receive bilateral GPi DBS for a segmental or focal dystonia can develop stimulation-induced bradykinesia in previously unaffected limbs.[36,92–94] Even in a prospective, double-blind study of GPi DBS in PGD, there was a nonsignificant trend toward slowed finger-taps in the stimulation group (9 fewer per minute) than the sham group (31 more per minute) compared with baseline (P = .24).[16]

Our center[36] reported that 4 of 6 patients who underwent GPi DBS for craniocervical dystonia (Meige syndrome) reported new difficulty with coordination and slowness of movement in sites previously without dystonia. Despite proper lead placement in these patients, this stimulation-induced bradykinesia was difficult to avoid with programming changes without loss of the antidystonic effects.[36] In a survey of primary cervical or craniocervical dystonia treated with GPi DBS, this phenomenon was common (worsening of handwriting [82%], difficulty rising from a chair [73%], difficulty holding items above head [55%], and trouble rolling over in bed [45%]).[93] These effects were not secondary to pyramidal tract stimulation, because of the insidious onset and lack of involvement of muscles typically activated with capsular stimulation, such as facial pulling. There was a positive correlation between the improvement in dystonia and degree of stimulation-induced bradykinesia experienced.

In the most recent prospective trial showing benefit in primary CD with GPi DBS,[31] 2 patients reported new hand bradykinesia, and stimulation-induced micrographia was documented in 1 of the patients. Volkman and colleagues[21] also reported 1 case of stimulation-induced parkinsonism, although this was not routinely screened for so this could be an underestimation. Zauber and colleagues[94] reported a patient with DYT1− craniocervical dystonia who experienced a good motoric benefit (70% improvement in BFMDRS-m score) but also had significant axial and appendicular bradykinesia with stimulation of the dorsal GPi. Stimulation in the ventral GPi led to resolution of this bradykinesia but allowed return of dystonia. In 71 patients with GPi DBS for various types of dystonia, 6 patients presented with a dramatic hypokinetic gait associated with freezing of gait despite improvement in BFMDRS-m score by 54%.[95] Again, both the dystonia control and bradykinesia were reversible when stimulation was turned off.

Increased risk of hemorrhage The pallidal target is a more vascularized nucleus compared with the STN or thalamus. In a report on the incidence of hemorrhage associated with DBS surgery for PD and dystonia,[96] the only statistically significant predictor of hemorrhage risk was brain target (P = .001), with hemorrhage in 7.0% of GPi cases versus 2.2% in STN cases. Although the number of microelectrode recording penetrations was higher for GPi, this was not a predictive factor in the multivariate analysis, suggesting that the difference in hemorrhage rate was inherent to the target itself.

Delayed benefit of stimulation The beneficial effects of pallidal DBS on dystonia can be delayed for weeks, months, or even years. As indicated by the recent 5-year follow-up of the German study,[21] patients with PGD continue to experience improvement in motor symptoms between 3 and 5 years. This situation complicates programming, especially in patients who live remotely from the closest center for movement disorders. It is unclear if patients with another brain target may have earlier symptom improvement but some have suggested that this may be the case.

Overall, GPi DBS for dystonia is the only procedure supported by class I evidence for efficacy, although potential limitations include stimulation-induced bradykinesia, possibly higher hemorrhage rate than other targets, and delayed benefit of stimulation. There may also be a nonresponder rate of up to 19%,[2] which could be treated using other brain targets.

STN

The STN has been well studied as a brain target for DBS in PD, associated with treatment of PD-associated dyskinesia and dystonia. The literature is still limited, with fewer than 50 cases reported to date of using STN as a brain target in dystonia, but the data are promising. STN stimulation has been applied to various types of dystonia, including primary dystonia,[97–99] dopa-responsive dystonia,[100] dystonia and essential tremor,[101] and NBIA.[102,103] In our original series of 9 patients with primary CD, we reported a 62.9% (P<.001) improvement in the total TWSTRS score higher than baseline as assessed by a blinded rater, with most of the improvement being reached after 3 months (50.6% improvement in total TWSTRS).[104] To date, we have studied a total of 20 patients with primary dystonia and continue to show a similar response in this larger cohort (article under review for publication). Included in this cohort of patients are 4 patients with DYT1+ dystonia who have also shown significant improvement. None of our patients has experienced stimulation-induced bradykinesia, as can be seen with GPi DBS.

Pahapill and O'Connell[97] reported 2 cervical patients with dystonia implanted with bilateral STN DBS and reported favorable outcomes. Another series of 4 patients with STN DBS for dystonia[98] reported a significant 5-point mean improvement on the TWSTRS severity score.

Potential limitations

Dyskinesia All of the patients predominantly with CD in our pilot study of STN DBS experienced stimulation-induced dyskinesia during the study as voltage was increased. Dyskinesia could be overcome by slower up-titration of the voltage or sometimes by activation of the dorsal electrode contacts.[99]

Possible weight gain Weight gain was also seen in some patients. A retrospective chart review of 36 patients with dystonia (9 with STN DBS and 27 with GPi DBS) showed that the STN was the only statistically significant predictor of postoperative weight gain in a multivariate regression analysis controlling for sex, age, preoperative body mass index, follow-up time, and change in BFMDRS-m score.[105] In our now larger cohort of patients, patients with STN DBS have not shown a significant weight gain after surgery (article under review for publication).

Mood We have not seen a worsening of depression in our larger cohort of patients (article under review for publication). The BDI did not show statistically significant worsening, and depressive symptoms were improved with titration of an antidepressant or removal of a medication known to cause depression in some patients.

Cognition Of interest is also the difference in specific cognitive outcomes seen between patients with GPi and STN DBS PD, such as decreased verbal fluency in patients with PD with STN DBS.[106] In the 9 studies published so far on STN DBS for patients with dystonia, and in 7 other unpublished cases, we have not seen changes in thorough neuropsychological testing postoperatively[99] (Ostrem, personal communication, 2013). Only 1 other study has reported neuropsychological outcomes after surgery and no significant differences were found.[98] To thoroughly address the possibility of cognitive decline/change after STN (as has been seen in PD) a larger study is needed.

Although few studies exist regarding the efficacy of subthalamic stimulation for dystonia, it deserves further study as a target. In our experience, patients treated with STN DBS are at a lower risk of developing stimulation-induced bradykinesia in body segments unaffected by dystonia. However, they are at risk of developing transient stimulation-induced dyskinesia, and programming parameters may need to be carefully tailored.

Thalamus

After a report of successful treatment of focal, task-specific hand dystonia (writer's cramp) with a ventro-oralis (Vo) thalamotomy,[107] the Vo was explored as a DBS target for medication-refractory writer's cramp.[108] In this case report, both GPi and Vo were implanted, and stimulation at either site led to immediate and complete relief of the focal hand dystonia. Another series[109] reported outcomes in 5 patients with writer's cramp who received Vo DBS and experienced immediate and complete response with stimulation. One patient who was implanted with both GPi and Vo electrodes experienced greater benefit with Vo than GPi stimulation. The thalamus could also serve as an alternative target in secondary dystonia when the normal basal ganglia architecture is disturbed or missing.[110]

Thalamic stimulation might also be useful when dystonia is seen in association with other movement disorders that respond favorably to thalamic stimulation such as myoclonus-dystonia.[111] Dystonic tremor, defined as an irregular tremor with variable frequency seen in an extremity or body part that is affected by dystonia,[112] has also been reported to improve by about 50% with ventral intermediate nucleus (Vim) stimulation.[113] In another patient, Vim DBS, GPi DBS, and thalamotomy were combined for a dramatic improvement in symptoms.[108]

Potential issues

There exist almost no data on thalamic DBS in PGD or segmental dystonia. Thalamotomy was once a commonly used procedure in the treatment of generalized dystonia,[114] although later series reported a lower rate of sustained success (4 of 16 patients).[115] For patients with bilateral segmental or generalized disease, bilateral thalamic stimulation could potentially lead to dysarthria or gait abnormalities, as has been seen in patients with essential tremor.

Thalamic DBS for dystonia deserves more study, especially in patients with complex movement disorders, including tremor or dystonic tremor and in the setting of focal, task-specific limb dystonia.

Cortex

There is evidence that the pathophysiology of dystonia probably involves the cortex through disordered surround inhibition,[116] sensorimotor integration, and plasticity.[117] It is possible that augmentation of one or more of these processes at the cortical level could lead to symptomatic treatment of dystonic contractions. Repetitive transcortical magnetic stimulation (rTMS) at low (theta) frequencies in motor areas may augment abnormal cortical inhibition,[118] and rTMS has provided transient improvement in focal hand dystonia.[119,120] Furthering this approach, a trial of 10 patients showed a 30% improvement in the Disability of the Arm, Shoulder, and Hand scale after epidural stimulation over the motor cortex contralateral to a fixed dystonia.[121]

Cortical stimulation has the potential to be especially useful in patients who are not candidates for implantation of a device, have disrupted basal ganglia anatomy, are at high risk for hemorrhage, or who are interested in a less invasive approach.

SUMMARY

DBS continues to be refined as an important therapeutic intervention offered in medication-refractory dystonia, and probably exerts an effect through modulation of basal ganglia-thalamic-cortical circuits, although the exact therapeutic effect on physiology is unclear. With the greater understanding of factors that influence the degree of therapeutic response to DBS, including type of dystonia, genetic cause, target symptoms (eg, movement type, pain), age at the time of surgery, disease duration, and presence of fixed skeletal deformities, we can determine patient candidacy for this surgery and counsel patients more accurately about expected outcome after surgery. There may be less concern over certain premorbid conditions such as psychiatric illness and cognitive impairment than in DBS for other neurodegenerative conditions such as PD. Although primary dystonia generally shows a robust response with GPi DBS, emerging evidence suggests a reasonable response in certain types of secondary dystonia such as tardive dystonia, dyskinetic CP, and even NBIA. Genetic factors may also improve prognostication, because there is suggestion of a potentially less robust response in a recently described dystonia related to the THAP1 mutation (DYT6).

Target selection is an emerging issue in DBS for dystonia now that other deep and cortical targets are being explored. Although strong evidence exists for the use of GPi DBS in primary dystonia, the STN is a new promising alternative stimulation target deserving of more study.

REFERENCES

1. Fahn S. Classification of movement disorders. Mov Disord 2011;26(6):947–57.
2. Vidailhet M, Vercueil L, Houeto JL, et al. Bilateral, pallidal, deep-brain stimulation in primary generalised dystonia: a prospective 3 year follow-up study. Lancet Neurol 2007;6(3):223–9.
3. Fahn S, Jankovic J. Principles and practice of movement disorders. Philadelphia: Churchill Livingstone/Elsevier; 2007.
4. Ozelius LJ, Hewett JW, Page CE, et al. The early-onset torsion dystonia gene (DYT1) encodes an ATP-binding protein. Nat Genet 1997;17(1):40–8.
5. Fuchs T, Gavarini S, Saunders-Pullman R, et al. Mutations in the THAP1 gene are responsible for DYT6 primary torsion dystonia. Nat Genet 2009;41(3): 286–8.
6. Vercueil L, Pollak P, Fraix V, et al. Deep brain stimulation in the treatment of severe dystonia. J Neurol 2001;248(8):695–700.
7. Yianni J, Bain PG, Gregory RP, et al. Post-operative progress of dystonia patients following globus pallidus internus deep brain stimulation. Eur J Neurol 2003;10(3):239–47.
8. Cif L, El Fertit H, Vayssiere N, et al. Treatment of dystonic syndromes by chronic electrical stimulation of the internal globus pallidus. J Neurosurg Sci 2003;47(1):52–5.
9. Kupsch A, Klaffke S, Kuhn AA, et al. The effects of frequency in pallidal deep brain stimulation for primary dystonia. J Neurol 2003;250(10):1201–5.
10. Katayama Y, Fukaya C, Kobayashi K, et al. Chronic stimulation of the globus pallidus internus for control of primary generalized dystonia. Acta Neurochir Suppl 2003;87:125–8.
11. Coubes P, Cif L, El Fertit H, et al. Electrical stimulation of the globus pallidus internus in patients with primary generalized dystonia: long-term results. J Neurosurg 2004;101(2):189–94.
12. Vayssiere N, van der Gaag N, Cif L, et al. Deep brain stimulation for dystonia confirming a somatotopic organization in the globus pallidus internus. J Neurosurg 2004;101(2):181–8.
13. Eltahawy HA, Saint-Cyr J, Giladi N, et al. Primary dystonia is more responsive than secondary dystonia to pallidal interventions: outcome after pallidotomy or pallidal deep brain stimulation. Neurosurgery 2004; 54(3):613–9 [discussion: 619–21].
14. Krause M, Fogel W, Kloss M, et al. Pallidal stimulation for dystonia. Neurosurgery 2004;55(6):1361–8 [discussion: 1368–70].
15. Vidailhet M, Vercueil L, Houeto JL, et al. Bilateral deep-brain stimulation of the globus pallidus in primary generalized dystonia. N Engl J Med 2005; 352(5):459–67.
16. Kupsch A, Benecke R, Muller J, et al. Pallidal deep-brain stimulation in primary generalized or segmental dystonia. N Engl J Med 2006;355(19): 1978–90.
17. Valldeoriola F, Regidor I, Minguez-Castellanos A, et al. Efficacy and safety of pallidal stimulation in primary dystonia: results of the Spanish multicentric study. J Neurol Neurosurg Psychiatry 2010; 81(1):65–9.
18. Loher TJ, Capelle HH, Kaelin-Lang A, et al. Deep brain stimulation for dystonia: outcome at long-term follow-up. J Neurol 2008;255(6):881–4.

19. Isaias IU, Alterman RL, Tagliati M. Deep brain stimulation for primary generalized dystonia: long-term outcomes. Arch Neurol 2009;66(4):465–70.
20. Cif L, Vasques X, Gonzalez V, et al. Long-term follow-up of DYT1 dystonia patients treated by deep brain stimulation: an open-label study. Mov Disord 2010;25(3):289–99.
21. Volkmann J, Wolters A, Kupsch A, et al. Pallidal deep brain stimulation in patients with primary generalised or segmental dystonia: 5-year follow-up of a randomised trial. Lancet Neurol 2012; 11(12):1029–38.
22. Hung SW, Hamani C, Lozano AM, et al. Long-term outcome of bilateral pallidal deep brain stimulation for primary cervical dystonia. Neurology 2007; 68(6):457–9.
23. Yamada K, Hamasaki T, Hasegawa Y, et al. Long disease duration interferes with therapeutic effect of globus pallidus internus pallidal stimulation in primary cervical dystonia. Neuromodulation 2012; 16(3):219–25.
24. Krauss JK, Pohle T, Weber S, et al. Bilateral stimulation of globus pallidus internus for treatment of cervical dystonia. Lancet 1999;354(9181):837–8.
25. Krauss JK, Loher TJ, Pohle T, et al. Pallidal deep brain stimulation in patients with cervical dystonia and severe cervical dyskinesias with cervical myelopathy. J Neurol Neurosurg Psychiatry 2002; 72(2):249–56.
26. Bittar RG, Yianni J, Wang S, et al. Deep brain stimulation for generalised dystonia and spasmodic torticollis. J Clin Neurosci 2005;12(1):12–6.
27. Starr PA, Turner RS, Rau G, et al. Microelectrode-guided implantation of deep brain stimulators into the globus pallidus internus for dystonia: techniques, electrode locations, and outcomes. J Neurosurg 2006;104(4):488–501.
28. Cacciola F, Farah JO, Eldridge PR, et al. Bilateral deep brain stimulation for cervical dystonia: long-term outcome in a series of 10 patients. Neurosurgery 2010;67(4):957–63.
29. Skogseid IM, Ramm-Pettersen J, Volkmann J, et al. Good long-term efficacy of pallidal stimulation in cervical dystonia: a prospective, observer-blinded study. Eur J Neurol 2012;19(4):610–5.
30. Moro E, Piboolnurak P, Arenovich T, et al. Pallidal stimulation in cervical dystonia: clinical implications of acute changes in stimulation parameters. Eur J Neurol 2009;16(4):506–12.
31. Walsh RA, Sidiropoulos C, Lozano AM, et al. Bilateral pallidal stimulation in cervical dystonia: blinded evidence of benefit beyond 5 years. Brain 2013;136(Pt 3):761–9.
32. Capelle HH, Weigel R, Krauss JK. Bilateral pallidal stimulation for blepharospasm-oromandibular dystonia (Meige syndrome). Neurology 2003;60(12): 2017–8.
33. Foote KD, Sanchez JC, Okun MS. Staged deep brain stimulation for refractory craniofacial dystonia with blepharospasm: case report and physiology. Neurosurgery 2005;56(2):E415 [discussion: E415].
34. Houser M, Waltz T. Meige syndrome and pallidal deep brain stimulation. Mov Disord 2005;20(9): 1203–5.
35. Opherk C, Gruber C, Steude U, et al. Successful bilateral pallidal stimulation for Meige syndrome and spasmodic torticollis. Neurology 2006;66(4): E14.
36. Ostrem JL, Marks WJ Jr, Volz MM, et al. Pallidal deep brain stimulation in patients with cranial-cervical dystonia (Meige syndrome). Mov Disord 2007;22(13):1885–91.
37. Reese R, Gruber D, Schoenecker T, et al. Long-term clinical outcome in Meige syndrome treated with internal pallidum deep brain stimulation. Mov Disord 2011;26(4):691–8.
38. Lyons MK, Birch BD, Hillman RA, et al. Long-term follow-up of deep brain stimulation for Meige syndrome. Neurosurg Focus 2010;29(2):E5.
39. Ghang JY, Lee MK, Jun SM, et al. Outcome of pallidal deep brain stimulation in Meige syndrome. J Korean Neurosurg Soc 2010;48(2):134–8.
40. Sako W, Morigaki R, Mizobuchi Y, et al. Bilateral pallidal deep brain stimulation in primary Meige syndrome. Parkinsonism Relat Disord 2011;17(2): 123–5.
41. Inoue N, Nagahiro S, Kaji R, et al. Long-term suppression of Meige syndrome after pallidal stimulation: a 10-year follow-up study. Mov Disord 2010; 25(11):1756–8.
42. Trottenberg T, Volkmann J, Deuschl G, et al. Treatment of severe tardive dystonia with pallidal deep brain stimulation. Neurology 2005;64(2): 344–6.
43. Damier P, Thobois S, Witjas T, et al. Bilateral deep brain stimulation of the globus pallidus to treat tardive dyskinesia. Arch Gen Psychiatry 2007;64(2): 170–6.
44. Sako W, Goto S, Shimazu H, et al. Bilateral deep brain stimulation of the globus pallidus internus in tardive dystonia. Mov Disord 2008;23(13): 1929–31.
45. Gruber D, Trottenberg T, Kivi A, et al. Long-term effects of pallidal deep brain stimulation in tardive dystonia. Neurology 2009;73(1):53–8.
46. Chang EF, Schrock LE, Starr PA, et al. Long-term benefit sustained after bilateral pallidal deep brain stimulation in patients with refractory tardive dystonia. Stereotact Funct Neurosurg 2010; 88(5):304–10.
47. Capelle HH, Blahak C, Schrader C, et al. Chronic deep brain stimulation in patients with tardive dystonia without a history of major psychosis. Mov Disord 2010;25(10):1477–81.

48. Spindler MA, Galifianakis NB, Wilkinson JR, et al. Globus pallidus interna deep brain stimulation for tardive dyskinesia: case report and review of the literature. Parkinsonism Relat Disord 2013;19(2): 141–7.
49. Krauss JK, Loher TJ, Weigel R, et al. Chronic stimulation of the globus pallidus internus for treatment of non-dYT1 generalized dystonia and choreoathetosis: 2-year follow up. J Neurosurg 2003;98(4): 785–92.
50. Zorzi G, Marras C, Nardocci N, et al. Stimulation of the globus pallidus internus for childhood-onset dystonia. Mov Disord 2005;20(9):1194–200.
51. Air EL, Ostrem JL, Sanger TD, et al. Deep brain stimulation in children: experience and technical pearls. J Neurosurg Pediatr 2011;8(6):566–74.
52. Marks WA, Honeycutt J, Acosta F Jr, et al. Dystonia due to cerebral palsy responds to deep brain stimulation of the globus pallidus internus. Mov Disord 2011;26(9):1748–51.
53. Vidailhet M, Yelnik J, Lagrange C, et al. Bilateral pallidal deep brain stimulation for the treatment of patients with dystonia-choreoathetosis cerebral palsy: a prospective pilot study. Lancet Neurol 2009;8(8):709–17.
54. Gimeno H, Tustin K, Selway R, et al. Beyond the Burke-Fahn-Marsden dystonia rating scale: deep brain stimulation in childhood secondary dystonia. Eur J Paediatr Neurol 2012;16(5):501–8.
55. Koy A, Hellmich M, Pauls KA, et al. Effects of deep brain stimulation in dyskinetic cerebral palsy: a meta-analysis. Mov Disord 2013;28(5): 647–54.
56. Ma Y, Ge M, Meng F, et al. Bilateral deep brain stimulation of the subthalamic nucleus effectively relieves dystonia secondary to Fahr's disease: a case report. Int J Neurosci 2013;123(8):582–6.
57. Fuller J, Prescott IA, Moro E, et al. Pallidal deep brain stimulation for a case of hemidystonia secondary to a striatal stroke. Stereotact Funct Neurosurg 2013;91(3):190–7.
58. Witt J, Starr PA, Ostrem JL. Use of pallidal deep brain stimulation in postinfarct hemidystonia. Stereotact Funct Neurosurg 2013;91(4):243–7.
59. Cif L, Biolsi B, Gavarini S, et al. Antero-ventral internal pallidum stimulation improves behavioral disorders in Lesch-Nyhan disease. Mov Disord 2007; 22(14):2126–9.
60. Roze E, Navarro S, Cornu P, et al. Deep brain stimulation of the globus pallidus for generalized dystonia in GM1 Type 3 gangliosidosis: technical case report. Neurosurgery 2006;59(6):E1340 [discussion: E1340].
61. Evidente VG, Lyons MK, Wheeler M, et al. First case of X-linked dystonia-parkinsonism ("Lubag") to demonstrate a response to bilateral pallidal stimulation. Mov Disord 2007;22(12):1790–3.
62. Wadia PM, Lim SY, Lozano AM, et al. Bilateral pallidal stimulation for x-linked dystonia parkinsonism. Arch Neurol 2010;67(8):1012–5.
63. Kemmotsu N, Price CC, Oyama G, et al. Pre- and post- GPi DBS neuropsychological profiles in a case of X-linked dystonia-parkinsonism. Clin Neuropsychol 2011;25(1):141–59.
64. Kilbane C, Glass GA, Witt J, et al. Clinical outcomes in a series of X-linked dystonia parkinsonism treated with bilateral pallidal DBS. San Francisco (CA): American Society for Stereotactic and Functional Neurosurgery; 2012.
65. Oyama G, Fernandez HH, Foote KD, et al. Differential response of dystonia and parkinsonism following globus pallidus internus deep brain stimulation in X-linked dystonia-parkinsonism (Lubag). Stereotact Funct Neurosurg 2010; 88(5):329–33.
66. Lim BC, Ki CS, Cho A, et al. Pantothenate kinase-associated neurodegeneration in Korea: recurrent R440P mutation in PANK2 and outcome of deep brain stimulation. Eur J Neurol 2012;19(4):556–61.
67. Castelnau P, Cif L, Valente EM, et al. Pallidal stimulation improves pantothenate kinase-associated neurodegeneration. Ann Neurol 2005;57(5): 738–41.
68. Timmermann L, Pauls KA, Wieland K, et al. Dystonia in neurodegeneration with brain iron accumulation: outcome of bilateral pallidal stimulation. Brain 2010;133(Pt 3):701–12.
69. Coubes P, Roubertie A, Vayssiere N, et al. Treatment of DYT1-generalised dystonia by stimulation of the internal globus pallidus. Lancet 2000; 355(9222):2220–1.
70. Borggraefe I, Mehrkens JH, Telegravciska M, et al. Bilateral pallidal stimulation in children and adolescents with primary generalized dystonia–report of six patients and literature-based analysis of predictive outcomes variables. Brain Dev 2010;32(3): 223–8.
71. Andrews C, Aviles-Olmos I, Hariz M, et al. Which patients with dystonia benefit from deep brain stimulation? A metaregression of individual patient outcomes. J Neurol Neurosurg Psychiatry 2010; 81(12):1383–9.
72. Jech R, Bares M, Krepelova A, et al. DYT 6–a novel THAP1 mutation with excellent effect on pallidal DBS. Mov Disord 2011;26(5):924–5.
73. Miyamoto R, Ohta E, Kawarai T, et al. Broad spectrum of dystonia associated with a novel thanatosis-associated protein domain-containing apoptosis-associated protein 1 mutation in a Japanese family with dystonia 6, torsion. Mov Disord 2012;27(10):1324–5.
74. Panov F, Tagliati M, Ozelius LJ, et al. Pallidal deep brain stimulation for DYT6 dystonia. J Neurol Neurosurg Psychiatry 2012;83(2):182–7.

75. Jeong SG, Lee MK, Kang JY, et al. Pallidal deep brain stimulation in primary cervical dystonia with phasic type: clinical outcome and postoperative course. J Korean Neurosurg Soc 2009;46(4):346–50.
76. Isaias IU, Alterman RL, Tagliati M. Outcome predictors of pallidal stimulation in patients with primary dystonia: the role of disease duration. Brain 2008;131(Pt 7):1895–902.
77. Bereznai B, Steude U, Seelos K, et al. Chronic high-frequency globus pallidus internus stimulation in different types of dystonia: a clinical, video, and MRI report of six patients presenting with segmental, cervical, and generalized dystonia. Mov Disord 2002;17(1):138–44.
78. Yianni J, Wang SY, Liu X, et al. A dominant bursting electromyograph pattern in dystonic conditions predicts an early response to pallidal stimulation. J Clin Neurosci 2006;13(7):738–46.
79. Kiss ZH, Doig-Beyaert K, Eliasziw M, et al. The Canadian multicentre study of deep brain stimulation for cervical dystonia. Brain 2007;130(Pt 11):2879–86.
80. Mueller J, Skogseid IM, Benecke R, et al. Pallidal deep brain stimulation improves quality of life in segmental and generalized dystonia: results from a prospective, randomized sham-controlled trial. Mov Disord 2008;23(1):131–4.
81. Alterman RL, Tagliati M. Deep brain stimulation for torsion dystonia in children. Childs Nerv Syst 2007;23(9):1033–40.
82. Isaias IU, Volkmann J, Kupsch A, et al. Factors predicting protracted improvement after pallidal DBS for primary dystonia: the role of age and disease duration. J Neurol 2011;258(8):1469–76.
83. Holloway KL, Baron MS, Brown R, et al. Deep brain stimulation for dystonia: a meta-analysis. Neuromodulation 2006;9(4):253–61.
84. Markun LC, Starr PA, Air EL, et al. Shorter disease duration correlates with improved long-term deep brain stimulation outcomes in young-onset DYT1 dystonia. Neurosurgery 2012;71(2):325–30.
85. Witt J, Moro E, Ash R, et al. Predictive factors of outcome in primary cervical dystonia following pallidal deep brain stimulation. Mov Disord 2013;28(10):1451–5.
86. Lumsden DE, Kaminska M, Gimeno H, et al. Proportion of life lived with dystonia inversely correlates with response to pallidal deep brain stimulation in both primary and secondary childhood dystonia. Dev Med Child Neurol 2013;55(6):567–74.
87. Lewis L, Butler A, Jahanshahi M. Depression in focal, segmental and generalized dystonia. J Neurol 2008;255(11):1750–5.
88. Foncke EM, Schuurman PR, Speelman JD. Suicide after deep brain stimulation of the internal globus pallidus for dystonia. Neurology 2006;66(1):142–3.
89. Burkhard PR, Vingerhoets FJ, Berney A, et al. Suicide after successful deep brain stimulation for movement disorders. Neurology 2004;63(11):2170–2.
90. Halbig TD, Gruber D, Kopp UA, et al. Pallidal stimulation in dystonia: effects on cognition, mood, and quality of life. J Neurol Neurosurg Psychiatry 2005;76(12):1713–6.
91. Pillon B, Ardouin C, Dujardin K, et al. Preservation of cognitive function in dystonia treated by pallidal stimulation. Neurology 2006;66(10):1556–8.
92. Tisch S, Zrinzo L, Limousin P, et al. Effect of electrode contact location on clinical efficacy of pallidal deep brain stimulation in primary generalised dystonia. J Neurol Neurosurg Psychiatry 2007;78(12):1314–9.
93. Berman BD, Starr PA, Marks WJ Jr, et al. Induction of bradykinesia with pallidal deep brain stimulation in patients with cranial-cervical dystonia. Stereotact Funct Neurosurg 2009;87(1):37–44.
94. Zauber SE, Watson N, Comella CL, et al. Stimulation-induced parkinsonism after posteroventral deep brain stimulation of the globus pallidus internus for craniocervical dystonia. J Neurosurg 2009;110(2):229–33.
95. Schrader C, Capelle HH, Kinfe TM, et al. GPi-DBS may induce a hypokinetic gait disorder with freezing of gait in patients with dystonia. Neurology 2011;77(5):483–8.
96. Binder DK, Rau GM, Starr PA. Risk factors for hemorrhage during microelectrode-guided deep brain stimulator implantation for movement disorders. Neurosurgery 2005;56(4):722–32 [discussion: 722–32].
97. Pahapill PA, O'Connell B. Long-term follow-up study of chronic deep brain stimulation of the subthalamic nucleus for cervical dystonia. Neuromodulation 2010;13(1):26–30.
98. Kleiner-Fisman G, Liang GS, Moberg PJ, et al. Subthalamic nucleus deep brain stimulation for severe idiopathic dystonia: impact on severity, neuropsychological status, and quality of life. J Neurosurg 2007;107(1):29–36.
99. Ostrem JL, Racine CA, Glass GA, et al. Subthalamic nucleus deep brain stimulation in primary cervical dystonia. Neurology 2011;76(10):870–8.
100. Tormenti MJ, Tomycz ND, Coffman KA, et al. Bilateral subthalamic nucleus deep brain stimulation for dopa-responsive dystonia in a 6-year-old child. J Neurosurg Pediatr 2011;7(6):650–3.
101. Chou KL, Hurtig HI, Jaggi JL, et al. Bilateral subthalamic nucleus deep brain stimulation in a patient with cervical dystonia and essential tremor. Mov Disord 2005;20(3):377–80.
102. Benabid AL, Koudsie A, Benazzouz A, et al. Deep brain stimulation of the corpus luysi (subthalamic nucleus) and other targets in Parkinson's disease.

Extension to new indications such as dystonia and epilepsy. J Neurol 2001;248(Suppl 3):III37–47.
103. Ge M, Zhang K, Ma Y, et al. Bilateral subthalamic nucleus stimulation in the treatment of neurodegeneration with brain iron accumulation type 1. Stereotact Funct Neurosurg 2011;89(3):162–6.
104. Ostrem JL, Starr PA. Treatment of dystonia with deep brain stimulation. Neurotherapeutics 2008; 5(2):320–30.
105. Mills KA, Scherzer R, Starr PA, et al. Weight change after globus pallidus internus or subthalamic nucleus deep brain stimulation in Parkinson's disease and dystonia. Stereotact Funct Neurosurg 2012; 90(6):386–93.
106. Follett KA, Weaver FM, Stern M, et al. Pallidal versus subthalamic deep-brain stimulation for Parkinson's disease. N Engl J Med 2010;362(22): 2077–91.
107. Goto S, Tsuiki H, Soyama N, et al. Stereotactic selective Vo-complex thalamotomy in a patient with dystonic writer's cramp. Neurology 1997;49(4): 1173–4.
108. Goto S, Shimazu H, Matsuzaki K, et al. Thalamic Vo-complex vs pallidal deep brain stimulation for focal hand dystonia. Neurology 2008;70(16 Pt 2): 1500–1.
109. Fukaya C, Katayama Y, Kano T, et al. Thalamic deep brain stimulation for writer's cramp. J Neurosurg 2007;107(5):977–82.
110. Ghika J, Villemure JG, Miklossy J, et al. Postanoxic generalized dystonia improved by bilateral Voa thalamic deep brain stimulation. Neurology 2002; 58(2):311–3.
111. Kuncel AM, Turner DA, Ozelius LJ, et al. Myoclonus and tremor response to thalamic deep brain stimulation parameters in a patient with inherited myoclonus-dystonia syndrome. Clin Neurol Neurosurg 2009;111(3):303–6.
112. Deuschl G, Bain P, Brin M. Consensus statement of the movement disorder society on tremor. Ad Hoc Scientific Committee. Mov Disord 1998; 13(Suppl 3):2–23.
113. Morishita T, Foote KD, Haq IU, et al. Should we consider Vim thalamic deep brain stimulation for select cases of severe refractory dystonic tremor. Stereotact Funct Neurosurg 2010;88(2): 98–104.
114. Cooper IS. 20-year followup study of the neurosurgical treatment of dystonia musculorum deformans. Adv Neurol 1976;14:423–52.
115. Andrew J, Fowler CJ, Harrison MJ. Stereotaxic thalamotomy in 55 cases of dystonia. Brain 1983; 106(Pt 4):981–1000.
116. Hallett M. Neurophysiology of dystonia: the role of inhibition. Neurobiol Dis 2011;42(2):177–84.
117. Tamura Y, Ueki Y, Lin P, et al. Disordered plasticity in the primary somatosensory cortex in focal hand dystonia. Brain 2009;132(Pt 3):749–55.
118. Huang YZ, Edwards MJ, Bhatia KP, et al. One-Hz repetitive transcranial magnetic stimulation of the premotor cortex alters reciprocal inhibition in DYT1 dystonia. Mov Disord 2004;19(1):54–9.
119. Lefaucheur JP, Fenelon G, Menard-Lefaucheur I, et al. Low-frequency repetitive TMS of premotor cortex can reduce painful axial spasms in generalized secondary dystonia: a pilot study of three patients. Neurophysiol Clin 2004;34(3–4):141–5.
120. Havrankova P, Jech R, Walker ND, et al. Repetitive TMS of the somatosensory cortex improves writer's cramp and enhances cortical activity. Neuro Endocrinol Lett 2010;31(1):73–86.
121. Messina G, Cordella R, Dones I, et al. Improvement of secondary fixed dystonia of the upper limb after chronic extradural motor cortex stimulation in 10 patients: first reported series. Neurosurgery 2012; 70(5):1169–75 [discussion: 1175].
122. Diamond A, Shahed J, Azher S, et al. Globus pallidus deep brain stimulation in dystonia. Mov Disord 2006;21(5):692–5.
123. Alterman RL, Miravite J, Weisz D, et al. Sixty hertz pallidal deep brain stimulation for primary torsion dystonia. Neurology 2007;69(7):681–8.
124. Cersosimo MG, Raina GB, Piedimonte F, et al. Pallidal surgery for the treatment of primary generalized dystonia: long-term follow-up. Clin Neurol Neurosurg 2008;110(2):145–50.
125. Groen JL, Ritz K, Contarino MF, et al. DYT6 dystonia: mutation screening, phenotype, and response to deep brain stimulation. Mov Disord 2010;25(14): 2420–7.

Central Neuromodulation for Refractory Pain

Nina Z. Moore, MD, MSE[a], Scott F. Lempka, PhD[b], Andre Machado, MD, PhD[a,*]

KEYWORDS

- Deep brain stimulation (DBS) • Motor cortex stimulation (MCS) • Pain • Neuromatrix
- Neuromodulation

KEY POINTS

- Motor cortex stimulation (MCS) and deep brain stimulation (DBS) have been used for the treatment of refractory pain with good early results.
- MCS and DBS are used off label for pain applications because conclusive effectiveness studies are still needed to prove therapeutic value.
- New targets are being evaluated with new clinical trials that will explore pain with regard to the afferent component.

INTRODUCTION

Chronic neuropathic pain affects 8.2% of adults, extrapolated to roughly 18 million people every year in the United States.[1,2] Patients who have pain that cannot be controlled with pharmacologic management or less invasive techniques can be considered for deep brain stimulation (DBS) or motor cortex stimulation (MCS).[3] These techniques are not currently approved by the American Food and Drug Administration for chronic pain and are, thus, considered off-label use of medical devices for this patient population. Conclusive effectiveness studies are still needed to demonstrate the best targets as well as the reliability of the results with these approaches.

MCS

In the early 1990s, stimulation of feline and rodent cortex via epidural leads was found to modulate thalamic hyperactivity in a model of deafferentation.[4,5] This concept, when applied to patients with chronic central or peripheral deafferentation pain, demonstrated initial success.[6] However, subsequent studies have exhibited mixed clinical outcomes of MCS.[7,8] MCS has been explored as an option to treat trigeminal neuralgia, poststroke central pain, spinal cord injury pain, and other pain disorders.[7,9,10] In a review of 22 chronic pain studies, Lima and Fregni[11] found that epidural MCS showed a significant effect in chronic pain and recommended further clinical trials to elucidate the role of MCS. It is important to note that, as for all meta-analysis, the conclusions are limited by the level of evidence of the literature included. Because there is no large, randomized placebo-controlled trial to date, the meta-analysis included mostly uncontrolled case series with various technical approaches. A recent randomized, double-blind, placebo-controlled, crossover trial examined the efficacy of MCS in a small number of patients with a variety of peripheral neuropathies.[12] Although MCS efficacy was considered good or satisfactory in 60% of the patients during the open phase, no significant differences in pain ratings were detected between the ON and OFF stimulation groups when adjusting for multiple comparisons.[12] The mixed clinical outcomes of MCS indicate that the therapy would benefit from a multicenter, prospective, randomized controlled trial with systematic patient

[a] Department of Neurosurgery, Center for Neurological Restoration, Neurological Institute, Cleveland Clinic, 9500 Euclid Avenue, Desk S31, Cleveland, OH 44195, USA; [b] Center for Neurological Restoration, Neurological Institute, Cleveland Clinic, Cleveland, OH, USA
* Corresponding author.
E-mail address: machada@ccf.org

Neurosurg Clin N Am 25 (2014) 77–83
http://dx.doi.org/10.1016/j.nec.2013.08.011
1042-3680/14/$ – see front matter

selection, surgical technique, programing methodology, and follow-up. In the meantime, it is likely that MCS will continue to be used sporadically for selected patients in need of alternatives for refractory pain. MCS has risks that are typical of most craniotomies, including infection, hemorrhage, and neurologic deficits but is considered to be, overall, safe. MCS has been associated with seizures during stimulator programing and active stimulation; however, seizures and epilepsy do not seem to be a long-term complication.[13]

PAIN PATHWAYS

Pain transmission and its pathways are complex. It is thought that activity in two pathways, the lateral pain system and the medial pain system, can be modulated with DBS. The lateral pain system consists of spinothalamic tracts, which connect to the ventral posterior lateral (VPL), ventral posterior medial (VPM), and ventral posterior inferior nuclei of the thalamus, which then project to the primary and secondary somatosensory cortices. This pathway, thought to be involved in central pain, is seen in the Dejerine-Roussy syndrome (or thalamic pain syndrome) whereby damage to the thalamus or afferent and efferent fiber bundles can cause chronic pain with or without allodynia and hyperalgesia. The medial pain system consists of spinothalamic projections to the medial thalamic nuclei, limbic cortices, anterior cingulate cortex, and reticular formation and has been found to modulate emotional and affective perception with painful stimuli.[14,15] The periaqueductal gray (PAG) is part of a pain inhibitory pathway in which dopamine and serotonin signaling are linked with pain suppression and analgesia whereas norepinephrine facilitates pain transmission.[16,17]

DBS TARGETS

DBS for modulation of refractory pain goes back to studies beginning in the 1950s, with targets including the septal region, central medial, and parafascicular thalamic nuclei.[18–20] The most frequently reported targets are the sensory nucleus of the thalamus (ventral caudal or VPL/VPM) and the PAG and periventricular gray matter (PVG) (**Fig. 1**A).[17,21,22] New targets under exploration include the mesial thalamic nuclei and the area of the ventral anterior limb of the internal capsule (VC) and ventral striatum (VS) (see **Fig. 1**B).[23,24]

Sensory Nucleus of the Thalamus (VPL, VPM)

In the early 1970s, Mazars and colleagues[26] chronically implanted electrodes to stimulate the sensory thalamic relay nuclei based on prior work in

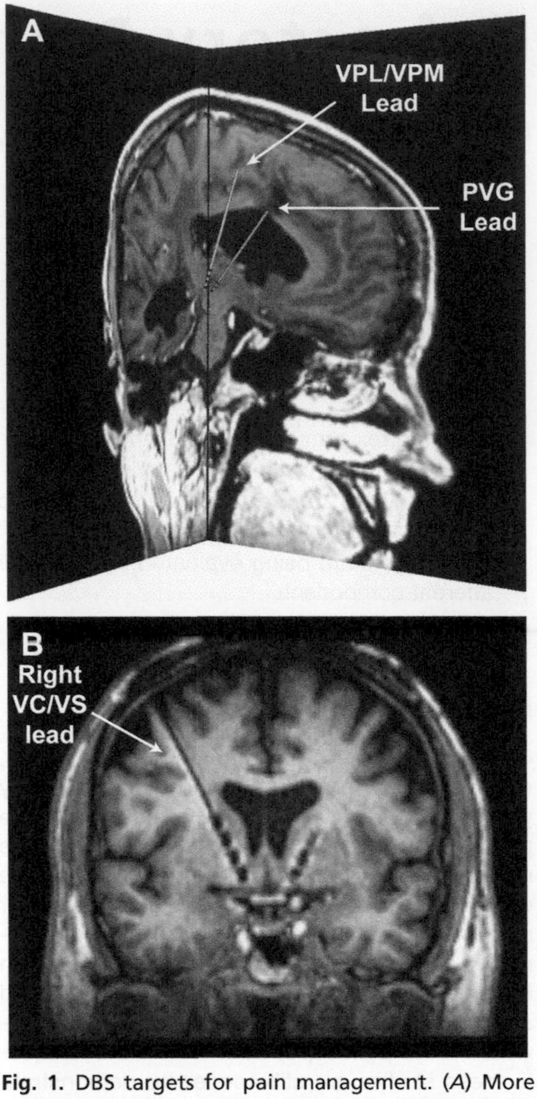

Fig. 1. DBS targets for pain management. (*A*) More traditional DBS targets aimed at treating the sensory-discriminative component of pain. The image shows the preoperative magnetic resonance imaging (MRI) and corresponding lead (model 3387, Medtronic, Minneapolis, MN) locations for a patient with one DBS lead in the VPL/VPM and a second DBS lead in the PVG. Both sagittal and coronal slices are shown near the distal ends of the leads. The patient-specific lead locations and trajectories were determined using the software Cicerone v1.3.[25] (*B*) A recently proposed DBS target aimed at treating the affective-motivational component of pain.[24] The image shows an oblique coronal view of the postoperative MRI for a patient with bilateral DBS leads (Medtronic model 3391) implanted in the ventral capsule and ventral striatal (VC/VS) area. It is possible to see the 4 electrodes in the right hemisphere as well as the distal end of the DBS lead implanted in the left hemisphere.

the 1960s in which they stimulated the ventral posterolateral thalamic relay nucleus. Hosobuchi and colleagues[21] chronically implanted electrodes in the sensory thalamus and were able to alleviate refractory facial pain in 4 of 5 patients for up to 2 years of follow-up. Turnbull and colleagues[27] studied 18 cases of sensory thalamic implantation, and they found 72% of successful pain relief over a 10-month average follow-up. In a retrospective evaluation of 76 patients implanted with chronic stimulators in the thalamic somatosensory area for deafferentation pain, 44 patients reported substantial pain relief for longer than 2 years.[28] Levy and colleagues[29] reviewed a series of 84 patients with deafferentation pain implanted in either the VPL (extremity deafferentation) or the VPM (facial deafferentation); they found that 61% had initial success (patients using stimulator regularly with pain relief), but only 30% had long-term success after at least 2 years. Patients with peripheral neuropathy had greater long-term success (50%) compared with central anesthesia dolorosa (18%) or pain associated with spinal cord injury (0%), demonstrating great variability of outcomes depending on the location of the precipitating injury. Ten years later, Kumar and colleagues[30] published a study in which they prospectively evaluated 20 patients who had a negative response to a morphine-naloxone test and were diagnosed with deafferentation pain and implanted with externalized DBS leads targeting the sensory thalamus, 3 of which had dual-implanted PVG and sensory thalamus electrodes. Twelve patients underwent chronic implantation, and 6 patients reported long-term relief at an average of 3.8 years. In a prospective, double-blind, placebo-controlled trial, Marchand and colleagues[31] evaluated the effect of sensory thalamic stimulation in 6 patients who had been implanted for at least 2 years. These patients reported a significant reduction in daily pain with DBS, but a strong placebo component was noted. Hamani and colleagues[32] demonstrated much less favorable results after implantation of 21 patients whereby only 5 patients (4 patients with DBS in the sensory thalamus and one patient with DBS in both the sensory thalamus and the PAG/PVG) experienced at least 1 year of pain relief.

PAG and PVG Matter

Reynolds described an application of focal stimulation to the PAG in rats that induced electroanesthesia via chronic monopolar stainless steel electrodes. The anesthetic effect was so profound that investigators were able to perform laparotomies under the analgesia provided by DBS.[33] This study helped serve as the groundwork to translate the concept of central gray matter stimulation to the human as seen in work by Richardson and Akil.[22] These studies initiated with a group of 5 patients who received a short period of acute stimulation before thalamic ablation. Monopolar stainless steel electrodes were stereotactically implanted into the PAG/PVG, transversing through other locations, which were tested. The 5 patients had diverse conditions, including phantom limb leg pain, abdominal cancer pain, brachial plexus pain, thalamic stroke pain, and intention tremor without pain. During stimulation, numerous side effects were seen, including nystagmus and dizziness. The best relief was seen around the nucleus parafascicularis in the medial thalamus with the least amount of side effects.[34] Based on these findings, the group then decided to test the effects of DBS at a site medial to the parafascicularis nucleus in the PVG, with externalized leads for 1 to 2 weeks. Eight patients with various pain syndromes, including cervical and lumbar back pain, brachial plexus pain, and cancer pain, were included. Six of the eight patients obtained significant pain relief with their implant.[34] The investigators then expanded their case series to include 30 patients, 27 of whom were chronically implanted. Of those implanted, 66% reported significant long-term relief with stimulation.[35] In agreement with these results, Hosobuchi[28] reported successful pain relief in 50 out of 65 patients (77%) with PAG stimulation for pain of peripheral origin. However, the investigator also noted a buildup of tolerance to DBS that was often accompanied by a tolerance to opiate analgesics. DBS analgesic efficacy was usually restored by intermittent stimulation breaks as well as concurrent use of L-tryptophan.[28] Young and colleagues[20] reported a 57% success rate in the stimulation of 26 patients over a 20-month mean follow-up period with implantation of PVG or PAG region alone with excellent pain relief.[10,29] Levy and colleagues[29] reported more modest results, with only a 32% rate of long-term relief in 57 patients at 7 years of follow-up, indicating that the long-term outcome was much less successful than initially anticipated in patients with nociceptive pain with PVG and VPL leads. Kumar and colleagues[30] implanted 49 patients with PVG electrodes who had positive responses to the morphine-naloxone test and were diagnosed with nociceptive pain. The study found that 71% of those who received a permanent implant after an externalized trial reported adequate pain relief at a mean follow-up of 7.1 years. Additional studies have suggested a benefit from targeting the PAG/PVG regions, but similar limitations of previous studies apply.[36] Recently, the group at Oxford led by Tipu Aziz[37] has reported on the combined targeting of sensory thalamic nucleus and PVG in series of patients with central or peripheral pain syndromes. Unlike prior studies, this group has tried PVG DBS in patients with pain of neuropathic characteristics, showing that the potential analgesic effects of this target are not limited to those with pain of nociceptive characteristics.[29,36]

A NEED FOR NEW TARGETS AND RIGOROUS STUDY DESIGN

Coffey[38] analyzed the results of 2 multicenter clinical trials investigating the effects of DBS for managing chronic pain of various causes. The study found that, although 46% of patients had greater than a 50% reduction of pain at 1 year, only 18% maintained pain relief at 2 years when an older lead model was used. The success rate was even lower for the second clinical trial with a newer electrode lead model. This low efficacy contributed to the manufacturer's choice to not pursue approval by the Food and Drug Administration for the use of DBS to treat chronic pain.[38] Coffey and Lozano[39] described the need for specific diagnosis and randomized, controlled, and double-blinded studies to more systematically evaluate potential stimulation targets.

NEW STIMULATION TARGETS

The Neuromatrix and the Link Between Neuropsychiatric Illness and Pain

In 1965, Melzack and Wall[40] proposed the gate-control theory of pain, which described the regulation or gating of pain signals at the level of the spinal dorsal horn. The gate-control theory led to advances in pain research and therapy and was a major driving force behind the development of spinal cord stimulation for pain management. However, in response to limitations of the gate-control theory, Melzack[41] proposed a modified theory, called the *neuromatrix theory*. Melzack described the neuromatrix as a widespread neural network that consisted of loops between the thalamus and cortex and the cortex and the limbic system.[41] The neuromatrix emphasized the multidimensional (ie, sensory-discriminative, affective-motivational, and evaluative-cognitive) nature of the pain with all components contributing equally to the overall pain experience.

The limbic circuits mentioned by Melzack were delineated by several anatomic studies, including seminal work by Nauta.[42] Initial surgeries to affect chronic pain and psychiatric illness involved radiofrequency ablation of these networks at the cingulate cortex.[43] Other targets, including the anterior limb of the internal capsule, were mainly targeted for treating obsessive-compulsive and anxiety disorders.[44,45] Broadmann areas 24/25 and the VC/VS have also been considered as possible targets for treating mood disorders.[46,47] Stimulation of these areas seems to be safe and is not associated with cognitive decline, as previously shown with ablative procedures.[47]

Ventral Striatum and Anterior Limb of the Internal Capsule

The orbitofrontal cortico-striato-pallido-thalamo-cortical system and the circuit of Papez are involved in the control of emotion and behavior. In addition to projections from frontal and prefrontal cortical areas into the dorsal striatum, there are also direct projections from the anterior frontal cortical areas and orbitofrontal cortical areas to the ventral striatum, as well as direct projections to the thalamus via the anterior limb of the internal capsule. The authors have previously shown that acute stimulation of the ventral striatum and ventral part of the anterior limb of the capsule is associated with changes in mood and anxiety and, in some patients, sensation of warmth, flushing, and, less commonly, dizziness.[46] Some patients were noted to smile and laugh. Stimulation in more dorsal areas of the internal capsule rarely produces the same effects. Chronic stimulation of these same areas is associated with improvements in patients with refractory major depressive disorder and obsessive-compulsive disorder.[47] These areas, although affecting mood, may in turn modulate the affective part of chronic pain.

A SYSTEMATIC APPROACH TO EXPLORE A NOVEL TARGET AND EVALUATE THERAPEUTIC EFFECTS

Intracranial neurostimulation for pain management has a strong history of case reports and clinical trials that were often uncontrolled, included multiple pain causes, and considered multiple brain targets. The mixed results of these studies illustrate the need for systematic evaluation of these therapies and the need for novel research and exploration of novel targets. As discussed earlier, future research will be more informative if performed with a sham-controlled phase and allowed investigators to quantify the placebo effect, which has been shown to be significant in intracranial neurostimulation for pain.[31,48] In the authors' ongoing work for evaluating the effects of VC/VS stimulation, they chose a multiphase design, including a prolonged titration phase and a 6-month sham-controlled phase.

STUDY DESIGN

In a prospective, double-blind, controlled trial under Institutional Review Board approval and a physician-sponsored Food and Drug Administration Investigational Device Exemption, 10 patients with refractory intractable hemibody pain secondary to a lesion of the contralateral thalamic area (or related afferent and efferent pathways) are enrolling. The main phase of the pilot study is randomized and sham-controlled, with a 2-group crossover. The exclusion criteria include patients with severe, unmanaged psychiatric or cognitive comorbidities and usual contraindications for DBS or intracranial procedures. The details can be seen at the study's page in clinicaltrials.gov.[49] In a 6-phase study, the patients are initially enrolled (phase I) after meeting the selection criteria and then undergo baseline evaluation, which includes functional neuroimaging and neurologic, cognitive, and behavioral assessments (phase II). Phase III involves the implantation of the DBS electrodes bilaterally in the VC/VS area and implantation of the implantable pulse generator. Phase IV involves initial programing, which will occur at least one 1 month after implantation to allow for healing after surgery and to minimize the influence of the microlesional effects.[32,50] A 1-month break occurs before proceeding to the (main) phase V portion of the study to washout possible carryover effects of titration. The patients are then randomized to either the sham DBS control group or the active stimulation group and, after 3 months, will cross over to the other group. The final phase (VI) will allow all patients to receive active, unblinded stimulation and follow-up through 24 months. Functional neuroimaging is acquired during each part of the blinded phase and is then repeated at 12 and 24 months. This imaging is an explorative part of the research, aimed at identifying possible mechanisms underlying the observed effects. The primary outcome measure for the study is the pain disability index, matching the authors' primary hypothesis that stimulation of this novel target area will reduce pain-related disability via modulation of the affective sphere of neuropathic pain.

SUMMARY

DBS and MCS can alleviate chronic pain in select patients, particularly those with peripheral neuropathies. Common targets are the sensory thalamic nuclei and PVG/PAG areas. Given the vast amount of retrospective reports and uncontrolled case series, there is a paucity of reliable data in the literature, and the magnitude of the placebo effect is not well known. The future of this application depends on an organized, systematic approach with randomized studies in which the effects of stimulation can be differentiated from placebo and other confounding features. Novel approaches, including those targeting the networks related to the affective sphere of chronic pain, may show improvements in quality of life and reduce disability.

ACKNOWLEDGMENTS

Fig. 1 was generated with assistance from Angela M. Noecker, Case Western Reserve University.

REFERENCES

1. Torrance N, Smith BH, Bennett MI, et al. The epidemiology of chronic pain of predominantly neuropathic origin. Results from a general population survey. J Pain 2006;7(4):281–9.
2. United States Census Bureau. The 2012 statistical abstract. The national data book, "Table 7: resident population by sex and age: 1980 to 2010". 2013. Available at: http://www.census.gov/compendia/statab/2012/tables/12s0007.pdf. Accessed on May 16, 2013.
3. Machado A, Kopell BH, Rezai AR. Chronic electrical stimulation for refractory chronic pain. In: Star PA, Barbaro NM, Larson PS, editors. Neurosurgical operative atlas. Functional neurosurgery. 2nd edition. New York: Thieme Medical Publishers; 2009. p. 134.
4. Hirayama T, Tsubokawa T, Katayama Y, et al. Chronic changes in activity of thalamic lemniscal relay neurons following spino-thalamic tractotomy in cats: effects of motor cortex stimulation. Pain 1990;41:S273.
5. Yamasiro K, Mukawa J, Terada Y, et al. Neurons with high-frequency discharge in the central nervous system in chronic pain. Stereotact Funct Neurosurg 1994;62:290–4.
6. Tsubokawa T, Katayama Y, Yamamoto T, et al. Chronic motor cortex stimulation in patients with thalamic pain. J Neurosurg 1993;78(3):393–401.
7. Nguyen JP, Nizard J, Keravel Y, et al. Invasive brain stimulation for the treatment of neuropathic pain. Nat Rev Neurol 2011;7(12):699–709.
8. Meyerson BA, Lindblom U, Linderoth B, et al. Motor cortex stimulation as treatment of trigeminal neuropathic pain. Acta Neurochir Suppl (Wien) 1993;58:150–3.
9. Fontaine D, Hamani C, Lozano A. Efficacy and safety of motor cortex stimulation for chronic neuropathic pain: critical review of the literature. J Neurosurg 2009;110(2):251–6.

10. Levy R, Deer TR, Henderson J. Intracranial neurostimulation for pain control: a review Pain Physician 2010;13(2):157–65.
11. Lima MC, Fregni F. Motor cortex stimulation for chronic pain: systematic review and meta-analysis of the literature. Neurology 2008;70(24): 2329–37.
12. Lefaucheur JP, Drouot X, Cunin P, et al. Motor cortex stimulation for the treatment of refractory peripheral neuropathic pain. Brain 2009;132(Pt 6): 1463–71.
13. Henderson JM, Heit G, Fisher RS. Recurrent seizures related to motor cortex stimulator programming. Neuromodulation 2010;13(1):37–43.
14. Kandell ER, Schwartz JH, Jessell TM, editors. Principles of neural science. 4th edition. New York: McGraw-Hill; 2000. p. 472–91.
15. Ossipov MH, Dussor GO, Porreca F. Central modulation of pain. J Clin Invest 2010;120(11):3779–87.
16. Akil H, Mayer DJ. Antagonism of stimulation-produced analgesia by p-CPA, a serotonin synthesis inhibitor. Brain Res 1972;44(2):692–7.
17. Akil H, Liebeskind JC. Monoaminergic mechanisms of stimulation-produced analgesia. Brain Res 1975;94(2):279–96.
18. Heath RG. Electrical self-stimulation of the brain in man. Am J Psychiatry 1963;120:571–7.
19. Ervin FR, Brown CE, Mark VH. Striatal influence on facial pain. Confin Neurol 1966;27(1):75–90.
20. Young RF, Kroening R, Fulton W, et al. Electrical stimulation of the brain in treatment of chronic pain. Experience over 5 years. J Neurosurg 1985; 62(3):389–96.
21. Hosobuchi Y, Adams JE, Rutkin B. Chronic thalamic stimulation for the control of facial anesthesia dolorosa. Arch Neurol 1973;29(3):158–61.
22. Richardson DE, Akil H. Pain reduction by electrical brain stimulation in man. Part 1: acute administration in periaqueductal and periventricular sites. J Neurosurg 1977;47(2):178–83.
23. Kraus T, Hosl K, Kiess O, et al. BOLD fMRI deactivation of limbic and temporal brain structures and mood enhancing effect by transcutaneous vagus nerve stimulation. J Neural Transm 2007;114(11): 1485–93.
24. Machado AG, Baker KB, Plow E, et al. Cerebral stimulation for the affective component of neuropathic pain. Neuromodulation 2012. [Epub ahead of print].
25. Miocinovic S, Noecker AM, Maks CB, et al. Cicerone: stereotactic neurophysiological recording and deep brain stimulation electrode placement software system. Acta Neurochir Suppl 2007; 97(Pt 2):561–7.
26. Mazars G, Merienne L, Ciolocca C. Intermittent analgesic thalamic stimulation. Preliminary note. Rev Neurol (Paris) 1973;128(4):273–9.
27. Turnbull IM, Shulman R, Woodhurst WB. Thalamic stimulation for neuropathic pain. J Neurosurg 1980;52(4):486–93.
28. Hosobuchi Y. Subcortical electrical stimulation for control of intractable pain in humans. Report of 122 cases (1970-1984). J Neurosurg 1986;64(4): 543–53.
29. Levy RM, Lamb S, Adams JE. Treatment of chronic pain by deep brain stimulation: long term follow-up and review of the literature. Neurosurgery 1987; 21(6):885–93.
30. Kumar K, Toth C, Nath RK. Deep brain stimulation for intractable pain: a 15-year experience. Neurosurgery 1997;40(4):736–46 [discussion: 746–7].
31. Marchand S, Kupers RC, Bushnell MC, et al. Analgesic and placebo effects of thalamic stimulation. Pain 2003;105:481–8.
32. Hamani C, Schwalb JM, Rezai AR, et al. Deep brain stimulation for chronic neuropathic pain: long-term outcome and the incidence of insertional effect. Pain 2006;125(1–2):188–96.
33. Reynolds DV. Surgery in the rat during electrical analgesia induced by focal brain stimulation. Science 1969;164(3878):444–5.
34. Richardson DE, Akil H. Pain reduction by electrical brain stimulation in man. Part 2: Chronic self-administration in the periventricular gray matter. J Neurosurg 1977;47:184–94.
35. Richardson DE, Akil H. Long term results of periventricular gray self-stimulation. Neurosurgery 1977;1(2):199–202.
36. Boccard SG, Pereira EA, Moir L, et al. Long-term outcomes of deep brain stimulation for neuropathic pain. Neurosurgery 2013;72(2):221–30 [discussion: 231].
37. Owen SLF, Green AL, Stein JF, et al. Deep brain stimulation for the alleviation of post-stroke neuropathic pain. Pain 2006;120(1–2):202–6.
38. Coffey RJ. Deep brain stimulation for chronic pain: results of two multicenter trials and a structured review. Pain Med 2001;2(3):183–92.
39. Coffey RJ, Lozano AM. Neurostimulation for chronic noncancer pain: an evaluation of the clinical evidence and recommendations for future trial designs. J Neurosurg 2006;105(2):175–89.
40. Melzack R, Wall PD. Pain mechanisms: a new theory. Science 1965;150(3699):971–9.
41. Melzack R. From the gate to the neuromatrix. Pain 1999;(Suppl 6):S121–6.
42. Nauta WJ. Hippocampal projections and related neural pathways to the midbrain in the cat. Brain 1958;81(3):319–40.
43. Ballantine HT Jr, Cassidy WL, Flanagan NB, et al. Stereotaxic anterior cingulotomy for neuropsychiatric illness and intractable pain. J Neurosurg 1967;26(5):488–95.

44. Nyman H, Andreewitch S, Lundback E, et al. Executive and cognitive functions in patients with extreme obsessive-compulsive disorder treated by capsulotomy. Appl Neuropsychol 2001;8(2):91–8.
45. Lippitz B, Mindus P, Meyerson BA, et al. Obsessive compulsive disorder and the right hemisphere: topographic analysis of lesions after anterior capsulotomy performed with thermocoagulation. Acta Neurochir Suppl 1997;68:61–3.
46. Machado A, Haber S, Sears N, et al. Functional topography of the ventral striatum and anterior limb of the internal capsule determined by electrical stimulation of awake patients. Clin Neurophysiol 2009;120(11):1941–8.
47. Malone DA Jr, Dougherty DD, Rezai AR, et al. Deep brain stimulation of the ventral capsule/ventral striatum for treatment-resistant depression. Biol Psychiatry 2009;65(4):267–75.
48. Rasche D, Ruppolt M, Stippich C, et al. Motor cortex stimulation for long-term relief of chronic neuropathic pain: a 10 year experience. Pain 2006; 121(1–2):43–52.
49. Machado A. 2013. Available at: http://clinicaltrials.gov/ct2/show/NCT01072656?term=machado&rank=10. Accessed June 13, 2013.
50. Deuschl G, Herzog J, Kleiner-Fisman G, et al. Deep brain stimulation: postoperative issues. Mov Disord 2006;21(Suppl 14):S219–37.

Neuromodulation for Obsessive-Compulsive Disorder

Joshua P. Aronson, MD[1], Husam A. Katnani, PhD[1],
Emad N. Eskandar, MD*

KEYWORDS

- Obsessive-compulsive disorder • Deep brain stimulation • Neuromodulation
- Vagus nerve stimulation • Transcranial magnetic stimulation

KEY POINTS

- Obsessive-compulsive disorder (OCD) is refractory to standard psychotherapy and pharmacology in 40% to 60% of patients.
- In patients with OCD, corticostriatothalamocortical circuits show hyperactivity during resting states, which becomes further accentuated during symptom provocation, but can diminish after successful treatment.
- Neuromodulation targets have included the ventral capsule/ventral striatum (nucleus accumbens), subthalamic nucleus, and inferior thalamic peduncle.
- Studies examining the efficacy of deep brain stimulation for OCD report responder rates of 40% to 75%; however, these are mainly case series of fewer than 30 patients.
- There is a paucity of randomized, placebo-controlled, prospective trials of neuromodulation in the population with OCD.

INTRODUCTION

Obsessive-compulsive disorder (OCD) is a chronic psychiatric disorder defined by recurrent obsessions or compulsions that cause significant impairments in daily functioning. Global prevalence of OCD is 1% to 2%,[1,2] with slight female gender predominance among adults, but a 2:1 male/female ratio among pediatric patients.[2] The *Diagnostic and Statistical Manual of Mental Disorders, Fourth Edition, Text Revision* defines obsessions as recurrent and persistent thoughts or impulses that cause marked distress, with the person driven to perform repetitive, excessive compulsions to reduce or neutralize the distress or dreaded consequence. These obsessions and compulsions interfere with the person's normal functioning and social relationships.

OCD has a profound impact on the lives of patients. The severity of symptoms varies considerably between patients and during the course of the disease. Although most patients experience continuous symptoms, many suffer a relapsing/remitting course, with periods of only subclinical symptoms. In a prospective study of 293 patients with a diagnosis of OCD seeking treatment,[3] enrollment interviews revealed that 27% of patients were unable to work because of psychopathology and more than 70% were categorized as moderate to severe severity using the well-described Yale-Brown Obsessive Compulsive Scale (Y-BOCS). Quality-of-life research in patients with OCD shows lower marriage rates and significant interference with ability to study and work. Patients with OCD lose on average 3 full years of wages. Thirteen percent of patients

[1] Aronson and Katnani contributed equally to the preparation of this manuscript.
Disclosures: None.
Conflicts of Interest: None.
Department of Neurosurgery, Massachusetts General Hospital, 55 Fruit Street, Boston, MA 02114, USA
* Corresponding author.
E-mail address: eeskandar@partners.org

Neurosurg Clin N Am 25 (2014) 85–101
http://dx.doi.org/10.1016/j.nec.2013.08.003

carried out a suicide attempt. The direct and indirect costs attributable to OCD are significant; however, despite increased awareness of the disorder and its treatments, on average, 17 years pass from onset of symptoms and the start of appropriate treatment.[4]

COGNITIVE MODELS

Cognitive theories of OCD informed early pharmacologic and surgical interventions. Hobart Mowrer proposed a 2-factor avoidance learning theory in 1939.[2] In the first stage, a neutral cue becomes associated with a negative event, which is recalled on reexposure to the neutral cue. In the second stage, the anxiety aroused by the neutral cue is reduced by engaging in stereotyped behaviors. Thus, these behaviors are rewarding in the perceived avoidance of the anxiety-provoking event. In OCD, the behaviors reduce distress, and thus lead to maintenance of avoidance rituals.[2] This relationship between obsessions and compulsions became the definition of OCD.

In 1986, Foa and Kozak extended this cognitive model with their emotional processing theory.[2] Patients with OCD assign an erroneously high danger level to safe situations (eg, failing to scrub hands repeatedly and extensively after touching a door handle leads to serious disease). In addition, an exaggerated and often illogical negative repercussion is assigned to failing to assuage the obsession (eg, failing to turn a light switch on and off 4 times leads to a spouse's death). OCD sufferers presume that a situation is dangerous in the absence of evidence of safety. For example, this assumption may manifest in everyday life as refusal to eat at a restaurant without evidence of meticulous cleanliness, rather than a more typical assumption of cleanliness unless presented with evidence of unsanitary and dirty conditions.[2,5] These cognitive models support focusing treatment interventions on modifying the erroneous assumptions, leading to intense fear and altering the reward pathway that maintains compulsive behaviors.

CIRCUITS AND MECHANISMS OF OCD

Noninvasive techniques (eg, neuroimaging) used in modern neuroscience provided the capability of an in-depth examination of the brain basis of self-regulation and behavioral control. Converging evidence points to the involvement of corticostriatothalamocortical (CSTC) circuits as being fundamental to cognitive and motor functions.[6] CSTC circuits are organized in a common looplike fashion, in which circuits project from specific territories in frontal cortex, to targets within the striatum, and then via direct and indirect pathways project through specific areas in the basal ganglia to the thalamus, and back to the original frontal territory (**Fig. 1**).[7] Functional neuroimaging has been used to elucidate the pathophysiology of OCD by comparing the function and dysfunction of CSTC circuits at the level of the individual fiber tract, nucleus, or cortical region. The delineation of these brain circuits at different levels is necessary, because disorders resulting from the dysfunction of these circuits are unlikely to be explained solely by neurotransmitters, genetics, or brain region abnormalities.[8,9]

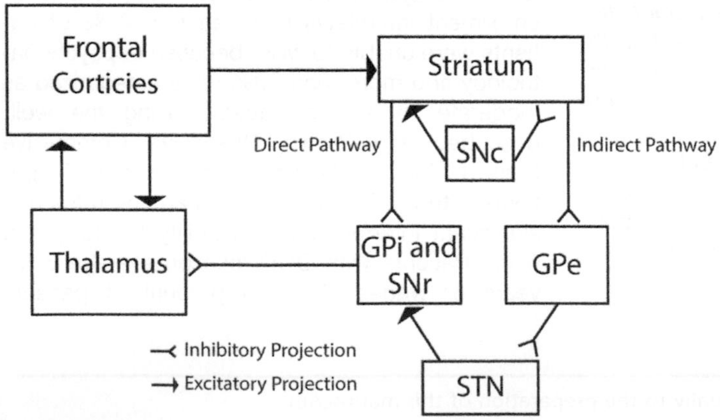

Fig. 1. Conceptual cortical-subcortical circuit. The block diagram shows direct and indirect loop pathways between cortical and subcortical structures. The direct pathway has projections from frontal cortex to the striatum, which then project to the internal segment of the globus pallidus and substantia nigra pars reticulata, which in turn projects back to the cortex via the thalamus. The indirect pathway differs by having projections from the striatum to the external segment of the globus pallidus, which then projects to the subthalamic nucleus before connecting with the globus pallidus and substantia nigra pars reticulate. Prefrontal cortex and thalamus have mutual excitatory projections. Under this framework, the direct pathway disinhibits the thalamus to generate a positive feedback loop, whereas the indirect pathway inhibits the thalamus to generate a negative feedback. Arrows indicate excitatory projections; inverse arrows indicate inhibitory projections. GPe, Globus Pallidus externa; GPi, Globus Pallidus interna; SNc, Substantia Nigra Pars Compacta; SNr, Substantia Nigra Pars reticulata; STN, subthalamic nucleus.

Within a broad framework, CSTC circuits convey information flow from cortical and limbic regions to modulate several processes, which include motivation, attention, and motor function.[10–12] Corrupting this information flow can result in disordered behavioral and emotional processing, which are core pathophysiologic features of OCD.[13] The key nodes within these circuits include: dorsal lateral prefrontal cortex (DLPFC), orbitofrontal cortex (OFC), anterior cingulate cortex (ACC), and striatum (specifically the caudate). Various imaging techniques have been used in mainly 4 different paradigm states in an attempt to focus on these key areas in order to understand the potential mechanisms that underlie OCD.

Comparing Patients with OCD with Healthy Controls in Neutral or Baseline States

Baxter and colleagues[14] conducted one of the first studies to quantify the different neural signatures of OCD by using positron emission tomography (PET) to compare a group of patients suffering from the disease with a sample of healthy participants. These investigators reported compelling results, which showed drastic differences in the neural profiles of each group when at a resting state. Patients with OCD showed bilateral hyperactivity in the OFC, in addition to predominantly right-sided hyperactivity in the caudate nucleus. Outside these key areas, the investigators also found that the glucose-metabolic rates in parietal and occipitoparietal regions were lower in patients with OCD. Similar studies have replicated these findings, in addition to showing that patients with OCD also have increased metabolic rates in the DLPFC, ACC, and thalamus.[14–18]

It has been discovered that along with showing different neural baseline states, patients with OCD also show differences in the neuroanatomic structures. For example, morphometric magnetic resonance imaging (MRI) and spectroscopy imaging, used to compare patients with OCD with healthy controls, have shown subtle differences in the caudate nucleus characterized by decreased tissue volume as well as decreased levels of *N*-acetyl aspartate, a marker of neuronal density.

Measuring Cerebral Activity Changes that Correspond to Treatment Response

Many studies have examined the changes in overall brain activity before and after patients with OCD have received a variety of different treatments, including serotonin (5-HT) reuptake inhibitors, cognitive behavioral therapy, or neurosurgery. The consensus of such studies shows that after treatment a significant reduction of glucose metabolism or regional cerebral blood flow (rCBF) can be found across the CSTC circuits.[14,16,19–25] Specifically, PET results have revealed that responders commonly showed significant decreases in bilateral OFC, bilateral caudate, and cingulate gyri metabolism.[18,19,21,23,26] Furthermore, the observed regional activity levels in patients with OCD has been shown to shift closer to healthy controls.[26]

The Differences Between OCD Symptoms During Provocation Versus a Neutral State

Hyperactivity in CSTC circuits is observed in patients with OCD during a neutral state, but there remains a question of how that baseline activity changes during symptom provocation. Breiter and colleagues[27] scanned patients with OCD with PET during both a resting state, in which patients were presented with a nonprovoking stimulus, and during a symptomatic state, in which patients were provoked by a specific stimulus that induced OCD symptoms. During the symptomatic state, PET scans showed a significant increase in rCBF in the OFC, ACC, and caudate nucleus. The same study repeated with functional MRI (fMRI) confirmed the finding in addition to revealing activation in lateral frontal, anterior temporal, insular cortex, amygdala, and lenticular nucleus. Another study[28] also showed that the striatum, globus pallidus, thalamus, and left hippocampus have higher rCBF in a symptomatic state.

Patients with OCD During Performance of a Cognitive Task and Comparison Conditions

Experimental studies that have used neuroimaging in combination with specific cognitive tasks have shed a great deal of light on the pathophysiology of OCD by showing abnormalities in neural profiles associated with the performance of cognitive tasks. Brain activation patterns studied with both PET and fMRI have shown that patients with OCD, compared with healthy controls, activate different brain structures during the performance of an implicit procedural learning task. Rauch and colleagues[29,30] reported that both patients and controls show learning of the task; however, patients with OCD showed bilateral mesial temporal activation, indicating that learning was occurring as a result of using brain systems implicated in explicit memory. In contrast, controls activated the bilateral inferior striatum, a brain region typically associated with implicit learning. These results suggest that patients with OCD have CSTC dysfunction that does not allow them to access brain systems that would process the task implicitly, as controls do without awareness. The brain activation of patients with OCD during a phonologically guided word-generation task has also been quantified with fMRI.[31] The study found that patients with OCD showed significantly greater frontal cortical activation during word generation and a defective suppression of this activation during the following rest period. The abnormal activation patterns provide further evidence of latent brain dysfunction associated with OCD during the performance of cognitive tasks. Continuing with this premise, Lucey and colleagues[32] used single-photon emission computed tomography (SPECT) during performance of the Wisconsin Card Sort Task to test the ability of patients with OCD to shift their cognitive set, compared with controls. The study found that patients with OCD not only made more errors but also had a high yield of null-sorts or responses that fail to match any of the possible cards. Furthermore, rCBF in left inferior frontal cortex and left caudate of patients with OCD was significantly correlated with the occurrence of null-sorts. No such activation patterns were observed in controls.

A plethora of imaging studies have focused on evaluating OCD to provide converging evidence that CSTC circuits show hyperactivity during resting or baseline states,[15,16] which becomes further accentuated during symptom provocation,[27,33,34] but can diminish after successful treatment.[19,26] These crucial findings can now be interpreted to speculate on mechanisms that underlie abnormal cognitive and motor behavior seen in patients with OCD.

Striatum

At the cellular level, the striatum is composed of 2 main neural components: smaller patchy compartments called striosomes, which are surrounded by a larger compartment called the matrix.[35] Ventral and anterior regions of the striatum are highly concentrated with striosomes[36] and receive cortical afferents from the OFC and ACC.[37] Studies that have evaluated the neuroanatomy of this frontal-subcortical circuit suggest that the striosomes are neurochemically specialized to exert a strong inhibitory influence on dopaminergic input,[38] thus influencing negative-feedback inhibition on the main frontal-subcortical circuits. A supposed function of the frontal projections that pass through the striatum is the execution of complex and emotional response behaviors that typically are executed quickly in response to stimuli.[19,39] Therefore, dysfunction involving striosomes, commonly quantified as hyperactivity in the caudate nucleus, might result in overactive inhibition of the negative-feedback processes that affect frontal cortices. Feedback of this nature allows for levels of cortical excitability that are higher than normal, leading to brain activation patterns in frontal-subcortical circuits that may underlie mechanisms for cognitive (eg, learning) and emotional deficits observed in patients with OCD.[40]

Prefrontal Cortices

The OFC plays an important role in emotion and social behavior. This brain region is involved in the mediation of emotional responses[41] as well as allowing for integration of emotional information.[42,43] Hyperactivity in the OFC can corrupt the weighing of emotional information, thereby skewing the consequences of immediate action to generate uncontrolled thoughts and behavior.[44] Different subregions of the OFC have also been evaluated in respect to OCD. Imaging studies have discovered that lateral orbital frontal cortex (LOFC) and medial orbital frontal cortex (MOFC) play distinct roles in processing behavioral control.[45] Specifically, activation in the LOFC seems to correlate with ritualized behavioral responses,[46–48] whereas the MOFC seems more involved in emotion regulation and reward processing.[49] Discovery of such regional distinction in the OFC provides a new level of detail, which can help elucidate the complexities of the disorder.

The DLPFC is a higher-order brain region that is implicated in executive processes needed for voluntary, goal-directed behavior. The region is also associated with different aspects of cognitive control, including the ability to focus thoughts or actions and the ability to flexibly shift that focus according to the environment.[50] Hyperactive brain patterns observed in the DLPFC of patients with OCD may corrupt these cognitive resources and impair executive function to cause compulsive behavior and obsessive thoughts.

The ACC is associated with cognitive processes such as attention, motivation, problem solving, detecting the presence of cognitive conflict, and error monitoring and detection.[44,51–53] Behavioral paradigms that use conflicting conditions, congruent or reflexive responses versus incongruent or responses that require the inhibition of reflexive behavior cause a large degree of activation in the ACC. Patients with OCD who are tested on such tasks show hyperactivation of the ACC in response to the incongruent relative to the congruent conditions.[54–57] A specific study[57] that used fMRI to examine the effective connectivity of frontal cortices while patients with OCD performed an error control task found significantly enhanced connectivity between ACC and the DLPFC. The study concluded that such connectivity supports the idea of abnormal corticocortical interactions affecting error processing in patients with OCD, and adversely affecting decision making. Hyperactivation of the ACC may facilitate faulty error detection, which contributes to cognitive difficulties and obsessions.

Other Brain Regions

Although many studies are dedicated to examining frontal cortex activation patterns associated with OCD, the disease is not an entirely prefrontal condition. Other regions have been found to be involved and may help to elucidate the complexity of the syndrome. Functional neuroimaging has revealed hypometabolism in the insula and the dorsoparietal cortex. The insular cortex is believed to be involved in processing emotional aspects such as empathy and compassion as well as characteristics such as fairness and cooperation. Areas of parietal cortex have been implicated in aspects such as attention, spatial perception, and response inhibition.[58] Accordingly, dysfunction in areas that process such information contributes to the OCD syndrome.

The cerebellum has also been implicated in OCD. The brain region is involved in a variety of cognitive functions, such as attention,[59,60] verbal learning and memory,[61] and cognitive planning.[62] Scans of patients with OCD using SPECT have revealed higher rCBF in the cerebellum than in controls.[63] Hyperactivity in such a critical cognitive processing center may underlie complex cognitive deficits observed in patients with OCD.

CURRENT TREATMENTS FOR OCD

Psychotherapy

Psychotherapy via exposure and response cognitive behavioral therapy (CBT) is considered first-line treatment. In a randomized control study,[64] 21 patients with OCD randomly assigned to the therapy arm completed 12 weeks of intensive CBT (daily visits for 4 weeks, followed by 8 weeks of weekly visits), resulting in a 55% decrease in Y-BOCS score. Response rates were 86% for the therapy arm. The intensive therapy regime in this study is atypical, with a usual outpatient treatment regime consisting of weekly therapy sessions. Outcomes after typical weekly sessions outside clinical trials show less effectiveness, with Y-BOCS reductions of 24% to 44% reported.[65,66]

Pharmacology

Several trials have examined effects of serotonergic medications, primarily the tricyclic antidepressant clomipramine and selective serotonin reuptake inhibitors. Multiple placebo-controlled randomized trials confirm the efficacy of serotonergic medications, with mean Y-BOCS reductions of 31% to 40%.[67–71] Most studies define partial responders as experiencing a decrease in Y-BOCS score greater than 25% and full responders at experiencing a decrease in Y-BOCS score greater than 35%; however, nonresponse to OCD treatment is common. The rate of nonresponders is 40% to 60%, with an additional fraction experiencing only partial response (Y-BOCS reduction of 25%–35%).[67,72] Although there is debate about how to define nonresponders, there is a definitive, substantial population of patients for whom therapy and pharmacologic treatments are inadequate.

Targeted Therapy

Guided by neuroanatomic and neuroimaging studies, new treatments target distinct brain circuits associated with OCD in an attempt to modulate disease state activation patterns and improve symptoms in resistant patients. There are many neuromodulatory techniques, which range in their degree of invasiveness. Some of these neurosurgical approaches include stereotactic lesioning, deep brain stimulation (DBS), vagus nerve stimulation (VNS), and transcranial magnetic stimulation (TMS). In the following section, the current state of each therapeutic intervention, in association with treating OCD, is discussed.

Stereotactic Lesioning

Stereotactic lesions or localized ablation of the human brain is the oldest method for treating psychiatric illness. In 1888, the Swiss psychiatrist Gottlieb Burkhardt carried out what is likely the first series of psychiatric neurosurgical procedures in the modern era. He removed focal regions of cortex to alter behavior in 6 patients: 1 with mania, 1 with dementia, and 4 described as suffering from paranoia. His surgical results were modest, with 1 patient dying postoperatively after developing status epilepticus, 1 improved (although later committed suicide), 2 stable, and 2 subdued.[73] The first broad use of neurosurgery for psychiatric conditions may be attributed to the Portuguese neurologist Egas Moniz. Inspired by the American neuroscientists Carlyle Jacobsen and John Fulton, who performed frontal lobectomies in primates, Moniz proposed frontal cortex ablation for psychiatric patients. With the assistance of the Portuguese neurosurgeon Pedro Almeida Lima, he popularized the frontal leukotomy, aiming to sever white matter connections within the frontal lobes. He introduced the leukotome, a rod with a retractable wire loop that could be inserted via a burr hole and rotated to carry out the procedure quickly and reproducibly. For his efforts, he was awarding the Nobel Prize in Medicine or Physiology in 1949.[74–76] Walter Freeman and James Watts introduced the transorbital leukotomy in 1946, enabling the procedure to be performed in an office setting rather than an operating room. They devised the orbitoclast, an ice pick–like tool that was driven through the orbital roof bilaterally into the brain and swept across white matter tracts. Frontal leukotomy expanded as a treatment of various psychiatric illnesses, with an estimated 60,000 procedures performed between 1936 and 1956.[77] However, with relative indiscriminate application of frontal leukotomy came increasing complications and public outcry around the world.[78] The advent of effective neuroleptic medications and increasing popularity of psychoanalysis cemented the decline of the frontal leukotomy era.[75,77]

In the late 1940s, a coordinate system devised by Jean Talairach combined with the development of stereotactic targeting systems by Ernest Spiegel and Henry Wycis in America and Lars Leksell in Sweden allowed for precise targeting of intracranial structures.[75,76] This system allowed surgeons to create small, focal lesions and thereby reduce complications. Stereotactic ablation procedures, including anterior cingulotomy, capsulotomy, subcaudate tractotomy, and limbic leukotomy, were developed in the decades after the prefrontal leukotomy era.

Modern ablative psychiatric neurosurgical procedures are performed using stereotactic open surgical approaches or often by using radiofrequency or Gamma Knife methodologies.[79] With converging evidence pointing to hyperactivity in CSTC as the cause of OCD, the logic of stereotactic intervention, pertaining to OCD, stems from reducing hyperactivity through targeted ablation.

Cingulotomies and capsulotomies are common neurosurgical lesioning procedures used to treat OCD (**Fig. 2**).[80,81] Small bilateral lesions in the cingulum bundle (**Fig. 3**A) or anterior limb of the internal capsule (ALIC) sever fibers from the white matter of the cingulate gyrus or internal capsule, respectively, in an attempt to disrupt hyperactive CSTC circuits. These interventions have shown moderate efficacy in severe, treatment-refractory OCD and have been reported to decrease the state of anxiety in patients.[82–87] Other stereotactic procedures include subcaudate tractotomies and limbic leukotomies (see **Fig. 3**B), which are also geared toward disrupting white matter fibers in CSTC circuits. A lesion is made in the substantia innominate, a small region located beneath the head of the caudate, during a subcaudate tractotomy,[88] whereas a lesion in both the frontal lobe and cingulum is made during a leukotomy.[89] Both procedures have been shown to relieve symptoms of anxiety and obsession in OCD, presumably through the interruption of frontothalamic circuits.[90,91] Multiple studies have examined the efficacy of these various procedures, with reported responder rates of 27% to 86% (**Table 1**).[84,85,87,89,91–95]

DBS

Because of the resulting success of DBS in movement disorders (eg, Parkinson disease [PD]) as well as the low-risk reversible nature of the intervention, DBS has become an attractive and prominent therapeutic intervention for therapy-refractory psychiatric disorders. The underlying mechanism of DBS was first believed to be similar to stereotactic lesioning, by which inhibitory DBS created a functional lesion through a depolarization blockage of neural circuits close to the electrodes.[96] Nevertheless, through modeling and imaging studies, stimulation has been discovered to work in a more complicated fashion, which activates neural circuitry in the brain to modulate activation patterns.[97–99] How this modulation works to alleviate motor and cognitive deficits it difficult to interpret, because several variables (eg, proximal cytoarchitecture and neuropil, stimulation parameters, electrode impedance) have been shown to affect the efficacy of DBS. However, in general, there exists an overarching interpretation that DBS alleviates deficits by increasing the fidelity of neural signaling to modulate disease state activation patterns and allow for better functionality.[100,101]

From successful ablative procedures for treating OCD, early DBS cases focused on exploring similar brain regions in the hope of replicating the success without the severity. The first studies chose DBS implantation sites within the ALIC, based on the success of the capsulotomy (see **Fig. 2**). Nuttin and colleagues[102,103] first published findings from patients with bilateral ALIC DBS. The initial study used only clinical observations, reporting a decrease of complaints and a progression away from being seriously disabled. Further studies from the group used the Y-BOCS questionnaire, to find an average 40% symptom decrease, and PET scans, to find a decrease in

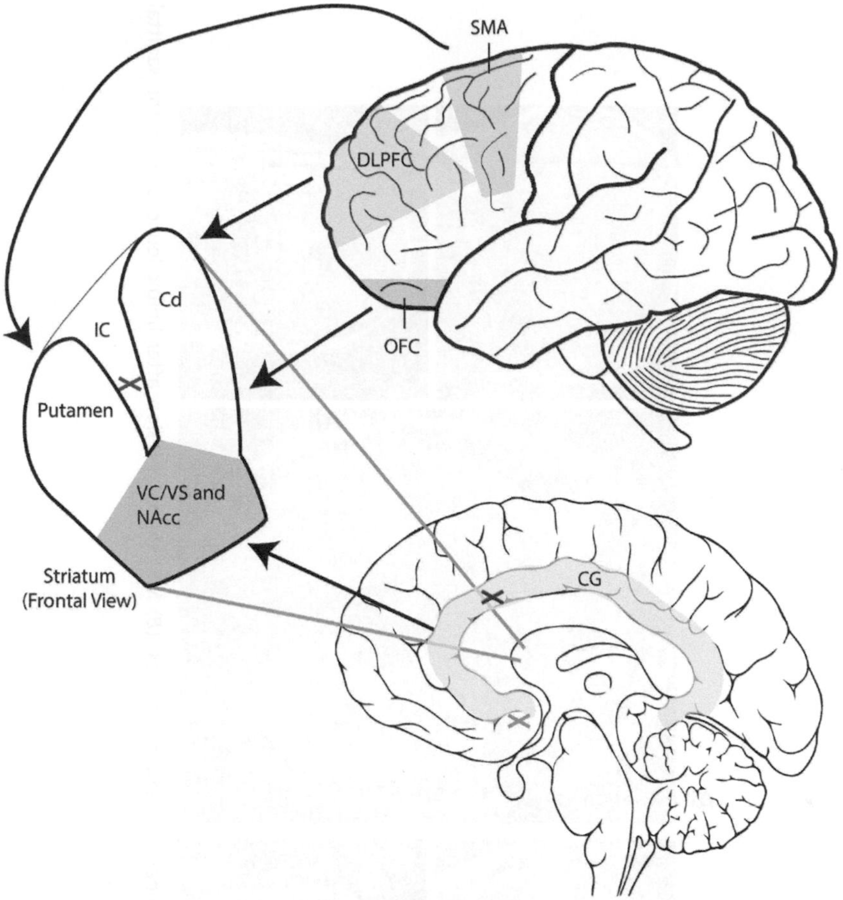

Fig. 2. Cortical-striatal regions and projections targeted for treatment of OCD. Sagittal views (*top and bottom, right*) show key cortical structures and their projections to specific striatal regions, shown in the coronal view (*middle, left*). Shaded or marked regions indicate regions targeted for the treatment of OCD. The supplementary motor areas (*green*), the dorsolateral prefrontal cortex (*light blue*), and the OFC (*light red*) project to the putamen, dorsolateral head of the caudate, and ventromedial head of the caudate, respectively, and are targets for TMS treatment. The ventral capsule/ventral striatum (VC/VS) and nucleus accumbens (NAc) (*light purple*) receive projections from the cingulate gyrus (CG) (*yellow*) and are targets for DBS treatment. The internal capsule, substantia innominate, and anterior cingulate (*blue, green, and red cross marks*, respectively) are targets for lesioning treatment. Cd, caudate; IC, internal capsule; SMA, supplementary motor area.

frontal cortex activity. Overall, the work was the first to robustly quantify the effects of ALIC DBS in patients with OCD. Subsequently, investigations using DBS expanded to explore the rostral-caudal extent of the ALIC, focusing on the ventral aspect of the anterior limb of the ventral capsule (VC) and the ventral striatum (VS).[104] In 2006, Greenberg and colleagues[105] reported a 3-year observation on 8 of 10 patients with OCD implanted with bilateral DBS systems targeting the VC/VS. The study found that, on average, complaints decreased 30% in the group and symptoms changed from severe to moderate. Furthermore, 4 patients were found to be responders and on average showed 35% reduction in symptoms. A more recent study reported by the same group[106] found that by refining the implantation site toward the VS, more patients with OCD had positive responses as well as needing lower-parameter settings (ie, pulse width, voltage). The use of PET imaging in certain patients also showed that DBS increased perfusion in areas such as the OFC, ACC, and thalamus. Several other studies have also reported benefit in targeting the VC/VS to treat OCD (**Table 2**).[107–110]

The nucleus accumbens (NAc), which lies within the VS, has becomes a major area of focus for treating OCD (see **Fig. 2**). Strum and colleagues[111] reported results from 4 patients implanted with unilateral NAc DBS for more than 2 years. Open stimulation was found to cause a near-complete recovery in 3 of the 4 patients; however, no validated questionnaire was used to quantify results.

A B

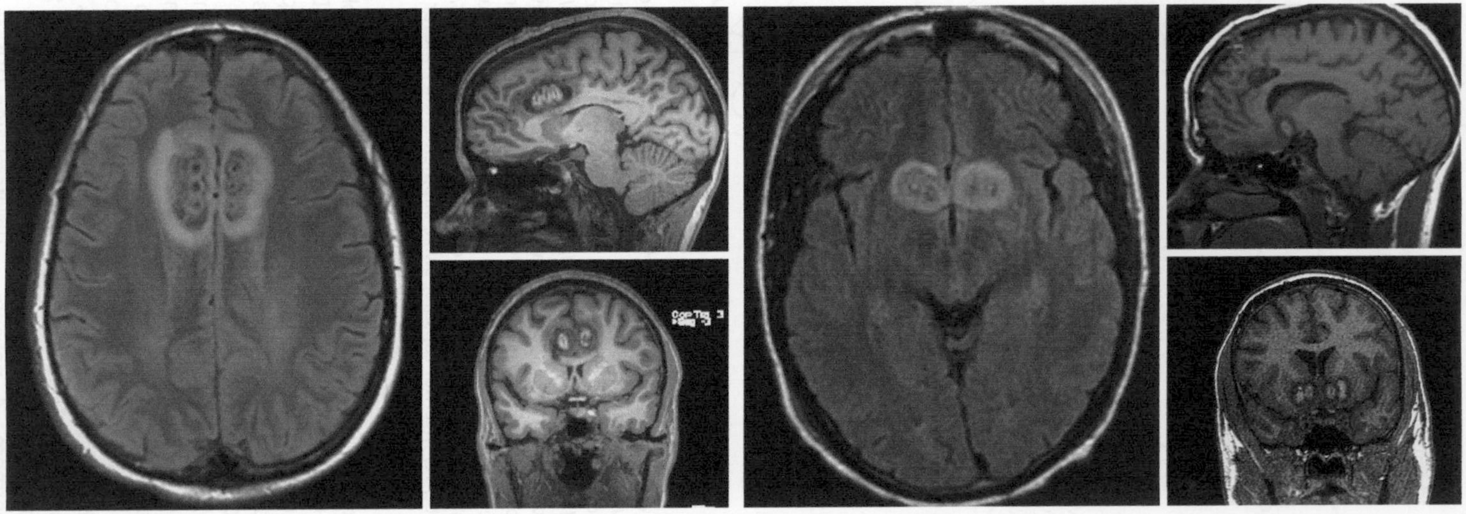

Fig. 3. (*A*) MRI showing lesion after stereotactic cingulotomy in axial, coronal, and sagittal planes. (*B*) MRI showing lesion after limbic leukotomy. In the sagittal projection, a previous cingulotomy lesion can also be seen.

Table 1
Case studies of lesioning procedures for OCD. Percentage responders is as defined in the study

Study	Procedure	n	Responders (%)
Liu et al,[87] 2008	Anterior capsulotomy	35	86[a]
Rück et al,[92] 2008	Anterior capsulotomy	25	48[b]
Ballantine et al,[85] 1987	Cingulotomy	32	25[c]
Jenike et al,[84] 1991	Cingulotomy	33	27[d]
Dougherty et al,[93] 2002	Cingulotomy	44	32[e]
Sheth et al,[94] 2013	Cingulotomy	34	38[e]
Hodgkiss et al,[95] 1995	Subcaudate tractotomy	15	33[f]
Mitchell-Heggs et al,[91] 1976	Limbic leukotomy	27	67[f]
Kelly et al,[89] 1973	Limbic leukotomy	17	41[f]

Responder defined as decrease in Y-BOCS of:
[a] ≥50%.
[b] ≥33%.
[c] Investigators' determination of normal with or without pharmacologic or behavioral treatment.
[d] Y-BOCS reduction of ≥25% or investigators' determination of at-least moderate improvement based on clinical record review.
[e] ≥35%.
[f] Investigators' determination of completely recovered or only mild residual symptoms.

Nevertheless, the same group reported quantified data from a 1-year follow-up on 10 more patients with OCD implanted with unilateral NAc DBS systems.[112] Only 1 of 10 patients manifested a Y-BOCS score reduction of 35% or more. On average, the study found Y-BOCS symptom decrease of 21%. Some of the most promising results for NAc DBS were reported by Denys and colleagues,[113] who examined 16 patients with OCD implanted with DBS targeting the NAc. The study reported an average 46% symptom decrease after 8 months of open treatment, with

Table 2
Studies of DBS procedures for OCD. Responders defined as decrease in Y-BOCS of 35% or greater

Study	Number of Patients	Target	Follow-up (mo)	Responders (%)
Nuttin et al,[102] 1999	4	ALIC	N/A	N/A
Nuttin et al,[103] 2003	6	ALIC	21	50
Goodman et al,[104] 2010	6	VC/VS	12	67
Greenberg et al,[105] 2006	10	VC/VS	36	40
Greenberg et al,[106] 2010	26	ALIC-VC/VS	3–36	62
Abelson et al,[107] 2005	4	ALIC	3–23	50
Anderson & Ahmed,[108] 2003	1	ALIC	10	100
Plewnia et al,[110] 2008	1	ALIC-NAc	24	0
Sturm et al,[111] 2003	4	NAc	24–30	75
Huff et al,[112] 2010	10	NAc	12	10
Denys et al,[113] 2010	16	NAc	21	56
Aouizerate et al,[109] 2004	1	NAc	15	100
Franzini et al,[147] 2010	2	NAc	24–27	50
Mallet et al,[114] 2002	2	STN	6	100
Fontaine et al,[115] 2004	1	STN	12	100
Mallet et al,[116] 2008	16	STN	3	75[a]
Jimenez-Ponce et al,[117] 2009	5	ITP	12	100

Abbreviations: ITP, inferior thalamic peduncle; NAc, nucleus accumbens; STN, subthalamic nucleus.
[a] Study defined responders as Y-BOCS reduction of ≥25%.

9 of the 16 patients found to be responders. Of those patients, there was an average Y-BOCS decrease of 72%. In addition, at a near 2-year follow-up, results were found to remain consistent.

Several DBS case studies have also successfully targeted other brain regions for the treatment of OCD (see **Table 2**). Electrode implantation in the subthalamic nucleus (STN), a predominant target for treating PD, has shown a great deal of promise in regards to OCD. Mallet and colleagues[114] and Fontaine and colleagues[115] found that when treating patients for PD, who also had OCD, all patients responded in regards to OCD, with an average Y-BOCS decrease of 82% after 6 months of treatment, and 97% after 12 months of treatment, respectively. Following up on this finding, Mallet and colleagues[116] reported results of a study that examined 16 patients with OCD implanted with bilateral STN DBS. Twelve of 16 patients were found to be responders; however, the criterion to be classified a responder for the study was only a 25% decrease in Y-BOCS score.

The inferior thalamic peduncle (ITP) is a white matter bundle that connects thalamic nuclei with areas of prefrontal cortex. Because of the presumed role of thalamic-prefrontal connections in the pathophysiology of OCD, 1 group[117] has tested ITP DBS to treat the psychiatric disorder. After 12 months of open-label DBS, the study reported 5 of 5 responders with an average 49% decrease in Y-BOCS score. However, the inclusion criteria of the study were not as stringent as in other studies, and only open series testing was observed. Therefore, although this study was promising, more studies are needed to determine the effective nature of ITP DBS.

VNS

Sensory afferents in the vagus nerve project and terminate in the nucleus tractus solitarius, a brain region that has direct and indirect connections throughout the limbic system.[118] As a result, VNS presents itself as a therapeutic intervention that can modulate key limbic regions associated with OCD.[119] These regions include the dorsal raphe nuclei and the locus ceruleus, regions associated with serotonin and norepinephrine production, respectively, as well as the amygdala, hypothalamus, thalamus, and OFC.[120] Accordingly, studies have found that VNS increases serotonergic transmission and decreases rCBF in the hippocampus, amygdala, and cingulate gyrus, thereby mimicking the mechanisms of antidepressant drugs (eg, serotonin reuptake inhibitors) used to treat OCD.[121,122] Furthermore, the vagus nerve plays a major role in the parasympathetic components of the autonomic nervous system. Signals for autonomic arousal, transmitted via the vagus nerve, are believed to be abnormal in patients with OCD, thus contributing to a state of high anxiety associated with the disorder. Modulation of this signal via VNS may provide another potential mechanism by which the therapeutic intervention can decrease anxiety in OCD.[123]

TMS

TMS is a noninvasive therapeutic technique, largely regarded as safe, and most recently used to treat and investigate OCD. The technique exploits the concept that when electrical current is passed through an electromagnetic coil, a depolarizing magnetic pulse is induced.[124] When this coil is placed on the scalp, these magnetic pulses have the ability to modulate superficial local neurons. Moreover, controlling the frequency of pulsed current through the coil modulates local neurons differently, in which low frequency TMS (0–5 Hz) results in decreased neural excitability and rCBF, and high-frequency TMS (5–20 Hz) results in the increase of both neural excitability and rCBF.[125] Under this framework, it has been hypothesized that the inhibitory effect of TMS may be useful in treating OCD symptoms caused by hypermetabolic orbitofrontal brain regions.

More than 100 patients with OCD have been studied and treated with TMS. Both high-frequency and low-frequency TMS has been used to explore the effects of individually modulating the OFC, DLPFC, and supplementary motor area (SMA) (see **Fig. 2**). Open-label studies using high-frequency TMS over the right or left DLPFC or low-frequency TMS over the right or left OFC have shown the greatest benefit for effectively reducing OCD symptoms.[126–128] Such effects were found to only acutely alleviate symptoms (first hours after stimulation), because patient improvement was not observed during follow-up studies. More importantly, TMS did not show any advantage in alleviating OCD symptoms in a double-blind, sham-controlled format.[127,129–131]

The use of TMS to modulate local neuronal activity in SMA has been more promising for the treatment of OCD. In regards to motor activity, studies have found that patients with OCD show decreased intracortical inhibition and lower resting and active motor thresholds.[132,133] Therefore, the inhibitory effect of low-frequency TMS has been explored as a potential means to decrease motor cortex excitability in patients with OCD. Specifically, the SMA has been targeted with TMS as a result of the role that the region plays in conveying information from limbic to cognitive and motor circuits.[134] Inhibitory stimulation in SMA was found to cause a clinically significant improvement in patients with OCD, alleviating both depression and anxiety for more than 3 months.[135] Nevertheless, the effects of TMS in SMA have not been explored in a double-blind, sham-controlled format, which is necessary to truly determine the impact of the treatment.

In severe cases of OCD, TMS has been used at extremely high frequencies in order to induce controlled seizures in targeted superficial brain structures.[136,137] This treatment is known as magnetic convulsion therapy and has been used to disrupt abnormal activity patterns in prefrontal cortex of patients with OCD without the spread of disruption into medial temporal structures. As a result, the treatment limits cognitive side effects and presents less risk for cognitive impairment, which can be seen with similar but more severe techniques such as stereotactic lesioning and electroconvulsive therapy.

Overall, TMS is still a new therapeutic tool to treat psychiatric illness. More studies are needed in order to explore and elucidate optimal brain region targets, effective parameter settings, and potential mechanisms by which the intervention works.

FUTURE DIRECTIONS

DBS and TMS rely on spatial targeting, with their effects encompassing thousands of neurons and axons, rendering them blunt tools. Optogenetics is a new methodology for driving neuronal activity not with electric current but with light. Light-sensitive microbial channels can be delivered into and expressed within an individual neuron.[138] Initially, 2 channels were developed: channelrhodopsin, a cation channel that produces a depolarizing sodium current when illuminated by blue light, and halorhodopsin, an anion channel that produces a hyperpolarizing chloride current when illuminated by yellow light.[139] Subsequent developments have led to color-shifted channels, channels with high-amplitude and low-amplitude currents, and channels that have different turnoff speeds after illumination.[140] A third class of light-activated channel has been developed, outward proton pumps, enabling hyperpolarization of cells, leading to 100% neural silencing.[140] Targeted delivery of illumination to neurons expressing these channels can function as a binary on/off switch or as a graded modulator of the activity of the cells. Light can be precisely delivered to the desired location using small stereotactically placed optical fibers attached to a light source, which could be implanted subcutaneously, similar to a DBS battery.

Optogenetics has already been used successfully to control and study dopaminergic neurons in parkinsonian mice.[141] Furthermore, recent efforts have expanded optogenetic therapy to a primate model, showing that optical stimulation of the arcuate sulcus alters behavior in a visually guided saccade task.[142] The development of optoXRs, opsin-receptor chimeras, which include intracellular loops from G protein coupled receptors, allows targetable, temporal control of light-activated control of G protein coupled signal cascades in vivo.[143] As a result of this development, optogenetics may have the potential to be a less severe alternative to ablation treatments and a more precise alternative to DBS. For example, the success of the anterior capsulotomy for treating severe OCD suggests that a reduction in firing in the ALIC may be therapeutic for the disorder. As an alternative to creating a lesion or placing a macroscopic DBS lead to achieve this goal, anion channels could be precisely delivered to cells in the ALIC. Activation of the channel would then decrease firing output of the targeted region. In a recent report, Burguière described optogenetic stimulation in a mouse model of OCD. Focused optogenetic stimulation of the lateral OFC restored response inhibition, suppressing compulsive behaviors.[144]

An optogenetic approach simultaneously reduces nonspecific stimulation to surrounding cells and allows superior spatial and temporal control over the frequency and amplitude of stimulation. Challenges remain in delivery and expression of the light-sensitive channels and in the transmission of light to the appropriate structure; however, recent successes in using optogenetics in the primate model provide a solid foundation to generate efforts toward developing a safe implantable optical stimulation device.

PATIENT CONSIDERATIONS

The early history of psychiatric neurosurgery led to ethical objections over the indiscriminate application of procedures to a vulnerable population, as well as concerns over affecting individual behavioral control. It is this legacy that led to the decline of historical procedures including frontal lobotomy and the establishment of standards for modern interventions. The attention on psychosurgery led to the passage of the National Research Act in 1974, establishing the National Commission for the Protection of Human Subjects of Biomedical and Behavioral Research. The Commission issued its Report and Recommendations on Psychosurgery in 1977, affirming that psychosurgery should be allowed to continue, but with appropriate safeguards in place. These safeguards include establishment of an institutional review board, which must approve all procedures performed based on the ability of the surgeon to carry out the procedure, the appropriateness of the patient, adequacy of preoperative and postoperative evaluations, and informed consent, which has been obtained from the patient or from the patient's guardian (if the patient does not object).[145,146] In following these principles, psychiatric neurosurgery may continue to be judiciously applied to patients who have failed medical management.

SUMMARY

Over the last few decades, neurosurgical treatment of psychiatric conditions has expanded, with advances in neuromodulation and the understanding of the circuitry involved in these disorders. New techniques in delivery of neuromodulation will likely improve the targeting and reliability of these interventions. This objective will require additional clinical trials to determine the population of patients with OCD most likely to respond to neuromodulation, ensuring that this vulnerable patient population is protected from undue risk. Given the degree of disability that patients with severe OCD suffer, expanded and perhaps novel neurosurgical interventions may provide an effective therapeutic option.

REFERENCES

1. Sasson Y, Zohar J, Chopra M, et al. Epidemiology of obsessive-compulsive disorder: a world view. J Clin Psychiatry 1997;58(Suppl 12):7–10.
2. Franklin ME, Foa EB. Treatment of obsessive compulsive disorder. Annu Rev Clin Psychol 2011;7:229–43.
3. Pinto A, Mancebo MC, Eisen JL, et al. The Brown Longitudinal Obsessive Compulsive Study: clinical features and symptoms of the sample at intake. J Clin Psychiatry 2006;67:703–11.
4. Hollander E. Obsessive-compulsive disorder: the hidden epidemic. J Clin Psychiatry 1997;58(Suppl 12):3–6.
5. Foa EB, Kozak MJ. Emotional processing of fear: exposure to corrective information. Psychol Bull 1986;99:20–35.
6. Di Filippo M, Picconi B, Tantucci M, et al. Short-term and long-term plasticity at corticostriatal synapses: implications for learning and memory. Behav Brain Res 2009;199:108–18.
7. Alexander GE, DeLong MR, Strick PL. Parallel organization of functionally segregated circuits linking basal ganglia and cortex. Annu Rev Neurosci 1986;9:357–81.
8. Nestler EJ, Barrot M, DiLeone RJ, et al. Neurobiology of depression. Neuron 2002;34:13–25.
9. Ressler KJ, Mayberg HS. Targeting abnormal neural circuits in mood and anxiety disorders: from the laboratory to the clinic. Nat Neurosci 2007;10:1116–24.
10. Llinas RR, Leznik E, Urbano FJ. Temporal binding via cortical coincidence detection of specific and nonspecific thalamocortical inputs: a voltage-dependent dye-imaging study in mouse brain slices. Proc Natl Acad Sci U S A 2002;99:449–54.
11. Goto Y, Grace AA. Limbic and cortical information processing in the nucleus accumbens. Trends Neurosci 2008;31:552–8.
12. Redgrave P, Gurney K, Reynolds J. What is reinforced by phasic dopamine signals? Brain Res Rev 2008;58:322–39.
13. Saxena S, Rauch SL. Functional neuroimaging and the neuroanatomy of obsessive-compulsive disorder. Psychiatr Clin North Am 2000;23:563–86.
14. Baxter LR, Schwartz JM, Mazziotta JC, et al. Cerebral glucose metabolic rates in nondepressed patients with obsessive-compulsive disorder. Am J Psychiatry 1988;145:1560–3.
15. Nordahl TE, Benkelfat C, Semple WE, et al. Cerebral glucose metabolic rates in obsessive compulsive disorder. Neuropsychopharmacology 1989;2:23–8.
16. Swedo SE, Schapiro MB, Grady CL, et al. Cerebral glucose metabolism in childhood-onset obsessive-compulsive disorder. Arch Gen Psychiatry 1989;46:518–23.
17. Kwon JS, Kim JJ, Lee DW, et al. Neural correlates of clinical symptoms and cognitive dysfunctions in obsessive-compulsive disorder. Psychiatry Res 2003;122:37–47.
18. Perani D, Colombo C, Bressi S, et al. [18F]FDG PET study in obsessive-compulsive disorder. A clinical/metabolic correlation study after treatment. Br J Psychiatry 1995;166:244–50.
19. Benkelfat C, Nordahl TE, Semple WE, et al. Local cerebral glucose metabolic rates in obsessive-compulsive disorder. Patients treated with clomipramine. Arch Gen Psychiatry 1990;47:840–8.
20. Rubin RT, Ananth J, Villanueva-Meyer J, et al. Regional 133xenon cerebral blood flow and cerebral 99mTc-HMPAO uptake in patients with obsessive-compulsive disorder before and during treatment. Biol Psychiatry 1995;38:429–37.
21. Schwartz JM, Stoessel PW, Baxter LR, et al. Systematic changes in cerebral glucose metabolic rate after successful behavior modification treatment of obsessive-compulsive disorder. Arch Gen Psychiatry 1996;53:109–13.
22. Brody AL, Saxena S, Schwartz JM, et al. FDG-PET predictors of response to behavioral therapy and

pharmacotherapy in obsessive compulsive disorder. Psychiatry Res 1998;84:1–6.

23. Saxena S, Brody AL, Maidment KM, et al. Localized orbitofrontal and subcortical metabolic changes and predictors of response to paroxetine treatment in obsessive-compulsive disorder. Neuropsychopharmacology 1999;21:683–93.
24. Kang DH, Kwon JS, Kim JJ, et al. Brain glucose metabolic changes associated with neuropsychological improvements after 4 months of treatment in patients with obsessive-compulsive disorder. Acta Psychiatr Scand 2003;107:291–7.
25. Nakatani E, Nakgawa A, Ohara Y, et al. Effects of behavior therapy on regional cerebral blood flow in obsessive-compulsive disorder. Psychiatry Res 2003;124:113–20.
26. Baxter LR, Schwartz JM, Bergman KS, et al. Caudate glucose metabolic rate changes with both drug and behavior therapy for obsessive-compulsive disorder. Arch Gen Psychiatry 1992; 49:681–9.
27. Breiter HC, Rauch SL, Kwong KK, et al. Functional magnetic resonance imaging of symptom provocation in obsessive-compulsive disorder. Arch Gen Psychiatry 1996;53:595–606.
28. McGuire PK, Bench CJ, Frith CD, et al. Functional anatomy of obsessive-compulsive phenomena. Br J Psychiatry 1994;164:459–68.
29. Rauch SL, Savage CR, Alpert NM, et al. Probing striatal function in obsessive-compulsive disorder: a PET study of implicit sequence learning. J Neuropsychiatry Clin Neurosci 1997;9:568–73.
30. Rauch SL, Whalen PJ, Curran T, et al. Probing striato-thalamic function in obsessive-compulsive disorder and Tourette syndrome using neuroimaging methods. Adv Neurol 2001;85:207–24.
31. Pujol J, Torres L, Deus J, et al. Functional magnetic resonance imaging study of frontal lobe activation during word generation in obsessive-compulsive disorder. Biol Psychiatry 1999;45:891–7.
32. Lucey JV, Burness CE, Costa DC, et al. Wisconsin Card Sorting Task (WCST) errors and cerebral blood flow in obsessive-compulsive disorder (OCD). Br J Med Psychol 1997;70(Pt 4):403–11.
33. Rauch SL, Jenike MA, Alpert NM, et al. Regional cerebral blood flow measured during symptom provocation in obsessive-compulsive disorder using oxygen 15-labeled carbon dioxide and positron emission tomography. Arch Gen Psychiatry 1994; 51:62–70.
34. Adler CM, McDonough-Ryan P, Sax KW, et al. fMRI of neuronal activation with symptom provocation in unmedicated patients with obsessive compulsive disorder. J Psychiatr Res 2000;34:317–24.
35. Graybiel AM. Neurotransmitters and neuromodulators in the basal ganglia. Trends Neurosci 1990;13: 244–54.
36. Desban M, Kemel ML, Glowinski J, et al. Spatial organization of patch and matrix compartments in the rat striatum. Neuroscience 1993;57:661–71.
37. Eblen F, Graybiel AM. Highly restricted origin of prefrontal cortical inputs to striosomes in the macaque monkey. J Neurosci 1995;15:5999–6013.
38. Besson MJ, Graybiel AM, Nastuk MA. [3H]SCH 23390 binding to D1 dopamine receptors in the basal ganglia of the cat and primate: delineation of striosomal compartments and pallidal and nigral subdivisions. Neuroscience 1988;26: 101–19.
39. Baxter LR, Saxena S, Brody AL, et al. Brain mediation of obsessive-compulsive disorder symptoms: evidence from functional brain imaging studies in the human and nonhuman primate. Semin Clin Neuropsychiatry 1996;1:32–47.
40. Rossi S, Bartalini S, Ulivelli M, et al. Hypofunctioning of sensory gating mechanisms in patients with obsessive-compulsive disorder. Biol Psychiatry 2005;57:16–20.
41. Zald DH, Kim SW. Anatomy and function of the orbital frontal cortex, I: anatomy, neurocircuitry; and obsessive-compulsive disorder. J Neuropsychiatry Clin Neurosci 1996;8:125–38.
42. Rolls ET. The orbitofrontal cortex and reward. Cereb Cortex 2000;10:284–94.
43. Krawczyk DC. Contributions of the prefrontal cortex to the neural basis of human decision making. Neurosci Biobehav Rev 2002;26:631–64.
44. Aouizerate B, Guehl D, Cuny E, et al. Pathophysiology of obsessive-compulsive disorder: a necessary link between phenomenology, neuropsychology, imagery and physiology. Prog Neurobiol 2004;72:195–221.
45. Milad MR, Rauch SL. The role of the orbitofrontal cortex in anxiety disorders. Ann N Y Acad Sci 2007;1121:546–61.
46. Elliott R, Agnew Z, Deakin JF. Hedonic and informational functions of the human orbitofrontal cortex. Cereb Cortex 2010;20:198–204.
47. O'Doherty J, Critchley H, Deichmann R, et al. Dissociating valence of outcome from behavioral control in human orbital and ventral prefrontal cortices. J Neurosci 2003;23:7931–9.
48. Hollerman JR, Tremblay L, Schultz W. Involvement of basal ganglia and orbitofrontal cortex in goal-directed behavior. Prog Brain Res 2000;126: 193–215.
49. Graham BM, Milad MR. The study of fear extinction: implications for anxiety disorders. Am J Psychiatry 2011;168:1255–65.
50. Kunde W, Reuss H, Kiesel A. Consciousness and cognitive control. Adv Cogn Psychol 2012;8:9–18.
51. Bush G, Luu P, Posner MI. Cognitive and emotional influences in anterior cingulate cortex. Trends Cogn Sci 2000;4:215–22.

52. Bush G, Vogt BA, Holmes J, et al. Dorsal anterior cingulate cortex: a role in reward-based decision making. Proc Natl Acad Sci U S A 2002;99:523–8.
53. van Veen V, Carter CS. The anterior cingulate as a conflict monitor: fMRI and ERP studies. Physiol Behav 2002;77:477–82.
54. Fitzgerald KD, Welsh RC, Gehring WJ, et al. Error-related hyperactivity of the anterior cingulate cortex in obsessive-compulsive disorder. Biol Psychiatry 2005;57:287–94.
55. Fitzgerald KD, Stern ER, Angstadt M, et al. Altered function and connectivity of the medial frontal cortex in pediatric obsessive-compulsive disorder. Biol Psychiatry 2010;68:1039–47.
56. Ursu S, Carter CS. Outcome representations, counterfactual comparisons and the human orbitofrontal cortex: implications for neuroimaging studies of decision-making. Brain Res Cogn Brain Res 2005;23:51–60.
57. Schlosser RG, Wagner G, Schachtzabel C, et al. Fronto-cingulate effective connectivity in obsessive compulsive disorder: a study with fMRI and dynamic causal modeling. Hum Brain Mapp 2010;31:1834–50.
58. Culham JC, Kanwisher NG. Neuroimaging of cognitive functions in human parietal cortex. Curr Opin Neurobiol 2001;11:157–63.
59. Courchesne E, Townsend J, Akshoomoff NA, et al. Impairment in shifting attention in autistic and cerebellar patients. Behav Neurosci 1994;108:848–65.
60. Allen G, Buxton RB, Wong EC, et al. Attentional activation of the cerebellum independent of motor involvement. Science 1997;275:1940–3.
61. Andreasen NC, O'Leary DS, Cizadlo T, et al. Schizophrenia and cognitive dysmetria: a positron-emission tomography study of dysfunctional prefrontal-thalamic-cerebellar circuitry. Proc Natl Acad Sci U S A 1996;93:9985–90.
62. Kim SG, Ugurbil K, Strick PL. Activation of a cerebellar output nucleus during cognitive processing. Science 1994;265:949–51.
63. Busatto GF, Zamignani DR, Buchpiguel CA, et al. A voxel-based investigation of regional cerebral blood flow abnormalities in obsessive-compulsive disorder using single photon emission computed tomography (SPECT). Psychiatry Res 2000;99:15–27.
64. Foa EB, Liebowitz MR, Kozak MJ, et al. Randomized, placebo-controlled trial of exposure and ritual prevention, clomipramine, and their combination in the treatment of obsessive-compulsive disorder. Am J Psychiatry 2005;162:151–61.
65. Houghton S, Saxon D, Bradburn M, et al. The effectiveness of routinely delivered cognitive behavioural therapy for obsessive-compulsive disorder: a benchmarking study. Br J Clin Psychol 2010;49:473–89.
66. Anderson RA, Rees CS. Group versus individual cognitive-behavioural treatment for obsessive-compulsive disorder: a controlled trial. Behav Res Ther 2007;45:123–37.
67. Denys D. Pharmacotherapy of obsessive-compulsive disorder and obsessive-compulsive spectrum disorders. Psychiatr Clin North Am 2006;29:553–84, xi.
68. Hollander E, Koran LM, Goodman WK, et al. A double-blind, placebo-controlled study of the efficacy and safety of controlled-release fluvoxamine in patients with obsessive-compulsive disorder. J Clin Psychiatry 2003;64:640–7.
69. Hollander E, Allen A, Steiner M, et al. Acute and long-term treatment and prevention of relapse of obsessive-compulsive disorder with paroxetine. J Clin Psychiatry 2003;64:1113–21.
70. Kamijima K, Murasaki M, Asai M, et al. Paroxetine in the treatment of obsessive-compulsive disorder: randomized, double-blind, placebo-controlled study in Japanese patients. Psychiatry Clin Neurosci 2004;58:427–33.
71. Montgomery SA, Kasper S, Stein DJ, et al. Citalopram 20 mg, 40 mg and 60 mg are all effective and well tolerated compared with placebo in obsessive-compulsive disorder. Int Clin Psychopharmacol 2001;16:75–86.
72. Pallanti S, Hollander E, Bienstock C, et al. Treatment non-response in OCD: methodological issues and operational definitions. Int J Neuropsychopharmacol 2002;5:181–91.
73. Manjila S, Rengachary S, Xavier AR, et al. Modern psychosurgery before Egas Moniz: a tribute to Gottlieb Burckhardt. Neurosurg Focus 2008;25(1):E9. http://dx.doi.org/10.3171/FOC/2008/25/7/E9.
74. Heller AC, Amar AP, Liu CY, et al. Surgery of the mind and mood: a mosaic of issues in time and evolution. Neurosurgery 2008;62:921–40.
75. Mashour GA, Walker EE, Martuza RL. Psychosurgery: past, present, and future. Brain Res Brain Res Rev 2005;48:409–19.
76. Patel SR, Aronson JP, Sheth SA, et al. Lesion procedures in psychiatric neurosurgery. World Neurosurg 2012. http://dx.doi.org/10.1016/j.wneu.2012.11.038.
77. Feldman RP, Goodrich JT. Psychosurgery: a historical overview. Neurosurgery 2001;48:647–57 [discussion: 657–9].
78. Lichterman BL. On the history of psychosurgery in Russia. Acta Neurochir (Wien) 1993;125:1–4.
79. Kopell BH, Rezai AR. Psychiatric neurosurgery: a historical perspective. Neurosurg Clin N Am 2003;14:181–97, vii.
80. Whitty CW, Duffield JE, Tov PM, et al. Anterior cingulectomy in the treatment of mental disease. Lancet 1952;1:475–81.
81. Kihlstrom L, Hindmarsh T, Lax I, et al. Radiosurgical lesions in the normal human brain 17 years after

gamma knife capsulotomy. Neurosurgery 1997;41: 396–401 [discussion: 401–2].
82. Mindus P, Edman G, Andreewitch S. A prospective, long-term study of personality traits in patients with intractable obsessional illness treated by capsulotomy. Acta Psychiatr Scand 1999;99:40–50.
83. Freeman W, Watts JW. Prefrontal lobotomy: the surgical relief of mental pain. Bull N Y Acad Med 1942; 18:794–812.
84. Jenike MA, Baer L, Ballantine T, et al. Cingulotomy for refractory obsessive-compulsive disorder. A long-term follow-up of 33 patients. Arch Gen Psychiatry 1991;48:548–55.
85. Ballantine HT, Bouckoms AJ, Thomas EK, et al. Treatment of psychiatric illness by stereotactic cingulotomy. Biol Psychiatry 1987;22:807–19.
86. Greenberg BD, Price LH, Rauch SL, et al. Neurosurgery for intractable obsessive-compulsive disorder and depression: critical issues. Neurosurg Clin N Am 2003;14:199–212.
87. Liu K, Zhang H, Liu C, et al. Stereotactic treatment of refractory obsessive compulsive disorder by bilateral capsulotomy with 3 years follow-up. J Clin Neurosci 2008;15:622–9.
88. Knight G. Stereotactic tractotomy in the surgical treatment of mental illness. J Neurol Neurosurg Psychiatr 1965;28:304–10.
89. Kelly D, Richardson A, Mitchell-Heggs N. Stereotactic limbic leucotomy: neurophysiological aspects and operative technique. Br J Psychiatry 1973;123:133–40.
90. Bridges PK, Bartlett JR, Hale AS, et al. Psychosurgery: stereotactic subcaudate tractomy. An indispensable treatment. Br J Psychiatry 1994;165: 599–611 [discussion: 612–3].
91. Mitchell-Heggs N, Kelly D, Richardson A. Stereotactic limbic leucotomy–a follow-up at 16 months. Br J Psychiatry 1976;128:226–40.
92. Rück C, Karlsson A, Steele JD, et al. Capsulotomy for obsessive-compulsive disorder: long-term follow-up of 25 patients. Arch Gen Psychiatry 2008;65:914–21.
93. Dougherty DD, Baer L, Cosgrove GR, et al. Prospective long-term follow-up of 44 patients who received cingulotomy for treatment-refractory obsessive-compulsive disorder. Am J Psychiatry 2002;159:269–75.
94. Sheth SA, Neal J, Tangherlini F, et al. Limbic system surgery for treatment-refractory obsessive-compulsive disorder: a prospective long-term follow-up of 64 patients. J Neurosurg 2013;118:491–7.
95. Hodgkiss AD, Malizia AL, Bartlett JR, et al. Outcome after the psychosurgical operation of stereotactic subcaudate tractotomy, 1979-1991. J Neuropsychiatry Clin Neurosci 1995;7:230–4.
96. McIntyre CC, Savasta M, Goff LK, et al. Uncovering the mechanism(s) of action of deep brain stimulation: activation, inhibition, or both. Clin Neurophysiol 2004;115:1239–48.
97. Logothetis NK, Augath M, Murayama Y, et al. The effects of electrical microstimulation on cortical signal propagation. Nat Neurosci 2010; 13:1283–91.
98. Histed MH, Bonin VB, Reid RC. Direct activation of sparse, distributed populations of cortical neurons by electrical microstimulation. Neuron 2009;63: 508–22.
99. McIntyre CC, Grill WM, Sherman DL, et al. Cellular effects of deep brain stimulation: model-based analysis of activation and inhibition. J Neurophysiol 2004;91:1457–69.
100. Guo Y, Rubin JE, McIntyre CC, et al. Thalamocortical relay fidelity varies across subthalamic nucleus deep brain stimulation protocols in a data-driven computational model. J Neurophysiol 2008;99: 1477–92.
101. Johnson MD, Miocinovic S, McIntyre CC, et al. Mechanisms and targets of deep brain stimulation in movement disorders. Neurotherapeutics 2008;5: 294–308.
102. Nuttin B, Cosyns P, Demeulemeester H, et al. Electrical stimulation in anterior limbs of internal capsules in patients with obsessive-compulsive disorder. Lancet 1999;354:1526.
103. Nuttin BJ, Gabriels L, van Kuyck K, et al. Electrical stimulation of the anterior limbs of the internal capsules in patients with severe obsessive-compulsive disorder: anecdotal reports. Neurosurg Clin N Am 2003;14:267–74.
104. Goodman WK, Foote KD, Greenberg BD, et al. Deep brain stimulation for intractable obsessive compulsive disorder: pilot study using a blinded, staggered-onset design. Biol Psychiatry 2010;67: 535–42.
105. Greenberg BD, Malone DA, Friehs GM, et al. Three-year outcomes in deep brain stimulation for highly resistant obsessive-compulsive disorder. Neuropsychopharmacology 2006;31: 2384–93.
106. Greenberg BD, Gabriels LA, Malone DAJ, et al. Deep brain stimulation of the ventral internal capsule/ventral striatum for obsessive-compulsive disorder: worldwide experience. Mol Psychiatry 2010;15:64–79.
107. Abelson JL, Curtis GC, Sagher O, et al. Deep brain stimulation for refractory obsessive-compulsive disorder. Biol Psychiatry 2005;57:510–6.
108. Anderson D, Ahmed A. Treatment of patients with intractable obsessive-compulsive disorder with anterior capsular stimulation. Case report. J Neurosurg 2003;98:1104–8.
109. Aouizerate B, Cuny E, Martin-Guehl C, et al. Deep brain stimulation of the ventral caudate nucleus in the treatment of obsessive-compulsive disorder

and major depression. Case report. J Neurosurg 2004;101:682–6.
110. Plewnia C, Schober F, Rilk A, et al. Sustained improvement of obsessive-compulsive disorder by deep brain stimulation in a woman with residual schizophrenia. Int J Neuropsychopharmacol 2008; 11:1181–3.
111. Sturm V, Lenartz D, Koulousakis A, et al. The nucleus accumbens: a target for deep brain stimulation in obsessive-compulsive- and anxiety-disorders. J Chem Neuroanat 2003;26:293–9.
112. Huff W, Lenartz D, Schormann M, et al. Unilateral deep brain stimulation of the nucleus accumbens in patients with treatment-resistant obsessive-compulsive disorder: outcomes after one year. Clin Neurol Neurosurg 2010;112:137–43.
113. Denys D, Mantione M, Figee M, et al. Deep brain stimulation of the nucleus accumbens for treatment-refractory obsessive-compulsive disorder. Arch Gen Psychiatry 2010;67:1061–8.
114. Mallet L, Mesnage V, Houeto JL, et al. Compulsions, Parkinson's disease, and stimulation. Lancet 2002;360:1302–4.
115. Fontaine D, Mattei V, Borg M, et al. Effect of subthalamic nucleus stimulation on obsessive-compulsive disorder in a patient with Parkinson disease. Case report. J Neurosurg 2004;100:1084–6.
116. Mallet L, Polosan M, Jaafari N, et al. Subthalamic nucleus stimulation in severe obsessive-compulsive disorder. N Engl J Med 2008;359:2121–34.
117. Jimenez-Ponce F, Velasco-Campos F, Castro-Farfan G, et al. Preliminary study in patients with obsessive-compulsive disorder treated with electrical stimulation in the inferior thalamic peduncle. Neurosurgery 2009;65:203–9 [discussion: 209].
118. Barnes A, Duncan R, Chisholm JA, et al. Investigation into the mechanisms of vagus nerve stimulation for the treatment of intractable epilepsy, using 99mTc-HMPAO SPET brain images. Eur J Nucl Med Mol Imaging 2003;30:301–5.
119. George MS, Sackeim HA, Rush AJ, et al. Vagus nerve stimulation: a new tool for brain research and therapy. Biol Psychiatry 2000;47:287–95.
120. Rutecki P. Anatomical, physiological, and theoretical basis for the antiepileptic effect of vagus nerve stimulation. Epilepsia 1990;31(Suppl 2):S1–6.
121. Ben-Menachem E, Hamberger A, Hedner T, et al. Effects of vagus nerve stimulation on amino acids and other metabolites in the CSF of patients with partial seizures. Epilepsy Res 1995;20:221–7.
122. Henry TR, Votaw JR, Pennell PB, et al. Acute blood flow changes and efficacy of vagus nerve stimulation in partial epilepsy. Neurology 1999;52: 1166–73.
123. Groves DA, Brown VJ. Vagal nerve stimulation: a review of its applications and potential mechanisms that mediate its clinical effects. Neurosci Biobehav Rev 2005;29:493–500.
124. Barker AT, Jalinous R, Freeston IL. Non-invasive magnetic stimulation of human motor cortex. Lancet 1985;1:1106–7.
125. Speer AM, Kimbrell TA, Wassermann EM, et al. Opposite effects of high and low frequency rTMS on regional brain activity in depressed patients. Biol Psychiatry 2000;48:1133–41.
126. Greenberg BD, George MS, Martin JD, et al. Effect of prefrontal repetitive transcranial magnetic stimulation in obsessive-compulsive disorder: a preliminary study. Am J Psychiatry 1997;154:867–9.
127. Ruffini C, Locatelli M, Lucca A, et al. Augmentation effect of repetitive transcranial magnetic stimulation over the orbitofrontal cortex in drug-resistant obsessive-compulsive disorder patients: a controlled investigation. Prim Care Companion J Clin Psychiatry 2009;11:226–30.
128. Sachdev PS, McBride R, Loo CK, et al. Right versus left prefrontal transcranial magnetic stimulation for obsessive-compulsive disorder: a preliminary investigation. J Clin Psychiatry 2001;62: 981–4.
129. Sachdev PS, Loo CK, Mitchell PB, et al. Repetitive transcranial magnetic stimulation for the treatment of obsessive compulsive disorder: a double-blind controlled investigation. Psychol Med 2007;37: 1645–9.
130. Prasko J, Paskova B, Zalesky R, et al. The effect of repetitive transcranial magnetic stimulation (rTMS) on symptoms in obsessive compulsive disorder. A randomized, double blind, sham controlled study. Neuro Endocrinol Lett 2006;27:327–32.
131. Sarkhel S, Sinha VK, Praharaj SK. Adjunctive high-frequency right prefrontal repetitive transcranial magnetic stimulation (rTMS) was not effective in obsessive-compulsive disorder but improved secondary depression. J Anxiety Disord 2010;24: 535–9.
132. Greenberg BD, Ziemann U, Cora-Locatelli G, et al. Altered cortical excitability in obsessive-compulsive disorder. Neurology 2000;54:142–7.
133. Greenberg BD, Ziemann U, Harmon A, et al. Decreased neuronal inhibition in cerebral cortex in obsessive-compulsive disorder on transcranial magnetic stimulation. Lancet 1998;352:881–2.
134. Haber SN. The primate basal ganglia: parallel and integrative networks. J Chem Neuroanat 2003;26: 317–30.
135. Mantovani A, Lisanby SH, Pieraccini F, et al. Repetitive transcranial magnetic stimulation (rTMS) in the treatment of obsessive-compulsive disorder (OCD) and Tourette's syndrome (TS). Int J Neuropsychopharmacol 2006;9:95–100.
136. Lisanby SH, Luber B, Schlaepfer TE, et al. Safety and feasibility of magnetic seizure therapy (MST)

in major depression: randomized within-subject comparison with electroconvulsive therapy. Neuropsychopharmacology 2003;28:1852–65.

137. Spellman T, McClintock SM, Terrace H, et al. Differential effects of high-dose magnetic seizure therapy and electroconvulsive shock on cognitive function. Biol Psychiatry 2008;63:1163–70.
138. Deisseroth K, Feng G, Majewska AK, et al. Next-generation optical technologies for illuminating genetically targeted brain circuits. J Neurosci 2006;26:10380–6.
139. Zhang F, Aravanis AM, Adamantidis A, et al. Circuit-breakers: optical technologies for probing neural signals and systems. Nat Rev Neurosci 2007;8:577–81.
140. Bernstein JG, Boyden ES. Optogenetic tools for analyzing the neural circuits of behavior. Trends Cogn Sci 2011;15:592–600.
141. Tsai HC, Zhang F, Adamantidis A, et al. Phasic firing in dopaminergic neurons is sufficient for behavioral conditioning. Science 2009;324:1080–4.
142. Gerits A, Farivar R, Rosen BR, et al. Optogenetically induced behavioral and functional network changes in primates. Curr Biol 2012;22(18):1722–6.
143. Airan RD, Thompson KR, Fenno LE, et al. Temporally precise in vivo control of intracellular signalling. Nature 2009;458:1025–9.
144. Burguière E, Monteiro P, Feng G, et al. Optogenetic stimulation of lateral orbitofronto-striatal pathway suppresses compulsive behaviors. Science 2013;340:1243–6.
145. U.S. Department of Health, Education, and Welfare. Protection of human subjects. Use of psychosurgery in practice and research: report and recommendations of National Commission for the Protection of Human Subjects. Fed Regist 1977;42:26318–32.
146. Wind JJ, Anderson DE. From prefrontal leukotomy to deep brain stimulation: the historical transformation of psychosurgery and the emergence of neuroethics. Neurosurg Focus 2008;25:E10.
147. Franzini A, Messina G, Gambini O, et al. Deep-brain stimulation of the nucleus accumbens in obsessive compulsive disorder: clinical, surgical and electrophysiological considerations in two consecutive patients. Neurol Sci 2010;31:353–9.

Neuromodulation for Depression

Invasive and Noninvasive (Deep Brain Stimulation, Transcranial Magnetic Stimulation, Trigeminal Nerve Stimulation)

Ian A. Cook, MD[a,*], Randall Espinoza, MD, MPH[b],
Andrew F. Leuchter, MD[c]

KEYWORDS

- Depression • Treatment-resistant depression • Neuromodulation • Deep brain stimulation
- Transcranial magnetic stimulation • Trigeminal nerve stimulation

KEY POINTS

- Despite best practices for the management of major depression with medications and psychotherapy, many patients do not fully recover and need other treatment options.
- Neuromodulation interventions span from surgically implanted devices to noninvasive systems.
- Neuromodulation interventions may have complementary mechanisms of action, and may offer new hope for recovery for patients with pharmacoresistant depression.
- Additional comparative research is needed to clarify how best to make use of these technologies.

INTRODUCTION: WHY WE NEED NEUROMODULATION FOR DEPRESSION

Major depressive disorder (MDD; codes 293.2 and 293.3 in *Diagnostic and Statistical Manual of Mental Disorders*, 5th edition and the International Classification of Diseases, 9th revision) is a common, disabling, and undertreated condition. With a lifetime prevalence of 1 in 6 and an annual prevalence of 6.6%, at least 20 million Americans will have an

Funding Sources: I.A. Cook: NIH, VA, NeoSync, Covidien, Shire Pharmaceuticals; R. Espinoza: NIH, UCLA intramural (Clinical Science Translational Institute, Cousins Center for Psychoneuroimmunology) St Jude Medical, Up To Date (royalties); A.F. Leuchter: NIH, Neuronetics, NeuroSigma, Shire Pharmaceuticals.
Conflicts of Interest: I.A. Cook: TNS patents (assigned to UCLA, licensed to NeuroSigma), research support (NeoSync), speakers bureau (Neuronetics), advisor & stock options (NeuroSigma); R. Epinoza: Research Support (St. Jude); A.F. Leuchter: Research Support (Neuronetics, NeuroSigma), consultant/advisor (NeoSync, Brain Cells, MedGenesis Therapeutics, Taisho Pharmaceutical, Lilly).
[a] UCLA Depression Research & Clinic Program, Semel Institute for Neuroscience and Human Behavior at UCLA, David Geffen School of Medicine at UCLA, Henry Samueli School of Engineering at UCLA, 760 Westwood Plaza, Los Angeles, CA 90095, USA; [b] Electroconvulsive Therapy Program, Resnick Neuropsychiatric Hospital at UCLA, UCLA Longevity Center, Semel Institute for Neurosciences and Human Behavior at UCLA, Department of Psychiatry and Biobehavioral Sciences, David Geffen School of Medicine at UCLA, 300 Medical Plaza, Los Angeles, CA 90095, USA; [c] Laboratory of Brain, Behavior, and Pharmacology, Semel Institute for Neuroscience and Human Behavior, David Geffen School of Medicine at UCLA, 760 Westwood Plaza, Los Angeles, CA 90095, USA
* Corresponding author.
E-mail address: icook@ucla.edu

Neurosurg Clin N Am 25 (2014) 103–116
http://dx.doi.org/10.1016/j.nec.2013.10.002
1042-3680/14/$ – see front matter

episode in 2013.[1] In middle-income and high-income countries, MDD already ranks above ischemic heart disease as causing annually the greatest disability for both men and women.[2] It has been estimated that more than 40% of North Americans with MDD do not receive any treatment.[1]

For those who do receive treatment, the landmark STAR*D study (Sequenced Treatment Alternatives to Relieve Depression) found that less than one-third of adults with MDD remitted with their first medication trial and, thus, a majority need to try something else to aid recovery.[3] The likelihood of achieving remission decreases with each successive pharmacologic treatment[3] while the 12-month rate of relapse increases (71% after 3 failures).[4] There clearly is a need for treatments that have both greater efficacy and durability of benefit.

Treatment-resistant depression generally refers to those patients who remain ill despite repeated vigorous attempts using adequate doses of medication for trials of an adequate duration[5–7]; this might better be termed pharmacoresistance than treatment resistance,[8] as it is generally applied in patient care to signify failures of medication treatments. Neuromodulation represents a family of interventions that may have complementary mechanisms of action, and therefore may offer new hope for recovery for patients with pharmacoresistant depression.

The use of neuromodulation for mood disorders is not itself a new idea, but there has been a recent proliferation of approaches. Electroconvulsive therapy (ECT, convulsive therapy) has been in use since the late 1930s,[9] and is believed to achieve a therapeutic alteration of brain activity by the use of electrical currents that pass through the brain and produce a seizure. This seizure activity has been hypothesized to be transduced into clinical benefits through such mechanisms (cf. Bolwig[10]) as affecting neurogenesis,[11,12] neuroendocrine regulation,[13] or cytokine levels[14]; normalizing patterns of cerebral metabolism[15] or glutamatergic neurotransmission[16,17]; or altering gene expression.[18] Recent efforts to address the cognitive side effects by focusing the stimulation have led to innovations such as focal electrically administered seizure therapy (FEAST[19]) and magnetic seizure therapy (MST[20,21]). At the other end of the spectrum, methods for nonconvulsive, low-energy stimulation of the brain have been examined, with approaches such as transcranial direct current stimulation (tDCS) and transcranial alternating current stimulation (tACS), as forms of cranial electrotherapy stimulation (CES), whereby current flux lines pass through brain tissue but no seizure is effected.[22–25]

From a long and expanding list of neuromodulation approaches with potential use in depression, the editors of this issue have asked the authors to focus on just 3: deep brain stimulation (DBS), transcranial magnetic stimulation (TMS), and trigeminal nerve stimulation (TNS). All 3 of these approaches have histories in which the developments of neurologic and psychiatric applications have gone hand in hand. One of these interventions (TMS) has regulatory approval by the US Food and Drug Administration (FDA) for use in depression, and is reimbursed by some insurance carriers in the United States, whereas the other approaches do not yet have US regulatory approval; these experimental devices are limited to investigational use in the United States, although they may have regulatory approval in other countries. These treatments differ notably in terms of their mode of delivery and risk profile: DBS involves a neurosurgical implantation procedure, whereas the TMS is noninvasive, and TNS can be administered either noninvasively or with a minimally invasive approach. This article describes salient features of each of these interventions. For each intervention, the authors primarily have surveyed controlled studies that have been completed or other peer-reviewed data that have been published and are widely accessible, and have noted where salient trials are ongoing or completed but for which published data are not available at the time of writing. Across all modalities, **Table 1** summarizes critical aspects of stimulation to consider in evaluating a clinical

Table 1
Parameters of neuromodulation stimulation

Anatomic Features	Features Related to the Stimulation Signal
Target structure	Signal waveform (pulse, sinusoidal)
Laterality (right, left, bilateral)	Frequency (pulses/s, Hz)
Estimated size of stimulated region (mm^3)	Pulse width (μs)
	Duty cycle (seconds signal is on vs seconds signal off)
	Signal amplitude (voltage, current, or magnetic field strength)

trial, namely, the anatomic target(s) being stimulated, and the nature of signal (electrical or magnetic) being used for stimulation.

DEEP BRAIN STIMULATION FOR DEPRESSION

DBS uses the stereotactic neurosurgical implantation of stimulating electrodes at 1 or more specific anatomic target locations in the brain, then applies electrical currents at controlled signal parameters to achieve the intended therapeutic effects. Direct stimulation of the brain was observed to affect complex behaviors in the mid-twentieth century (by, eg, Delgado[26,27]). However, societal fears regarding the adequacy of informed consent for neurosurgical procedures to treat mental illness prompted establishment of legal constraints in some jurisdictions (eg, California Welfare and Institutions Code § 5325 from 1967). The use of DBS for treating neurologic conditions, such as movement disorders, falls outside these legal considerations. Building on a pathophysiologic model of an electrically induced reversible or simulated lesion[28,29] that could be adjusted postoperatively, unlike once-only ablative surgical interventions (eg, pallidotomy, thalamotomy), DBS systems were approved by the FDA for essential tremor in 1997, for Parkinson disease in 2002, and for dystonia in 2003. A humanitarian device exemption (HDE) approval was granted by the FDA for use in obsessive-compulsive disorder (OCD) in 2009, as an initial psychiatric indication for a DBS system. (HDE is an FDA regulatory approval pathway for devices that will be used in a very limited number of patients each year and does not have the same level of clinical trial evidence to support safety and efficacy as a regular pathway [i.e., investigational device exemption pivotal study followed by a premarket approval to permit sales]. Some have drawn an analogy to orphan drugs.) CE Mark regulatory approval for OCD was issued the same year. (CE Mark [Conformité Européenne] is a requirement for certain medical [and other] devices to be made commercially available in the European Economic Area, namely, the 27 member states of the European Union plus Iceland, Norway, and Liechtenstein.)

Effects on mood were observed in many of the patients implanted for the treatment of neurologic conditions, prompting interest in developing DBS specifically for use in depression. Several different targets have been explored for potential in the management of depression (cf. Hauptman and colleagues,[30] Anderson and colleagues[31]), guided by different insights into structures implicated in the pathophysiology of mood disorders and the behavioral, cognitive, and affective symptoms of depression. These structures include: (1) subgenual (subcallosal) cingulate cortex, Brodmann area 25 (SCG); (2) ventral anterior internal capsule/ventral striatum (VC/VS); (3) nucleus accumbens (NAcc) and ventral striatum; (4) inferior thalamic peduncle (ITP); (5) lateral habenula (LH); (6) median forebrain bundle (MFB); and (7) internal globus pallidus (GP) (**Fig. 1**). Other targets have been proposed (cf. Hauptman and colleagues[30]),

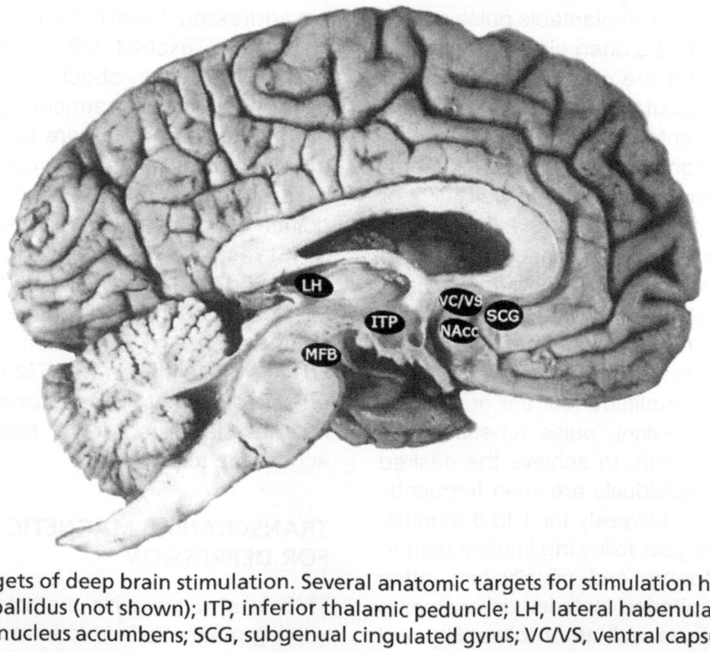

Fig. 1. Common targets of deep brain stimulation. Several anatomic targets for stimulation have been examined: GP, internal globus pallidus (not shown); ITP, inferior thalamic peduncle; LH, lateral habenula; MFB, median forebrain bundle; NAcc, nucleus accumbens; SCG, subgenual cingulated gyrus; VC/VS, ventral capsule/ventral striatum.

but no publications about clinical effects for these other locations could be found via online searches.

Table 2 summarizes key publications, findings, and considerations for each of these targets. Of note, none of these have used a parallel-group, double-blind, randomized controlled trial (RCT) model. A review of preclinical studies[32] and an accompanying commentary[33] amplified some of the rationale for the targets, and also highlight nuanced aspects of stimulation beyond the reversible lesion concept (eg, hyperpolarization of 1 part of a neuron while other portions are depolarized) that must be considered in trying to understand the potential mechanisms of action at work in DBS. A recent report by Ramasubbu and colleagues[34] examined the relationship between stimulation parameters and acute and chronic symptom responses using a systematic approach to explore variations in the type of stimulation (see **Table 1**). The investigators reported that clinical response was related more to pulse width than to frequency of stimulation, a finding that emphasizes that additional studies to explore different stimulation parameters may be important in improving clinical outcomes in patients using DBS to address depression.

Regardless of target or the particular device being used, treatment with DBS is generally undertaken by a multidisciplinary team, including psychiatrists and stereotactic neurosurgeons, working together with neuropsychologists and other support staff. Because implantation is conventionally performed bilaterally, it is common to place an electrode into the target of each hemisphere, and each is then connected to a programmable neurostimulator (also called an implantable pulse generator or IPG); the IPGs are often placed pectorally, near the clavicle, and are connected to the implanted leads via subcutaneously tunneled extension wires. Experimental protocols in depression have followed the example of those used for neurologic indications, and subjects often wait for 2 or more weeks postoperatively before the device is activated and a period of adjustment is begun to find the best settings. In this process, physicians select the specific electrode contact(s) to be stimulated (ie, to fine-tune the exact anatomic region being stimulated), and adjust key signal parameters such as signal amplitude (current or voltage, depending on the device), pulse repetition frequency, and pulse width, to achieve the desired symptom control. Individuals are seen frequently (commonly weekly or biweekly for 1 to 3 months, then monthly) in the year following implantation to allow close monitoring, and usually less often thereafter. This monitoring includes assessments of clinical response as well as of tolerability and side effects. It is worth noting that DBS is currently used adjunctively as an addition to ongoing pharmacotherapy and psychotherapy.

Complications of DBS affect a minority of individuals, and can best be conceptualized as those related to (1) the surgical procedure acutely (eg, intracranial hemorrhage, postoperative infection, stroke), (2) the chronic presence of the device in the body (eg, lead migration or erosion), or (3) the stimulation signal itself (eg, undesired behavioral or affective symptom changes). Adverse events in this last category have included the development of manic/hypomanic states, anxiety symptoms, and worsening of depression, but these generally have been found to respond to adjustments in the stimulation parameters. Suicides have been reported after DBS implantation (eg, Kennedy and colleagues[35]), but it is challenging to differentiate reliably the risk ascribed to device stimulation as opposed to the risk associated simply with chronic unremitting depression.

At present, no DBS system has received FDA approval for use with an indication for depression, either unipolar MDD or depression in bipolar-spectrum disorders, although trials for these indications are currently registered in the ClinicalTrials.gov database. Because clinical benefits only emerge over months to years of use,[35] DBS for treatment-resistant depression is not an acute intervention, and other approaches continue concomitantly at least until a response is obtained. Should regulatory approval occur, health economic factors will be considered as the questions of cost-benefit and cost-effectiveness that affect reimbursement and insurance coverage policies are addressed. Initial DBS device and implantation costs may exceed US$200,000 per patient,[36] raising questions about how this intervention might best fit into treatment algorithms in this era of attention to health care costs, some of which may be addressed through comparative effectiveness studies of at least 12 months' duration. As points of comparison, vagus nerve stimulation (VNS) received FDA regulatory approval in 2005, but in 2007 the Centers for Medicare and Medicaid Services issued a decision that VNS would not be a covered benefit, a decision which it reiterated in 2013.[37] The situation with TMS is discussed next, but it is clear that FDA approval is a necessary but not sufficient step for a treatment to become accessible to patients.

TRANSCRANIAL MAGNETIC STIMULATION FOR DEPRESSION

TMS is a noninvasive therapy that uses a time-varying magnetic field to induce a current in brain

Table 2
Studies of DBS for depression

Target	Study	Follow-up or Extension	Sample Size	Diagnosis	Outcome Measure	Response (ITT)	Remission (ITT)	Best Outcomes	Trial Duration
SCG	Mayberg,[101] 2005	—	6	5 MDD; 1 BPII	HDRS17	4/6	2/6	6 mo	6 mo
	Lozano,[102] 2008	x	20	19 MDD; 1 BPII	HDRS17	12/20	7/20	6 mo	12 mo
	Kennedy et al,[35] 2011	x	20	19 MDD; 1 BPII	HDRS17	12/20	8/20	3 y	3–6 y
	Neimat,[103] 2008	—	1	1 MDD	HDRS17	1/1	1/1	24 mo	30 mo
	Lozano,[104] 2012	—	21	21 MDD	HDRS17	12/21	n.r.	1 mo	12 mo
	Puigdemont,[105] 2012	—	8	8 MDD	HDRS17	5/8	3/8	12 mo	12 mo
	Holztheimer,[106] 2012	—	10	10 MDD; 7 BP	HDRS17	11/17	7/17	2 y	2 y
	Ramasubbu et al,[34] 2013	—	4	4 MDD	HDRS17	2/4	0/4	30 wk	38 wk
VC/VS	Malone,[107] 2009	—	15	14 MDD; 1 BP	HDRS24	6/15	5/15	LFU	51 mo
	Malone,[108] 2010	x	17	n.r.	MADRS	12/17	6/17	LFU	67 mo
NAcc	Schlaepfer,[109] 2008	—	3	3 MDD	HDRS24	n.r.	n.r.	Variable	6–22 wk
	Bewernick,[110] 2010	x	10	10 MDD	HDRS28	5/10	3/10	12 mo	12 mo
	Bewernick,[111] 2012	x	11	11 MDD	HDRS28	5/11	1/11	2 y	2 y
ITP	Jiménez,[112] 2005	—	1	1 MDD	HAM-D	n/a	n/a	n/a	24 mo
	Jiménez,[113] 2007	x	2	1 MDD; 1 OCD	HAM-D	n/a	n/a	n/a	18 mo
LH	Sartorius,[114] 2010	—	1	1 MDD	HAM-D21	n/a	n/a	n/a	60 wk
MFB	Schlaepfer,[115] 2013	—	7	6 MDD; 1 BP	MADRS	6/7	4/7	LFU	33 wk
GP	Kosel,[116] 2007	—	1	1 MDD	HRSD	n/a	n/a	18 mo	18 mo

Hamilton Depression Rating Scale: HDRS17, 17-item version; HDRS24, 24-item version; HAM-D21, 21-item version; HAM-D, HDRS unspecified form.

Abbreviations: BP, bipolar disorder; BPII, bipolar II disorder; GP, globus pallidus; ITP, inferior thalamic peduncle; ITT, intent-to-treat; LFU, last follow-up visit; LH, lateral habenula; MADRS, Montgomery-Åsberg Depression Rating Scale; MDD, unipolar major depressive disorder; MFB, median forebrain bundle; n/a, not applicable; NAcc, nucleus accumbens; n.r., not reported; OCD, obsessive-compulsive disorder; SCG, subgenual (subcallosal) cingulated gyrus; VC/VS, ventral anterior internal capsule/ventral striatum.

tissue. This magnetic field may be generated by a single coil, as with the 2 devices that currently have US regulatory clearance for use in treating MDD (NeuroStar TMS System from Neuronetics, Inc, Malvern, PA and Brainsway Deep TMS System from Brainsway Ltd, Jerusalem, Israel), or may use multiple coils or rotating permanent magnets (investigational devices). Although the induction of currents in the brain by magnetic fields traces back to the early twentieth century or earlier (cf. George and Belmaker[38]), the modern era of TMS is often connected to the introduction of a neurodiagnostic approach using single magnetic pulses to probe motor outflow,[39] and the use of repeated stimulations to achieve therapeutic benefits in MDD, using either high-frequency (>1 Hz) stimulation with a dorsolateral prefrontal target[40] or low-frequency (≤1 Hz) stimulation over a central (Cz) vertex location.[41] Originally described by some as electrodeless electrical stimulation,[42] the potential of a noninvasive, nonconvulsive neuromodulation approach spurred worldwide interest and a large number of research projects to examine this general approach.

Early reports of TMS in MDD explored a wide range of stimulation parameters, including anatomic target, pulse frequency, number of pulses per session and per course of treatment, and patterning of pulses into trains of different durations and different intertrain intervals; the findings from this dose-finding era were mixed, as is not unexpected with such heterogeneity of treatment paradigms,[43–48] but one consistent set of stimulation parameters that emerged as likely to be beneficial involved a target of the left dorsolateral prefrontal cortex (DLPFC) with pulses delivered at high frequency (10 Hz), in trains (4 seconds on, 26 seconds off), with daily sessions of 3000 pulses, for a course of treatment spanning 4 to 6 weeks. Under double-blind RCT conditions, the clinical efficacy of TMS with these parameters was shown in a 301-subject trial,[49,50] and confirmed in an independent double-blind RCT of 199 subjects.[51] The FDA granted regulatory clearance to one system in 2008 (Neuronetics) and to a second system in 2013 (Brainsway; registration trial data not yet published, with earlier open-label data reported by Harel and colleagues[52] and recent review of published data by Bersani and colleagues[53]).

Table 3 summarizes data from the peer-reviewed published literature on RCTs for TMS. As already noted, although 2 TMS systems have received FDA approval at this time, the trial results for 1 device (Brainsway) have not been published and so are not listed in the table. Based on the data available at the time, an effectiveness review performed for the US Agency for Healthcare Research and Quality[54] concluded that there was clear evidence of efficacy of TMS for pharmacoresistant MDD.

In clinical application, a course of treatment of TMS commonly takes between 4 and 6 weeks, although, anecdotally, some patients may remit sooner and some show a more gradual accrual of clinical benefit beyond this time frame. Treatments can be administered by a solo practitioner psychiatrist, but very often the treating physician is assisted by a system-operator staff person, who helps by monitoring the patient and treatment system during a session. For both approved devices, this begins with personalization of the treatment for the individual patient, in terms of determining how strong a magnetic field should be used and the coordinates of the anatomic target. The assessment of cortical excitability is performed by determining a motor threshold, conventionally relying on the field strength needed to elicit a motor movement in, for example, the abductor pollicis brevis (APB) muscle in the hand. Targeting can be performed as was done in the registration trial[49] using the APB portion of the motor strip as the primary landmark, and identifying the DLPFC region as a standard (5.5 cm)

Table 3
Double-blind, randomized, sham-controlled studies of TMS for depression

Coil Type	Study	Sample Size	Primary Outcome Measure and Time	Primary Response (%)	Primary Remission (%)	End of Trial Response (%)	End of Trial Remission (%)
Figure-of-8 coil	O'Reardon et al,[49] 2007	301	MADRS (wk 4)	18.1 vs 11.0	7.1 vs 6.2	23.9 vs 12.3	14.2 vs 5.5
Figure-of-8 coil	George et al,[51] 2010	199	HAM-D (wk 3)	15 vs 5	14.1 vs 5.1	n.r.	29.9 (open)

Abbreviations: HAM-D, Hamilton Depression Rating Scale; MADRS, Montgomery-Åsberg Depression Rating Scale; n.r., not reported; open, under open conditions at the end of trial (6 weeks).

distance anterior from there. The question has been raised as to whether a slightly different location might be preferable,[55] perhaps scaled to head size using the 10-20 system for electroencephalography electrode placement as a guide.[56,57] Indeed, recent studies have explored other neuronavigation methods to identify a DLPFC target position, either with structural or functional neuroimaging.[58–61] Although these methods may increase anatomic precision of target identification, or may focus target selection based on individual connectivity patterns between deep and superficial brain regions,[62] carefully designed and executed clinical trials will be needed to demonstrate the extent of additional clinical benefit to patients that may accrue from more complex targeting methods.

The course of treatment varies from individual to individual, but typically is in the 4- to 6-week range in real-world care,[63] and consists of in-office treatments 5 days per week, typically using 3000 or more pulses per session. Experimental work has shown that a larger number of stimulation pulses can be safely administered in a day (6800/d by Hadley and colleagues[64] vs the 3000/d in the studies by O'Reardon and colleagues[49] and George and colleagues[51]), and one study suggests that multiple treatment sessions in a single day may accelerate response.[65] Further research is necessary to establish whether the clinical benefits of more intensive courses of treatment are as great or sustained as those of longer, less intensive treatment.

The most commonly reported side effects include discomfort or pain at the stimulation site, tooth or eye pain, muscle twitching, and headache; nonetheless, less than 5% of subjects left the study by O'Reardon and colleagues[49] as a result of all-cause adverse events. A fairly rare but worrisome event is the possibility of a stimulus-driven seizure. No seizures occurred in the with the Neuronetics system in the trial by O'Reardon and colleagues,[49] and one is reported to have happened in the registration trial for Brainsway's H-coil TMS system (online reports and press releases but no peer-reviewed published information). In postmarketing use of the NeuroStar system, the risk of seizures is reported by Neuronetics to be 0.003% per treatment, or less than 1% per acute treatment course (data on file at Neuronetics). In addition, the few seizures that occurred all happened while the patient was observed and being stimulated, so that the treating team was able to intervene rapidly to stop the stimulation session and ensure safety.

Costs of treatment vary from practice to practice, but a course of treatment has been estimated to range between $8000 and $12,000, with the costs proportional to the number of treatments administered.[66] Cost projections for other approaches to TMS (Brainsway's and other devices) are not yet published. Insurance coverage is variable, and even within the Medicare system, TMS is a covered benefit in some regions but not in others. The Medicare Administrative Contractor for much of New England (NHIC Corp) issued a final local coverage decision granting first-in-the-nation Medicare coverage for TMS, effective in early 2012.[67] At present, several private insurers have adopted policies for covering patients who have had a minimum of several treatment failures with pharmacotherapy, while the FDA-approved indication is for adults with unipolar MDD who have had a single drug failure. The American Psychiatric Association's evidence-based Practice Guideline for the Treatment of Patients with Major Depression[68] described that TMS is an option to consider for patients with treatment-resistant depression, but did not clarify where in the treatment algorithm it might best be deployed. An analysis of data from the study by O'Reardon and colleagues[49] reported that higher prior treatment resistance, measured as the number of medications that had failed to be of benefit (ie, higher pharmacoresistance), was associated with poorer outcomes with TMS,[69] suggesting that it may be more usefully deployed earlier than later in the treatment algorithm. Overall, data from controlled trials and from real-world care-seeking patients support the efficacy of TMS in pharmacoresistant MDD, with remission in 30% to 40% of patients and a meaningful durability of remission (58% remain remitters at 3-month follow-up[70]).

TRIGEMINAL NERVE STIMULATION FOR DEPRESSION

The possibility of modulating brain activity via cranial nerve stimulation was demonstrated using stimulation of the vagus nerve (Cranial Nerve X),[71,72] with an initial clinical use for adjunctive treatment of drug-resistant epilepsy (DRE)[73,74] and later research in mood disorders.[75,76] To avoid the potential for cardiac and other vagally mediated adverse events,[77] as well as the need for surgical implantation, DeGiorgio and his colleagues at UCLA began to examine the potential of cranial nerve stimulation via the trigeminal nerve (cranial nerve V) for drug-resistant epilepsy. This structure is the largest cranial nerve and thus presents a high-bandwidth pathway for conveying information to the central nervous system. Unlike the vagus nerve, it contains no autonomic outflow fibers to pose a direct cardiac risk. Also unlike the vagus nerve, large branches can be stimulated transcutaneously using external surface electrodes (external or eTNS), or the identical branches can be stimulated using a minimally invasive, subcutaneously implanted electrodes (sTNS), so that clinical response to sTNS can be predicted with eTNS (as well as eTNS being used a noninvasive therapy in its own right). Because the trigeminal nerve is classically connected with pain (eg, trigeminal neuralgia, trigeminal autonomic cephalgias, dental pain), and prior studies of therapeutic trigeminal stimulation have primarily examined the management of pain,[78–80] the possibility of achieving therapeutic goals in other conditions by stimulation of this pathway was counterintuitive. Nonetheless, the trigeminal system reaches multiple targets of great relevance to psychiatric disorders: trigeminal afferent fibers carry sensory information from the face and project to the nucleus of the tractus solitarius (NTS), the locus coeruleus (LC), the raphe nuclei, the medullary reticular activation system (RAS), and thalamic structures, and from there to sensory, limbic, and other cortical and subcortical structures.[81–84] Neuroimaging data in humans[85] indicate that external transcutaneous stimulation of the V_1 branch of the trigeminal nerve leads acutely to: (1) significant increases in perfusion in structures including anterior cingulate (Brodmann areas [BA] 24, 32), inferior frontal gyrus (BA 44, 6, 22), and medial and middle frontal gyri DLPFC (BA 6, 8, 45, 46); and (2) robust perfusion decreases in primary sensorimotor cortex in the facial area (indicating target engagement), and areas of relevance to anticonvulsant effects, such as superior parietal and medial temporal areas.

Given the well-described projections of the trigeminal system and the benefits reported in DRE, including a double-blind sham-controlled trial,[86–88] an 8-week, proof-of-concept pilot study was undertaken at the University of California Los Angeles including 11 adults with pharmacoresistant MDD.[89,90] Each night, subjects applied the stimulating electrodes (electric patch) over the V_1 distribution of the forehead for approximately 8 hours of stimulation while sleeping. A significant reduction in depression severity was observed on all outcome measures,[90] with 4 of the 11 subjects (36%) remitting by trial end, despite an average of more than 5 treatment failures in the current episode. **Fig. 2**A (solid line) shows the time course of symptom change.

In a second study of 12 adults with combined pharmacoresistant recurrent MDD and posttraumatic stress disorder, a similar pattern of symptom improvement was seen (results presented in a poster[91]), but these results have not yet been disseminated in a peer-reviewed publication. The response trajectory in this sample is shown in **Fig. 2**A along with that from the treatment-resistant depression study,[90] and is remarkably similar in shape despite the comorbidity.

A third line of convergent evidence can be drawn from the phase II randomized clinical trial of TNS in DRE.[88] Under double-blind conditions, subjects were randomized to receive therapeutic

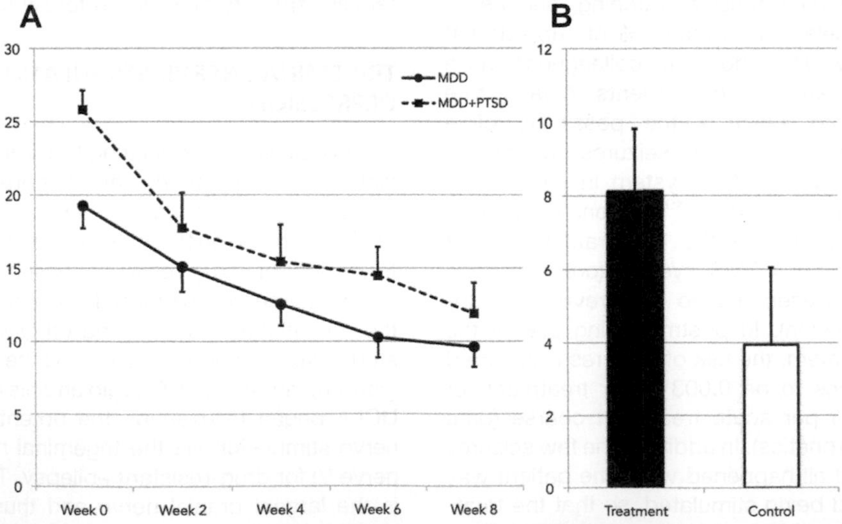

Fig. 2. Effects of eTNS on severity of depression. (*A*) Scores on the 17-item Hamilton Depression Rating Scale for the MDD trial (*solid line*, Cook and colleagues[90]) and the MDD + posttraumatic stress disorder trial (*dashed line*) described in the text.[91] (*B*) Changes in the Beck Depression Inventory for subjects in the two arms of the DRE trial (after DeGiorgio and coleagues[88]). *Data from* Refs.[88,90,91]

TNS at 120 Hz or an active sham with TNS stimulation at a very low frequency (2 Hz). The treatment group showed more than twice the improvement in Beck Depression Inventory score of the sham control group (**Fig. 2**B); interestingly, this improvement was not correlated with improvement in seizure frequency, and so cannot be simply attributed to subjects having fewer seizures and therefore being less depressed. Although depression in epilepsy cannot be assumed to be the same thing as MDD, these data under double-blind conditions are encouraging.

A dose-finding project in pharmacoresistant MDD is currently under way to identify contrasting stimulation conditions for use in a double-blind trial to seek FDA approval. In the meantime, regulatory approval has already been awarded for eTNS in the European Union (CE Mark) and in Canada (Health Canada). In clinical practice in these jurisdictions, eTNS is prescribed like a pharmaceutical product, and there are no device-programming procedures to consider. In an acute course of treatment, the system would be used nightly for 8 weeks. Pricing of the Monarch eTNS System (NeuroSigma, Inc, Los Angeles, CA) has been announced (www.Monarch-eTNS.com), with an 8-week course of treatment costing €1080 (less than US$1500). The durability of remission after an acute course is unknown at present, so it is not possible to forecast whether clinical-use patterns will be more like TMS, with an acute course and then retreatment of a minority of subjects,[92] or more like maintenance pharmacotherapy or maintenance ECT,[93] whereby continued treatment is used to prevent or delay subsequent episodes.

COMPARATIVE EFFICACY OF APPROACHES TO NEUROMODULATION

All of the approaches and devices discussed here must be viewed in the broader context of the rapidly evolving field of neuromodulation. There are several seemingly disparate trends in the development of novel neuromodulation techniques. Some approaches favor treatments that must be delivered to specific neuroanatomic targets, sometimes through invasive means (such as DBS). Other approaches use techniques that are delivered broadly to the brain using nonsignificant-risk devices (such as tDCS or tACS). There are published data to suggest that both highly targeted and nontargeted approaches are beneficial to patients. Although it is beyond the scope of this review, one recent study found that tDCS has efficacy comparable with that of antidepressant medication.[94] What is lacking are studies that compare the efficacy of these contrasting approaches, or that attempt to identify the patients for whom each approach may be the most useful. Given that some of these techniques are costly and proprietary (eg, DBS), whereas others are inexpensive and have little or no patent protection (ie, tDCS), it is unclear when, if ever, such studies will be undertaken.

Even for a single-step neuromodulation technique such as TMS, there is much that is unknown about comparative approaches. The magnetic fields generated by different coil configurations have been examined using finite-element-method models,[95] and the spatial characteristics of the magnetic field, and thus of the induced electric field, can vary considerably; the clinical implications of such variation are not yet well established with regard to either efficacy or safety. In addition, widely varying approaches to TMS are still under development for the treatment of MDD and other indications. These approaches include the use of multiple coils for stimulation[96] (Cervel, Inc, Foster City, CA), low-field magnetic stimulation (LFMS) with low-energy fields[97] (Tal Medical, Inc, Boston, MA), and subthreshold sinusoidal magnetic fields generated by permanent magnets set to rotate at patients' individual α frequency (synchronized TMS or sTMS)[98,99] (NeoSync, Inc, Newport Beach, CA). Trials using these approaches are listed in the ClinicalTrials.gov database. The development of TMS techniques again is marked by seemingly disparate trends between those methods that are predicated on focused delivery of high-field pulses (eg, conventional TMS) and those that use broad delivery of low-intensity energy (eg, sTMS, LFMS). It has been proposed that all forms of TMS may exert a therapeutic effect through a unitary mechanism, namely resetting of oscillators in thalamocortical networks,[99,100] a theory that could explain why all of these methods appear to be efficacious. Given the wide range of potential costs and risks of these devices, comparative efficacy studies would be very useful.

SUMMARY

Patients and clinicians need more therapeutic options for managing MDD, especially forms of the illness that are not responsive to the medications commonly used as first-line treatments. Neuromodulation interventions may have mechanisms of action that differ considerably from the pharmacotherapies, and thus may offer new hope and opportunity for recovery for patients with pharmacoresistant forms of depression. At present, neuromodulation treatments are considered second-line therapies for those who have failed pharmacotherapy and/or psychotherapy. It is possible, however, that these therapies may ultimately be shown to be as or more effective than pharmacotherapy. If less invasive and inexpensive technologies for neuromodulation treatments are proved to be effective, neuromodulation therapies may move to first-line status. Ongoing and future research will expand our knowledge so that physicians can offer patients safe and effective therapies across the clinical spectrum of need.

REFERENCES

1. Kessler RC, Berglund P, Demler O, et al. National Comorbidity Survey Replication. The epidemiology of major depressive disorder: results from the National Comorbidity Survey Replication (NCS-R). JAMA 2003;289:3095–105.
2. World Health Organization. The global burden of disease: 2004 update. WHO Press; 2008. Available at: http://www.who.int/healthinfo/global_burden_disease/GBD_report_2004update_full.pdf. Accessed October 25, 2013.
3. Warden D, Rush AJ, Trivedi MH, et al. The STAR*D Project results: a comprehensive review of findings. Curr Psychiatry Rep 2007;9:449–59.
4. Rush AJ, Trivedi MH, Wisniewski SR, et al. Acute and longer-term outcomes in depressed outpatients requiring one or several treatment steps: a STAR*D report. Am J Psychiatry 2006;163(11):1905–17.
5. Thase ME, Rush AJ. When at first you don't succeed: sequential strategies for antidepressant nonresponders. J Clin Psychiatry 1997;58(Suppl 13):23–9.
6. Sackeim HA. The definition and meaning of treatment-resistant depression. J Clin Psychiatry 2001;62(Suppl 16):10–7.
7. Fava M. Diagnosis and definition of treatment-resistant depression. Biol Psychiatry 2003;53:649–59.
8. Demitrack MA, Thase ME. Clinical significance of transcranial magnetic stimulation (TMS) in the treatment of pharmacoresistant depression: synthesis of recent data. Psychopharmacol Bull 2009;42:5–38.
9. Pallanti S. Images in Psychiatry: Ugo Cerletti 1877-1963. Am J Psychiatry 1999;156(4):630.
10. Bolwig TG. How does electroconvulsive therapy work? Theories on its mechanism. Can J Psychiatry 2011;56:13–8.
11. Taliaz D, Nagaraj V, Haramati S, et al. Altered brain-derived neurotrophic factor expression in the ventral tegmental area, but not in the hippocampus, is essential for antidepressant-like effects of electroconvulsive therapy. Biol Psychiatry 2013;74(4):305–12.
12. Ryan KM, O'Donovan SM, McLoughlin DM. Electroconvulsive stimulation alters levels of BDNF-associated microRNAs. Neurosci Lett 2013;549:125–9.
13. Fink M, Ottosson JO. A theory of convulsive therapy in endogenous depression: significance of hypothalamic functions. Psychiatry Res 1980;2:49–61.
14. Rotter A, Biermann T, Stark C, et al. Changes of cytokine profiles during electroconvulsive therapy in patients with major depression. J ECT 2013;29(3):162–9.
15. Lajoie C, Levasseur MA, Paquet N. Complete normalization of severe brain ^{18}F-FDG hypometabolism following electroconvulsive therapy in a major depressive episode. Clin Nucl Med 2013;38(9):735–6.
16. Pfleiderer B, Michael N, Erfurth A, et al. Effective electroconvulsive therapy reverses glutamate/glutamine deficit in the left anterior cingulum of unipolar depressed patients. Psychiatry Res 2003;122:185–92.
17. Zhang J, Narr KL, Woods RP, et al. Glutamate normalization with ECT treatment response in major depression. Mol Psychiatry 2013;18:268–70.
18. Sakaida M, Sukeno M, Imoto Y, et al. Electroconvulsive seizure-induced changes in gene expression in the mouse hypothalamic paraventricular nucleus. J Psychopharmacol 2013;27:1058–69.
19. Spellman T, Peterchev AV, Lisanby SH. Focal electrically administered seizure therapy: a novel form of ECT illustrates the roles of current directionality, polarity, and electrode configuration in seizure induction. Neuropsychopharmacology 2009;34:2002–10 [Erratum seems in 2012;37:1077].
20. Lisanby SH, Schlaepfer TE, Fisch HU, et al. Magnetic seizure therapy of major depression. Arch Gen Psychiatry 2001;58(3):303–5.
21. Kayser S, Bewernick BH, Hurlemann R, et al. Comparable seizure characteristics in magnetic seizure therapy and electroconvulsive therapy for major depression. Eur Neuropsychopharmacol 2013. http://dx.doi.org/10.1016/j.euroneuro.2013.04.011.
22. Zaghi S, Acar M, Hultgren B, et al. Noninvasive brain stimulation with low-intensity electrical currents: putative mechanisms of action for direct and alternating current stimulation. Neuroscientist 2010;16:285–307.
23. Kalu UG, Sexton CE, Loo CK, et al. Transcranial direct current stimulation in the treatment of major depression: a meta-analysis. Psychol Med 2012;42:1791–800.
24. Datta A, Dmochowski JP, Guleyupoglu B, et al. Cranial electrotherapy stimulation and transcranial pulsed current stimulation: a computer based high-resolution modeling study. Neuroimage 2013;65:280–7.

25. Berlim MT, Van den Eynde F, Daskalakis ZJ. Clinical utility of transcranial direct current stimulation (tDCS) for treating major depression: a systematic review and meta-analysis of randomized, double-blind and sham-controlled trials. J Psychiatr Res 2013;47(1):1–7.
26. Delgado JM. Free behavior and brain stimulation. Int Rev Neurobiol 1964;6:349–449.
27. Delgado JM, Mark V, Sweet W, et al. Intracerebral radio stimulation and recording in completely free patients. J Nerv Ment Dis 1968;147:329–40.
28. Andy OJ. Thalamic stimulation for control of movement disorders. Appl Neurophysiol 1983; 46:107–11.
29. Benabid AL, Pollak P, Louveau A, et al. Combined (thalamotomy and stimulation) stereotactic surgery of the VIM thalamic nucleus for bilateral Parkinson disease. Appl Neurophysiol 1987;50: 344–6.
30. Hauptman JS, DeSalles AA, Espinoza R, et al. Potential surgical targets for deep brain stimulation in treatment-resistant depression. Neurosurg Focus 2008;25:E3. http://dx.doi.org/10.3171/FOC/2008/25/7/E3.
31. Anderson RJ, Frye MA, Abulseoud OA, et al. Deep brain stimulation for treatment-resistant depression: efficacy, safety and mechanisms of action. Neurosci Biobehav Rev 2012;36:1920–33.
32. Hamani C, Nobrega JN. Preclinical studies modeling deep brain stimulation for depression. Biol Psychiatry 2012;72:916–23.
33. Dzirasa K, Lisanby SH. How does deep brain stimulation work? Biol Psychiatry 2012;72:892–4.
34. Ramasubbu R, Anderson S, Haffenden A, et al. Double-blind optimization of subcallosal cingulate deep brain stimulation for treatment-resistant depression: a pilot study. J Psychiatry Neurosci 2013; 38:325–32.
35. Kennedy SH, Giacobbe P, Rizvi SJ, et al. Deep brain stimulation for treatment-resistant depression: follow-up after 3 to 6 years. Am J Psychiatry 2011;168:502–10.
36. Cusin C, Dougherty DD. Somatic therapies for treatment-resistant depression: ECT, TMS, VNS, DBS. Biol Mood Anxiety Disord 2012;2:14 Correction: Biol Mood Anxiety Disord. 2013;3:1.
37. Reported by Cyberonics. Available at: http://ir.cyberonics.com/releasedetail.cfm?ReleaseID=767670. Accessed July 31, 2013.
38. George MS, Belmaker RH. Transcranial magnetic stimulation in clinical psychiatry. Arlington (VA): Amer Psychiatric Press; 2006.
39. Barker AT, Jalinous R, Freeston IL. Non-invasive magnetic stimulation of human motor cortex. Lancet 1985;1(8437):1106–7.
40. George MS, Wassermann EM, Williams WA, et al. Daily repetitive transcranial magnetic stimulation (rTMS) improves mood in depression. Neuroreport 1995;6:1853–6.
41. Kolbinger MH, Höflich1 G, Hufnagel A, et al. Transcranial magnetic stimulation (TMS) in the treatment of major depression—a pilot study. Hum Psychopharmacol Clin Exp 1995;10:305–10.
42. George MS, Lisanby SH, Sackeim HA. Transcranial magnetic stimulation: applications in neuropsychiatry. Arch Gen Psychiatry 1999;56:300–11.
43. George MS, Wassermann EM. Rapid-rate transcranial magnetic stimulation and ECT. Convuls Ther 1994;10:251–4.
44. George MS, Nahas Z, Molloy M, et al. A controlled trial of daily left prefrontal cortex TMS for treating depression. Biol Psychiatry 2000;48:962–70.
45. Martin JL, Barbanoj MJ, Schlaepfer TE, et al. Transcranial magnetic stimulation for treating depression. Cochrane Database Syst Rev 2002;(2):CD003493.
46. Slotema CW, Blom JD, Hoek HW, et al. Should we expand the toolbox of psychiatric treatment methods to include Repetitive Transcranial Magnetic Stimulation (rTMS)? A meta-analysis of the efficacy of rTMS in psychiatric disorders. J Clin Psychiatry 2010;71:873–84.
47. Berlim MT, Van den Eynde F, Jeff Daskalakis Z. Clinically meaningful efficacy and acceptability of low-frequency repetitive transcranial magnetic stimulation (rTMS) for treating primary major depression: a meta-analysis of randomized, double-blind and sham-controlled trials. Neuropsychopharmacology 2013;38:543–51.
48. Berlim MT, van den Eynde F, Tovar-Perdomo S, et al. Response, remission and drop-out rates following high-frequency repetitive transcranial magnetic stimulation (rTMS) for treating major depression: a systematic review and meta-analysis of randomized, double-blind and sham-controlled trials. Psychol Med 2013. http://dx.doi.org/10.1017/S0033291713000512.
49. O'Reardon JP, Solvason HB, Janicak PG, et al. Efficacy and safety of transcranial magnetic stimulation in the acute treatment of major depression: a multisite randomized controlled trial. Biol Psychiatry 2007;62:1208–16.
50. Janicak PG, O'Reardon JP, Sampson SM, et al. Transcranial magnetic stimulation in the treatment of major depressive disorder: a comprehensive summary of safety experience from acute exposure, extended exposure, and during reintroduction treatment. J Clin Psychiatry 2008;69:222–32.
51. George MS, Lisanby SH, Avery D, et al. Daily left prefrontal transcranial magnetic stimulation therapy for major depressive disorder: a sham-controlled randomized trial. Arch Gen Psychiatry 2010;67:507–16.
52. Harel EV, Rabany L, Deutsch L, et al. H-coil repetitive transcranial magnetic stimulation for treatment

resistant major depressive disorder: an 18-week continuation safety and feasibility study. World J Biol Psychiatry 2013. http://dx.doi.org/10.3109/15622975.2011.639802.

53. Bersani FS, Minichino A, Enticott PG, et al. Deep transcranial magnetic stimulation as a treatment for psychiatric disorders: a comprehensive review. Eur Psychiatry 2013;28:30–9.
54. Gaynes BN, Lux LJ, Lloyd SW, et al. AHRQ Comparative Effectiveness Review 33: nonpharmacologic interventions for treatment-resistant depression in adults. AHRQ Publication 11-EHC056-EF. Rockville (MD): Agency for Healthcare Research and Quality; 2011. Available at: http://effectivehealthcare.ahrq.gov/ehc/products/76/792/TRD_CER33_20111110.pdf. Accessed October 25, 2013.
55. Herbsman T, Avery D, Ramsey D, et al. More lateral and anterior prefrontal coil location is associated with better repetitive transcranial magnetic stimulation antidepressant response. Biol Psychiatry 2009;66:509–15.
56. Herwig U, Satrapi P, Schönfeldt-Lecuona C. Using the international 10-20 EEG system for positioning of transcranial magnetic stimulation. Brain Topogr 2003;16:95–9.
57. Beam W, Borckardt JJ, Reeves ST, et al. An efficient and accurate new method for locating the F3 position for prefrontal TMS applications. Brain Stimul 2009;2:50–4.
58. Herwig U, Padberg F, Unger J, et al. Transcranial magnetic stimulation in therapy studies: examination of the reliability of "standard" coil positioning by neuronavigation. Biol Psychiatry 2001;50:58–61.
59. Peleman K, Van Schuerbeek P, Luypaert R, et al. Using 3D-MRI to localize the dorsolateral prefrontal cortex in TMS research. World J Biol Psychiatry 2010;11:425–30.
60. Fitzgerald PB, Hoy K, McQueen S, et al. A randomized trial of rTMS targeted with MRI based neuro-navigation in treatment-resistant depression. Neuropsychopharmacology 2009;34:1255–62.
61. Trojak B, Meille V, Chauvet-Gelinier JC, et al. Further evidence of the usefulness of MRI-based neuronavigation for the treatment of depression by rTMS. J Neuropsychiatry Clin Neurosci 2011;23:E30–1.
62. Fox MD, Liu H, Pascual-Leone A. Identification of reproducible individualized targets for treatment of depression with TMS based on intrinsic connectivity. Neuroimage 2012;66C:151–60.
63. Carpenter LL, Janicak PG, Aaronson ST, et al. Transcranial magnetic stimulation (TMS) for major depression: a multisite, naturalistic, observational study of acute treatment outcomes in clinical practice. Depress Anxiety 2012;29:587–96.
64. Hadley D, Anderson BS, Borckardt JJ, et al. Safety, tolerability, and effectiveness of high doses of adjunctive daily left prefrontal repetitive transcranial magnetic stimulation for treatment-resistant depression in a clinical setting. J ECT 2011;27:18–25.
65. Holtzheimer PE 3rd, McDonald WM, Mufti M, et al. Accelerated repetitive transcranial magnetic stimulation for treatment-resistant depression. Depress Anxiety 2010;27:960–3.
66. URL Available at: http://www.usatoday.com/story/news/2012/11/30/magnets-zap-depression/1738621/. Accessed July 31, 2013.
67. URL Available at: http://www.icer-review.org/index.php/Announcements/maclcd.html. Accessed July 31, 2013.
68. American Psychiatric Association. Practice guideline for the treatment of patients with major depressive disorder. 3rd edition. Arlington (VA): Amer Psychiatric Press Inc; 2010. http://dx.doi.org/10.1176/appi.books.9780890423307.654001.
69. Lisanby SH, Husain MM, Rosenquist PB, et al. Daily left prefrontal repetitive transcranial magnetic stimulation in the acute treatment of major depression: clinical predictors of outcome in a multisite, randomized controlled clinical trial. Neuropsychopharmacology 2009;34:522–34.
70. George MS, Taylor JJ, Short EB. The expanding evidence base for rTMS treatment of depression. Curr Opin Psychiatry 2013;26(1):13–8.
71. Bailey P, Bremer F. A sensory cortical representation of the vagus nerve. J Neurophysiol 1938;1(5):405–12.
72. George MS, Sackeim HA, Rush AJ, et al. Vagus nerve stimulation: a new tool for brain research and therapy. Biol Psychiatry 2000;47:287–95.
73. Ben-Menachem E, Mañon-Espaillat R, Ristanovic R, et al. Vagus nerve stimulation for treatment of partial seizures: 1. A controlled study of effect on seizures. First International Vagus Nerve Stimulation Study Group. Epilepsia 1994;35:616–26.
74. Handforth A, DeGiorgio CM, Schachter SC, et al. Vagus nerve stimulation therapy for partial-onset seizures: a randomized active-control trial. Neurology 1998;51:48–55.
75. Rush AJ, George MS, Sackeim HA, et al. Vagus nerve stimulation (VNS) for treatment-resistant depressions: a multicenter study. Biol Psychiatry 2000;47:276–86.
76. Aaronson ST, Carpenter LL, Conway CR, et al. Vagus nerve stimulation therapy randomized to different amounts of electrical charge for treatment-resistant depression: acute and chronic effects. Brain Stimul 2013;6:631–40.

77. Matheny RG, Shaar CJ. Vagus nerve stimulation as a method to temporarily slow or arrest the heart. Ann Thorac Surg 1997;63:S28–9.
78. Reuter E, Krekeler G, Krainick JU, et al. Pain suppression in the trigeminal region by means of transcutaneous nerve stimulation. Dtsch Zahnarztl Z 1976;31:274–6 [in German].
79. Hellsing G. Transcutaneous neural stimulation (TNS) in chronic pain in patients with temporomandibular joint disorders. A clinical report. Tandlakartidningen 1976;68:789–93 [in Swedish].
80. Augustinsson LE, Bohlin P, Bundsen P, et al. Pain relief during delivery by transcutaneous electrical nerve stimulation. Pain 1977;4:59–65.
81. Caous CA, de Sousa Buck H, Lindsey CJ. Neuronal connections of the paratrigeminal nucleus: a topographic analysis of neurons projecting to bulbar, pontine and thalamic nuclei related to cardiovascular, respiratory and sensory functions. Auton Neurosci 2001;94:14–24.
82. de Sousa Buck H, Caous CA, Lindsey CJ. Projections of the paratrigeminal nucleus to the ambiguus, rostroventrolateral and lateral reticular nuclei, and the solitary tract. Auton Neurosci 2001;87:187–200.
83. Gura EV, Garkavenko VV, Limansky YuP. Influences of central gray matter stimulation on thalamic neuron responses to high- and low-threshold stimulation of trigeminal nerve structures. Neuroscience 1991;41:681–93.
84. Fanselow EE. Central mechanisms of cranial nerve stimulation for epilepsy. Surg Neurol Int 2012;3: S247–54.
85. Schrader LM, Geist CL, DeGiorgio CM, et al. Regional PET activations with trigeminal nerve stimulation (TNS) and correlation with therapeutic response. American Epilepsy Society Annual Meeting online abstract 2.279. Available at: http://www.aesnet.org/go/publications/aes-abstracts/abstract-search/mode/display?id=15012. Accessed October 25, 2013.
86. DeGiorgio CM, Murray D, Markovic D, et al. Trigeminal nerve stimulation for epilepsy: long-term feasibility and efficacy. Neurology 2009;72:936–8.
87. DeGiorgio CM, Fanselow EE, Schrader LM, et al. Trigeminal nerve stimulation: seminal animal and human studies for epilepsy and depression. Neurosurg Clin N Am 2011;22:449–56.
88. DeGiorgio CM, Soss J, Cook IA, et al. Randomized controlled trial of trigeminal nerve stimulation for drug-resistant epilepsy. Neurology 2013;80: 786–91.
89. Schrader LM, Cook IA, Miller PR, et al. Trigeminal nerve stimulation in major depressive disorder: first proof of concept in an open pilot trial. Epilepsy Behav 2011;22:475–8.
90. Cook IA, Schrader LM, Degiorgio CM, et al. Trigeminal nerve stimulation in major depressive disorder: acute outcomes in an open pilot study. Epilepsy Behav 2013;28:221–6.
91. Cook IA, DeGiorgio CM, Leuchter AF. Trigeminal nerve stimulation in post-traumatic stress disorder and major depression: a novel neuromodulation approach. NCDEU Annual Meeting. Poster I-7. Hollywood (FL), May 28-30, 2013.
92. Janicak PG, Nahas Z, Lisanby SH, et al. Durability of clinical benefit with transcranial magnetic stimulation (TMS) in the treatment of pharmacoresistant major depression: assessment of relapse during a 6-month, multisite, open-label study. Brain Stimul 2010;3:187–99.
93. Rabheru K. Maintenance electroconvulsive therapy (M-ECT) after acute response: examining the evidence for who, what, when, and how? J ECT 2012;28(1):39–47.
94. Brunoni AR, Valiengo L, Baccaro A, et al. The sertraline vs. electrical current therapy for treating depression clinical study: results from a factorial, randomized, controlled trial. JAMA Psychiatry 2013;70:383–91.
95. Deng ZD, Lisanby SH, Peterchev AV. Electric field depth-focality tradeoff in transcranial magnetic stimulation: simulation comparison of 50 coil designs. Brain Stimul 2013;6:1–13.
96. Tzabazis A, Aparici CM, Rowbotham MC, et al. Shaped magnetic field pulses by multi-coil repetitive transcranial magnetic stimulation (rTMS) differentially modulate anterior cingulate cortex responses and pain in volunteers and fibromyalgia patients. Mol Pain 2013;9:33.
97. Rohan M, Parow A, Stoll AL, et al. Low-field magnetic stimulation in bipolar depression using an MRI-based stimulator. Am J Psychiatry 2004;161: 93–8.
98. Jin Y, Potkin SG, Kemp AS, et al. Therapeutic effects of individualized alpha frequency transcranial magnetic stimulation (alphaTMS) on the negative symptoms of schizophrenia. Schizophr Bull 2006;32:556–61.
99. Leuchter AF, Cook IA, Jin Y, et al. The relationship between brain oscillatory activity and therapeutic effectiveness of transcranial magnetic stimulation in the treatment of major depressive disorder. Front Hum Neurosci 2013;7:37.
100. Fuggetta G, Noh NA. A neurophysiological insight into the potential link between transcranial magnetic stimulation, thalamocortical dysrhythmia and neuropsychiatric disorders. Exp Neurol 2013;245: 87–95.
101. Mayberg HS, Lozano AM, Voon V, et al. Deep brain stimulation for treatment-resistant depression. Neuron 2005;45:651–60.

102. Lozano AM, Mayberg HS, Giacobbe P, et al. Subcallosal cingulate gyrus deep brain stimulation for treatment-resistant depression. Biol Psychiatry 2008;64:461–7.
103. Neimat JS, Hamani C, Giacobbe P, et al. Neural stimulation successfully treats depression in patients with prior ablative cingulotomy. Am J Psychiatry 2008;165:687–93.
104. Lozano AM, Giacobbe P, Hamani C, et al. A multicenter pilot study of subcallosal cingulate area deep brain stimulation for treatment-resistant depression. J Neurosurg 2012;116:315–22.
105. Puigdemont D, Pérez-Egea R, Portella MJ, et al. Deep brain stimulation of the subcallosal cingulate gyrus: further evidence in treatment-resistant major depression. Int J Neuropsychopharmacol 2012;15:121–33.
106. Holtzheimer PE, Kelley ME, Gross RE, et al. Subcallosal cingulate deep brain stimulation for treatment-resistant unipolar and bipolar depression. Arch Gen Psychiatry 2012;69:150–8.
107. Malone DA Jr, Dougherty DD, Rezai AR, et al. Deep brain stimulation of the ventral capsule/ventral striatum for treatment-resistant depression. Biol Psychiatry 2009;65:267–75.
108. Malone DA Jr. Use of deep brain stimulation in treatment-resistant depression. Cleve Clin J Med 2010;77(Suppl 3):S77–80.
109. Schlaepfer TE, Cohen MX, Frick C, et al. Deep brain stimulation to reward circuitry alleviates anhedonia in refractory major depression. Neuropsychopharmacology 2008;33:368–77.
110. Bewernick BH, Hurlemann R, Matusch A, et al. Nucleus accumbens deep brain stimulation decreases ratings of depression and anxiety in treatment-resistant depression. Biol Psychiatry 2010;67:110–6.
111. Bewernick BH, Kayser S, Sturm V, et al. Long-term effects of nucleus accumbens deep brain stimulation in treatment-resistant depression: evidence for sustained efficacy. Neuropsychopharmacology 2012;37:1975–85.
112. Jiménez F, Velasco F, Salin-Pascual R, et al. A patient with a resistant major depression disorder treated with deep brain stimulation in the inferior thalamic peduncle. Neurosurgery 2005;57:585–93.
113. Jiménez F, Velasco F, Salín-Pascual R, et al. Neuromodulation of the inferior thalamic peduncle for major depression and obsessive compulsive disorder. Acta Neurochir Suppl. 2007;97(Pt 2):393–8.
114. Sartorius A, Kiening KL, Kirsch P, et al. Remission of major depression under deep brain stimulation of the lateral habenula in a therapy-refractory patient. Biol Psychiatry 2010;67:e9–11.
115. Schlaepfer TE, Bewernick BH, Kayser S, et al. Rapid effects of deep brain stimulation for treatment-resistant major depression. Biol Psychiatry 2013;73:1204–12.
116. Kosel M, Sturm V, Frick C, et al. Mood improvement after deep brain stimulation of the internal globus pallidus for tardive dyskinesia in a patient suffering from major depression. J Psychiatr Res. 2007;41:801–3.

Deep Brain Stimulation for Tourette Syndrome

Won Kim, MD[a,*], Nader Pouratian, MD, PhD[a,b,c,d]

KEYWORDS

• Deep brain stimulation • Tourette Syndrome • Tics • Neuromodulation

KEY POINTS

- Deep brain stimulation seems to be efficacious in reducing the frequency and severity of tics in many patients with medically refractory Tourette syndrome.
- The 2 most commonly accepted targets, based on clinical experience and expert opinion, are the centromedian-parafascicular nucleus of the thalamus and the internal globus pallidus.
- Patients with Tourette syndrome seem to be more prone to the infectious complications of deep brain stimulation surgery, including hardware and wound infections.
- Future multicenter clinical trials, and the sharing of the results thereof through the Tourette Syndrome Association online database (http://dbs.tsa-usa.org/), are necessary to determine the efficacy of stimulation at various target sites.

INTRODUCTION

Gilles de la Tourette syndrome (TS) is a movement disorder characterized by repetitive motor and phonic/vocal tics first described in 1885 by George Edouard Albert Brutus Gilles de la Tourette. The onset of the disease is typically during adolescence, with a natural history that consists of the waxing and waning of tics until the second decade of life, when many patients experience almost complete resolution of symptoms.[1] As such, the prevalence of the disease is higher in children, with nearly 1% of the pediatric population being affected, whereas only 0.05% of adults carry the diagnosis.[2] Although the severity and frequency of tics diminishes considerably in adulthood, most patients still have identifiable tics, albeit they are mild and infrequent enough to not require treatment.[3]

In addition to the motor features, TS commonly has multiple neuropsychiatric comorbidities including obsessive-compulsive disorder (OCD), attention-deficit/hyperactivity disorder (ADHD), autistic spectrum disorder, and many others, with almost 90% of patients showing some concomitant disorder.[4] As such, in addition to neuroleptic medications used to control tics, other medications including antidepressants are used to treat these psychiatric comorbidities as well.[5]

Despite advancements in behavioral and pharmacologic therapies, there remains a subset of patients with TS who are resistant to these management modalities.[6,7] As a result, there have been attempts to alter the underlying pathologic neural circuitry to alleviate, if not eliminate, tics by manipulating subcortical circuits. The first report of such methods was in 1970 by Hassler and colleagues,[8] who showed partial relief of tics through the ablative lesioning of thalamic nuclei including the median and rostral intralaminar nuclei and the internal ventral oral nucleus. Subsequent studies reproduced varying degrees of

[a] Department of Neurosurgery, University of California, Los Angeles 10945, Le Conte Avenue, Suite 2120, Los Angeles, CA 90095, USA; [b] Interdepartmental Program in Neuroscience, University of California, Los Angeles 10945, Le Conte Avenue, Suite 2120, Los Angeles, CA 90095, USA; [c] Department of Bioengineering, University of California, Los Angeles 10945, Le Conte Avenue, Suite 2120, Los Angeles, CA 90095, USA; [d] Brain Research Institute, University of California, Los Angeles 10945, Le Conte Avenue, Suite 2120, Los Angeles, CA 90095, USA
* Corresponding author.
E-mail address: wonism@gmail.com

Neurosurg Clin N Am 25 (2014) 117–135
http://dx.doi.org/10.1016/j.nec.2013.08.009
1042-3680/14/$ – see front matter

symptomatic relief, but at the cost of considerable, and frequent, postoperative morbidity including dysarthria, dystonia, and hemiparesis.[9,10]

In 1999, Vandewalle and colleagues[11] reported on the first deep brain stimulation (DBS) of a patient with medically refractory TS. The stereotactic target was the centromedian-parafascicular (CM-Pf) nucleus and the ventro-oral internus (Voi) of the thalamus based on the work by Hassler and colleagues.[8] The patient experienced a complete resolution of tics and tolerated the procedure well with only minimal neurologic sequelae from stimulation (excessive eye blinking). They and numerous other investigators have subsequently examined the effects of DBS at various targets within the corticostriatothalamocortical (CSTC) network thought to be implicated in the pathophysiology of TS, including the CM-Pf/Voi,[11–32] the globus pallidus internus (GPi),[14,16,17,22,30,33–40] globus pallidus externus (GPe),[41] the anterior limb of the internal capsule (ALIC),[21,22,42,43] the nucleus accumbens (NA),[21,22,44–46] and the subthalamic nucleus (STN).[47]

It is thought that through an aberrancy of the CSTC circuitry, the normal gating mechanisms of the basal ganglia in facilitating and inhibiting competing motor, limbic, and cognitive processes are disturbed, resulting in stereotyped behaviors or tics.[48–50] Although the various hubs within this network allow for a diverse selection of targets for neuromodulation, it has resulted in a collection of nearly 40 studies describing more than 100 patients with varying targets, stimulation parameters, and follow-up time. This article consolidates and summarizes the DBS experience for TS to date.

TARGETS FOR TS NEUROMODULATION

Methods for Literature Review

A PubMed search was conducted with the following terms alone or in combination: deep brain stimulation, DBS, Tourette syndrome, and Tourette's syndrome. Articles describing the implantation of patients with TS with DBS leads were identified, and their references used to acquire other articles not immediately found on initial PubMed query. Thirty-nine articles describing the experience of various groups with DBS for TS were found and included in our analysis. The results of the studies are reported here by target of stimulation.

CM-Pf Nucleus and the Voi Nucleus of the Thalamus

The initial target for DBS for TS was based on thalamic lesioning studies performed by Hassler and colleagues[8] in the late twentieth century. This target, namely the centromedian-parafascicular (CM-Pf) nucleus of the thalamus, along with the Voi, is thought to be situated in a unique position within the action-gating pathways of the basal ganglia.[51] Diffusion tensor imaging (DTI) studies in humans show structural connectivity between the CM-Pf nucleus and the putamen, pallidum, NA, amygdala, and hippocampus.[52] These findings corroborate primate studies that reveal sensorimotor projections from the ventrolateral GPi (motor pallidum) to the CM thalamus, and limbic projections from the ventral striatum/NA to the anteromedial GPi (limbic pallidum), which in turn projects to the rostral Pf thalamus and then back to the ventral striatum/NA region (**Fig. 1**).[53] Through

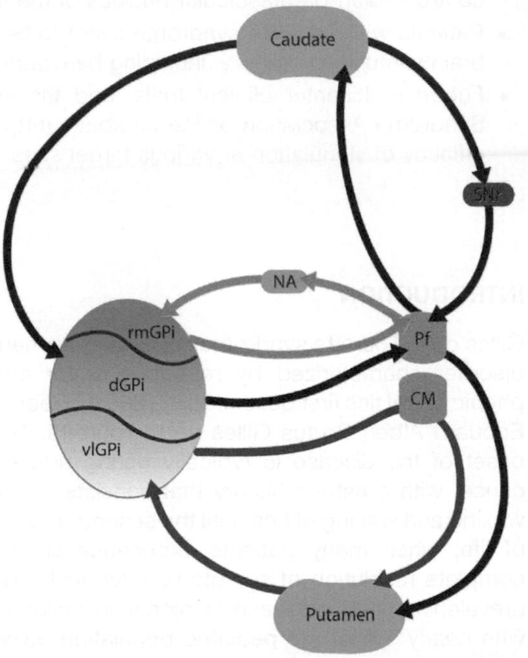

Fig. 1. The putative connectivity of the CSTC circuit in relation to TS DBS targets. The rostromedial (limbic) GPi has limbic projections to the Pf nucleus of the thalamus, which in turn projects to the NA/ventral striatum, which then projects back to the rostromedial GPi (*gray arrows*). The sensorimotor connectivity consists of projections from the ventrolateral (motor) GPi to the CM nucleus of the thalamus, which then projects to the putamen, which then projects back to the ventrolateral GPi (*red arrows*). The cognitive connectivity of the CSTC circuit consists of 2 loops. One consists of projections from the caudate to the dorsal GPi, which in turn projects to the Pf nucleus of the thalamus, which then projects to the putamen (*black arrows*). The other also arises from the caudate, but projects instead to the SNr, and then to the Pf nucleus of the thalamus (*black arrows*). Diagram based on primate studies performed by Sidibe and colleagues[53] (2002). dGPi, dorsal GPi; rmGPi, rostromedial GPi; SNr, substantia nigra pars reticulata; vlGPi, ventrolateral GPi.

modulating the excitatory feedback loops between the CM-Pf/Voi and the motor and limbic striatum, it is thought that the observed benefits of DBS for TS are achieved.[54]

To date there have been 20 published reports detailing approximately 68 distinct patients who have received DBS at the CM-Pf and Voi thalamus (**Table 1**). The initial report of the clinical success of CM-Pf/Voi DBS for TS was promising, with complete resolution of tics at 12 months.[11] However, on long-term follow-up (10 years), the patient had sustained only 78% tic reduction. Despite the decline in symptom improvement in this patient, another patient was found by the same group to have 93% tic reduction at 6 years, supporting the longevity of tic suppression with stimulation.[13] Other studies have reported similarly promising results using a well-regarded clinical measure for TS, the Yale Global Tic Severity Scale (YGTSS), which details patient severity by tics, functional impairment, and overall score.[55] At the last assessment (range 2–120 months), the reduction in the mean global YGTSS score for each study ranged from 19% to 78%,[11–28,31,32] although some individual patients had as little as 5% improvement.[20] Notable exceptions include 2 patients reported by Maciunas and colleagues[19] who did not experience any significant relief of their tics at 3 months' follow-up. In addition, Duits and colleagues[29] detailed their experience with 1 patient who experienced an increase in tics during double-blinded stimulation. This patient was thought to have severe concomitant psychiatric comorbidity that led to her refusal to eat and eventually to her death.

GPi

Soon after the success in stimulating the CM-Pf/Voi thalamus, parallel efforts were made to achieve similar results at other targets within the CSTC network. A total of 32 patients were implanted in the GPi, of whom 3 patients had simultaneous CM-Pf/Voi and GPi implantation and 1 patient had simultaneous ALIC/NA and GPi implantation. Houeto and colleagues[14] published one of the first reports in stimulating the GPi in a patient in whom bilateral thalamic as well as pallidal electrodes were implanted. The patient experienced similar reductions in YGTSS scores with CM-Pf/Voi and anteromedial GPi stimulation at various follow-up assessments in a double-blinded prospective study with a sham control period. The patient experienced these comparable results with stimulation at the limbic GPi, the portion of the pallidum not traditionally used in treating dystonia. However, long-term follow-up by the same group with an additional 2 patients revealed that GPi stimulation had more favorable results, with 78% YGTSS reduction, whereas CM-Pf stimulation provided only 45% reduction in scores.[16]

Following these initial promising results with the implantation and stimulation of the anteromedial GPi, numerous groups published their outcomes with stimulation of the posteroventral GPi, a region typically modulated in the DBS treatment of Parkinson disease and dystonia. Of the 16 patients who have received DBS of the posterolateral GPi for TS to date, 13 have received some benefit with 20% to 88% mean global reductions in YGTSS[33,34,36,37,39] and significant reductions in the number of observed tics,[17,30,35] even with unilateral lead placement.[56] These are comparable with the 38% to 78% mean global YGTSS reductions seen with anteromedial stimulation.[14,16,39,40] However, 3 patients from 2 different studies[37,38] did not experience any objective benefit from stimulation at the ventrolateral GPi. In one such case, in addition to being a pediatric patient, Dueck and colleagues[38] postulated that the lack of improvement could be attributed to the patient's intellectual impairment, which may have provided a baseline neurologic substrate distinct from those patients with TS who have concomitant psychiatric disease instead. The other 2 patients who failed to experience any significant reduction in YGTSS scores with ventrolateral GPi stimulation were part of a cohort in which 2 other patients received considerable benefit (64% and 88%).[37] These findings suggest that, at least for the GPi, there may be some patients who respond better than others, and some who receive no benefit.

Globus Pallidus Externus

Piedimonte and colleagues[41] describe the only report available in English regarding the implantation of the globus pallidus externus (GPe), although they credit the work done by Vilela Filho and colleagues[57] as the precedent for their study. With stimulation of the GPe, they were able to reduce the global YGTSS score by 70.5% at 6 months' follow-up.

ALIC and NA

The anterior limb of the internal capsule facilitates cognitive, motor, and limbic functions through its frontothalamic and frontostriatal connections, and has consequently been used as a target in the DBS treatment of medically refractory OCD.[58,59] Given the poorly understood involvement of TS in all of these domains, and the high incidence of comorbid OCD in patients with TS,

Table 1
Comprehensive summary of clinical studies involving TS DBS to date

Investigators	Patient Sex, Age (y)	Follow-up (mo)	Targets	Stimulation Parameters	Outcomes (Reduction in YGTSS/MRVRS)	Complications: Sequelae of Stimulation (Number of Patients)	Comments
Vandewalle et al,[11] 1999[a]	1 M (42)	12	CM-Pf, Voi	4 V, 130 Hz, 450 μs (at 1 y, 1.5 V was sufficient to abolish all tics)	Complete resolution of tics	Excessive eye blinking	—
Visser-Vandewalle et al,[12] 2003[a]	3 M (28, 42, 45)	8, 12, 60	CM-Pf, Voi	2.2–3 V, 65–100 Hz, 210 μs	82% mean reduction in number of tics	Decreased energy. Increased libido (1), decreased libido (1)	One pt is from Vandewalle et al,[11] 1999 study
Ackermans et al,[13] 2010[a]	2 M (42, 45)	72 and 120	CM-Pf, Voi	1–8 V, 100–130 Hz, 90–210 μs	85% mean reduction in number of tics	Reduction in energy	Long-term follow-up of Visser-Vandewalle et al,[12] 2003. Mild decrease in verbal fluency; transient worsening on Stroop task
Houeto et al,[14] 2005[b]	1 F (36)	24	CM-Pf and amGPi	1.5 V, 130 Hz, 60 μs	CM-Pf, 65% (global YGTSS)/77% (MRVRS); GPi, 65% (global YGTSS)/67% (MRVRS); CM-Pf + GPi stimulation, 60% (global YGTSS)/77% (MRVRS)	CM-Pf: weight loss. GPi: nausea, hypotonia and anxiety with increasing voltage	Implanted with both thalamic and GPi leads. Was not cumulative stimulation because they had different stimulation stages; prospective double-blinded study (with sham control)

Welter et al,[16] 2008[b]	2 F, 1 M (36, 30; 30)	60, 27, 20	CM-Pf and amGPi	CM-Pf, 1.5–1.7 V. 130 Hz, 60 μs. GPi, 1.5–3.5 V, 130 Hz, 60 μs	Mean reductions during blinded stimulation periods: GPi, 78% (global YGTSS); CM-Pf, 45% (global YGTSS). CM-Pf + GPi, 60% (global YGTSS)	Transient cheiro-oral or arm paresthesias (few minutes) or lethargy (3–4 d); nausea (2), vertigo (2), anxiety (1), decreased libido (1)	Implanted with both thalamic and GPi leads. Prospective, randomized, crossover trial using double-blind assessments comparing thalamic and GPi stimulation. Best improvement seen with GPi stimulation. Two of 3 were able to reintegrate socially
Flaherty et al,[22] 2005	1 M (27)	18	ALIC	4.1 V, 185 Hz, 210 μs	20% (global YGTSS), 17% (tic YGTSS), 25% (impairment YGTSS)	Hypomania when dorsal in body of capsule vs apathy/depression in NA	—
Diederich et al,[33] 2005	1 M (27)	14	pvlGPi	2 V, 185 Hz, 120–150 μs	47% (global YGTSS); 44% (tic YGTSS)	Small ICH in right pallidum; bradykinesia of left hand Transient fatigue for a few months	—
Ackermans et al,[17] 2006 Ackermans et al,[30] 2007	2 M (27, 45)	12	CM-Pf, Voi (1); pvlGPi (1)	CM-Pf, 6.4 V, 130 Hz, 120 μs; GPi, 3.1 V, 170 Hz, 210 μs	CM-Pf, 85% reduction in number of tics/min; GPi, 93% reduction in number of tics/min	Small ICH in midbrain; vertical gaze palsy Decreased energy, decreased libido (1); vertical gaze palsy (1)	—

(continued on next page)

Table 1
(continued)

Investigators	Patient Sex, Age (y)	Follow-up (mo)	Targets	Stimulation Parameters	Outcomes (Reduction in YGTSS/MRVRS)	Complications: Sequelae of Stimulation (Number of Patients)	Comments
Shahed et al,[34] 2006	1 M (16)	6	pvlGPi	5 V, 145–160 Hz, 90 μs	76% (global YGTSS), 72% (tics YGTSS)/21% (RVBTS)	—	First adolescent patient; YBOCS improved 69% (mostly obsessions). Neurocognitive testing indicated improvement in verbal reasoning, psychomotor speed, mental flexibility, and visual perception, with poorer memory
Gallagher et al,[35] (2006)	1 M (26)	Several months	pvlGPi	NA	Disappearance of vocal tics, improvement of motor tics	Infection requiring hardware removal (1)	—
Kuhn et al,[44] 2007	1 M (26)	30	NA	7 V, 130 Hz, 90 μs	41% (global YGTSS)/ 50% (MRVRS)	—	52% decrease in YBOCS
Bajwa et al,[18] 2007	1 M (48)	24	CM-Pf, Voi	2 V, 130 Hz, 90 μs	66% (tic YGTSS)	Occasional oozy feeling	Required numerous programing sessions; YBOCS improved 75%
Maciunas et al,[19] 2007	5 M (18–34)	3	CM-Pf, Voi	3.5–3.6 V, 130–185 Hz, 90–210 μs	44% (global YGTSS), 24% (tic YGTSS)	Acute psychosis	Prospective randomized crossover trial with On-Off stimulation periods; assessments done in double-blind fashion; 3 of 5 patients improved >50% (2 did not have any meaningful improvement)
Dehning et al,[36] 2008[c]	1 F (44)	12	pvlGPi	4.2 V, 145 Hz, 210 μs	88% (global YGTSS)	Depressive moods, vertigo, stomach aches	—

Dehning et al,[37] 2011[c]	1 M (38), 3 F (25, 28, 44)	5–48	pvlGPi	3.5–4.2 V, 130–145 Hz, 150–210 μs	Responders (2), 76% (global YGTSS). Other 2 patients had minimal response and discontinued stimulation	None	One patient from Dehning et al[36] (2008). Thought that responders had SIB and vocal tics as predominant symptoms and had some response to ECT
Shields et al,[15] 2008	1 F (40)	ALIC, 18; CM-Pf/Voi, 3	ALIC, then CM-Pf, Voi	ALIC, 4.1 V, 185 Hz, 210 μs; CM-Pf/Voi, 7 V, 185 Hz, 90 μs	ALIC (18 mo), 23% (global YGTSS), 21% (tic YGTSS); CM-Pf/Voi, 46% (global YGTSS), 41% (tic YGTSS)	Electrode connector fractures necessitating replacement of leads Hypomania when dorsal in body of capsule vs apathy/depression in NA	Moderate benefit with ALIC stimulation, did not completely suppress tics so thalamic stimulators placed when hardware was revised
Zabek et al,[45] 2008	1 M (31)	28	Right NA	3 V, 130 Hz, 210 μs	Reduction of vocal (88%) and motor tics (75%) during on stimulation at 28 mo	—	Unilateral DBS; kept stimulator on, but then evaluated in On-Off conditions separated by 12 h
Servello et al,[21] 2008[d]	15 M (18–47), 3 F (20–31)	3–17	CM-Pf, Voi	2.5–4 V, 120–130 Hz, 60–120 μs	65% (global YGTSS), 63% (tic YGTSS)	Wound healing problems requiring plastics repair (1), abdominal hematoma requiring evacuation (1) Transient vertigo, blurring of vision (4), abdominal discomfort (2), and upward ocular deviation (1)	9 of the patients underwent an On-Off blinded evaluation (8 of 9 deteriorated during Off state)
Porta et al,[24] 2009[d]	12 M, 3 F (17–46)	24	CM-Pf, Voi	—	52% (global YGTSS)	—	31% reduction in YBOCS; improvement of comorbid symptoms of depression, anxiety, and OCD behavior in 14 of 15 subjects

(*continued on next page*)

Table 1
(*continued*)

Investigators	Patient Sex, Age (y)	Follow-up (mo)	Targets	Stimulation Parameters	Outcomes (Reduction in YGTSS/MRVRS)	Complications: Sequelae of Stimulation (Number of Patients)	Comments
Servello et al,[23] 2009[d]	3 M (25, 37, 47), 1 F (31)	10–44	CM-Pf and ALIC/NA (3); ALIC/NA (1)	4–4.5 V, 130–160 Hz, 150–180 μs	Simultaneous CM-Pf and ALIC-NA (n = 1): 83% (global YGTSS), 60% (YBOCS). ALIC-NA alone (n = 1): 68% (global YGTSS), 54% (YBOCS). Rescue ALIC-NA (n = 2), 34% and 27% (global YGTSS) after CM-Pf DBS, failed to improve significantly in YBOCS following ALIC-NA DBS (9% and 21%); 49% and 62% (global YGTSS from baseline) following addition of ALIC-NA DBS	—	Two repeat patients from 2008 study; rescue therapy to help reduce OCD symptoms to improve quality of life that remained poor despite improvement in tics from thalamic DBS
Servello et al,[22] 2010[d]	28 M (17–57), 8 F (20–47) (only 30 included in analysis)	3 mo minimum (22 pts >2 y)	CM-Pf, Voi alone (30); unilateral CM-Pf, Voi (1); CM-Pf, Voi + rescue ALIC/NA (3); pvlGPi-ALIC/NA (1); ALIC/NA alone (1)		47% (YGTSS); 52% at 2 y for 19 pts who had long-term follow-up	3.2% needed leads repositioned; 19.3% rate of need for hardware replacement/wound revision because of infection	VAS, BDI, STAI, and YBOCS significantly decreased as well
Porta et al,[20] 2012[d]	15 M (17–47), 3 F (20–31)	60–72	CM-Pf, Voi	—	59% (YGTSS)	Wound healing problems and multiple infections (1); abdominal pouch hematoma (1) Blurring vision with >4 V stimulation (2)	Mean reductions of 22.9% (YBOCS), 25.6% (STAI), 27% (BDI). Not all individual patients had reductions in scores

Martinez-Torres et al,[47] (2009)	1 M (38)	12	STN	3–3.2 V, 130 Hz, 60 μs	Tic frequency reduced 89% at 6 mo and 97% at 1 y	—	Patient with Parkinson disease with concomitant untreated tics
Neuner et al,[46] 2009	1 M (38)	36	NA	6 V, 145 Hz, 90 μs	44% (global YGTSS); 58% (MRVRS); 56% (YBOCS)	—	—
Dueck et al,[38] 2009	1 M (16)	12	Ventral GPi	4 V, 130 Hz, 120 μs	No significant improvement (modified YGTSS)	Visual disturbances with ventral lead, nausea/dizziness when voltage increased	Negative report; comorbid mental retardation
Vernaleken et al,[60] 2009	1 M (22)	6	DM thalamus	4.4 V, 130 Hz, 180 μs	36% (global YGTSS), 33% (tic YGTSS)	—	Failed GPi DBS before thalamic DBS. Postoperative PET shows decreased thalamic dopamine release with stimulation
Idris et al,[26] 2010	1 M (24)	2	CM-Pf, Voi	3.5 V, 130 Hz, 120 ms	Improved	Bilateral ICH	Factor XIIIa deficiency, suggesting that patients with TS may be prone to factor XIIIa deficiency
Burdick et al,[43] 2010	1 M (33)	30	ALIC/NA	6.5 V, 135 Hz, 90 μs	No improvement objectively (subjective improvement stated by patient)	—	Negative report
Kaido et al,[25] 2011	1 M (20), 2 F (19, 21)	12	CM-Pf, Voi	2.1–3.2 V, 180–210 Hz, 80–130 μs	39% (global YGTSS), 35% (tic YGTSS)	Some visual disturbances with high voltage	Denied any YBOCS or wechsler adult intelligence scale changes. Cognition mildly improved
Lee et al,[27] 2011	1 M (31)	18	CM-Pf, Voi	3.5 V, 180 Hz, 180 ms	58% (global YGTSS)/ 39% (MRVRS)	—	Some improvement in neuropsychiatric testing caused by tic control

(continued on next page)

Table 1
(continued)

Investigators	Patient Sex, Age (y)	Follow-up (mo)	Targets	Stimulation Parameters	Outcomes (Reduction in YGTSS/MRVRS)	Complications: Sequelae of Stimulation (Number of Patients)	Comments
Ackermans et al,[28] 2011	6 M (35–48)	12	CM-Pf, Voi	1–7.3 V, 70–130 Hz, 60–210 μs	On-Off stimulation period: YGTSS score was 37% lower at end of On period compared with Off assessed at 1 y. Unblinded assessment: 49% (YGTSS)/35% (RVBRS)	ICH (1), infection of generator (1) Subjective gaze disturbances, reduction of energy level	Double-blind, randomized, crossover trial; after crossover period, 1 patient opted for intermittent stimulation. Secondary measures: no group differences in YBOCS, CAARS, BAI, BDI, SIB; but 1 pt had worse OCD and better depression and ADHD, but overall showed improvement at 1 year. Some mild decrease in Stroop task performance
Duits et al,[29] 2012	1 F (20)	36	CM-Pf, Voi	5 mV, 110 Hz, 60 μs	Off period, 71% (motor YGTSS); On period, 7% (motor YGTSS)	Disturbances in consciousness, mutism, and inability to tolerate food with refusal of intravenous hydration/alimentation resulting in death Hypertonia in extremities with or without stimulation	From the same trial reported in Ackermans et al[28] (2011); however, this patient's data were not included in that report because of unexplained complications. Paradoxic increase in tics when stimulation was on.

Martinez-Fernandez et al,[39] 2011	4 M (21–6), 1 F (35)	9–24	amGPi (2) vs pvlGPi (2) (see comment)	2.5–4.2 V, 20–170 Hz, 60–210 μs	All patients: 29% (global YGTSS)/26% (MRVRS). amGPi: 38% (global YGTSS)/54% (MRVRS). pvGPi: 20% (global YGTSS)/37% (MRVRS). One pt first had pvGPi: motor GPi (42% motor, and 60% phonic) and then amGPi (75% motor and 74% phonic tic reduction). Improved YBOCS (26%). 3 pts with preoperative and postoperative GTS-QOL measures showed improvement of 54.5%	Two hardware infections (1) Anxiety, agitation, constant tiredness (1); capsular effects when >2.8 V (1); weight gain with attempted smoking cessation (1)	amGPi (2), pvGPi (2), and pvGPi then amGPi (1). Comparison of amGPi and pvGPi stimulation
Cannon et al,[40] 2012	8 M (22–50), 3F (18–34)	4–30	amGPi	3–5 V, 100–160 Hz, 60–120 μs	49.6% (global YGTSS) at 3 mo. Reduction in YBOCS (59%) and HAM-D (74%)	Mechanical breakage necessitating lead repair/replacement (3); infection requiring bilateral lead replacement (1) Increased tics (1); anxiety/panic attack increased with changes in stimulation (2)	Open-label. Improvement in quality-of-life scale and global assessment of functioning as well
Savica et al,[32] 2012	2 M (17, 17), 1 F (35)	12	CM-Pf, Voi	2.5–4.1 V, 107–130 Hz, 90–120 μs	70% (global YGTSS); 60% (motor YGTSS)	Light headedness, mild paresthesias	Two pediatric patients
Piedimonte et al,[41] 2012	1 M (47)	6	GPe	3 V, 150 Hz, 300 μs	70.5% (global YGTSS)	—	Some improvement on HAM-A and HAM-D with stimulation
Dong et al,[56] 2012	2 M (22, 41)	12	Ventral GPi (unilateral right)	2.8–3.5 V, 130–160 Hz, 90 μs	55.8% (tic YGTSS)	—	—

(continued on next page)

Table 1
(continued)

Investigators	Patient Sex, Age (y)	Follow-up (mo)	Targets	Stimulation Parameters	Outcomes (Reduction in YGTSS/MRVRS)	Complications: Sequelae of Stimulation (Number of Patients)	Comments
Okun et al,[31] 2013	2 M (27, 35), 3 F (32–38)	6	CM region	0.5–4.5 mA, 125 Hz, 80–200 μs	19.4% (global YGTSS)/ 36% (MRTRS)	Paresthesias, dizziness, and subjective eye movements. Unable to tolerate stimulation requiring patient-controlled Off times (2)	Had assessments at different stimulation periods (continuous stimulation, off stimulation, schedule on stimulation) at 3 mo. No change in YBOCS or QOLAS scale

Abbreviations: ADHD, attention deficit hyperactivity disorder; ALIC, anterior limb of the internal capsule; amGPi, anteromedial GPi; BAI, Beck Anxiety Inventory; BDI, Beck Depression Inventory; CAARS, Conners Adult ADHD Rating Scale; CM, centromedian nucleus; DBS, deep brain stimulation; ECT, electroconvulsive therapy; GPe, globus pallidus externus; GTS-QOL, Gilles de la Tourette Syndrome Quality of Life Scale; HAM-A, Hamilton Anxiety Rating Scale; HAM-D, Hamilton Depression Rating Scale; ICH, intracranial hemorrhage; MRTRS, Modified Rush Tic Rating Scale; MRVRS, Modified Rush Videotape Rating Scale; OCD, obsessive-compulsive disorder; PET, positron emission tomography; Pf, parafascicular nucleus; pt, patient; pvlGPi, posteroventrolateral GPi; QOLAS, Quality of Life Assessment Schedule; SIB, self-injurious behavior; YGTSS, Yale Global Tic Severity Scale.

[a] Vandewalle and colleagues[11] (1999), Visser-Vandewalle and colleagues[12] (2003), and Ackermans and colleagues[13] (2010) shared common patients in their reports.

[b] Houeto and colleagues[14] (2005) and Welter and colleagues[16] (2008) shared common patients in their reports.

[c] Dehning and colleagues[36,37] (2008) and (2012) shared common patients in their reports.

[d] Servello and colleagues[21] (2008), Porta and colleagues[24] (2009), Servello and colleagues[23] (2009), Servello and colleagues[22] (2010), and Porta and colleagues[20] (2012) shared common patients in their reports.

Flaherty and colleagues[42] argued that the ALIC would be a reasonable target for the DBS treatment of TS. Although she did not have concomitant OCD, their patient experienced a 20% reduction in her global YGTSS score when assessed at 18 months following ALIC DBS. Including this first report, there have been 15 patients who have been implanted at either the ALIC alone (n = 2), ALIC and NA (n = 10), or NA alone (n = 3) (see **Table 1**). Most of the patients who underwent stimulation of the ALIC, with or without the NA, received modest benefit in the reduction of tics, with mean reductions in global YGTSS scores ranging from 20% to 68%.[20,48,49,54]

The NA, situated at the ventral aspect of the internal capsule, receives major dopaminergic afferents from mesolimbic regions of the brain. Because dopamine is implicated as the primary neurotransmitter involved in the pathophysiology of TS, the NA was thought to be an important target in modulating the course of the disease.[44] Patients who underwent solely NA stimulation received 41% to 44% reduction in global YGTSS,[44,46] with 1 study reporting benefit in the form of absolute tic reduction (88% vocal and 75% motor tics).[45] One notable exception was a patient reported by Burdick and colleagues[43] who received no objective improvement in tics, although the patient reported some subjective benefit.

Despite most centers using DBS for TS to control the number and severity of tics, the ALIC and NA targets were used by some groups as a rescue procedure in order to help reduce the severity of comorbid symptoms that were limiting improvements in quality of life despite improvements in tic symptoms.[22,23] In their original report, Servello and colleagues[23] identified 2 patients with previously implanted CM-Pf/Voi leads who experienced good tic reduction with stimulation, but were still functionally impaired by their obsessions, to be implanted with ALIC/NA DBS. An additional patient was recruited to receive simultaneous CM-Pf/Voi and ALIC/NA DBS on account of his severe comorbid OCD. The 2 patients who received rescue DBS at the ALIC/NA did not experience any significant improvement in their Yale-Brown Obsessive Compulsive Scale (YBOCS) score, although they did experience even further improvements in their global YGTSS scores (34% and 27% to 49% and 62%). However, it is difficult to determine whether this is a result of a new target of stimulation, or rather the cumulative effect of extended periods of stimulation. Despite these discouraging results in concomitantly treating tics and OCD symptoms in these two patients, the patient who underwent simultaneous de novo CM-Pf/Voi and ALIC/NA DBS experienced a significant reduction in his YBOCS score (60%) in addition to an 83% reduction in his YGTSS.

Subthalamic Nucleus

There is only 1 report to date of STN stimulation for the treatment of tics.[47] The patient was a 38-year-old man with Parkinson disease and a history of untreated tics that began in childhood. Following the implantation and stimulation of the STN, the patient's tics reduced by 97% and he had significant improvement in his Unified Parkinson's Disease Rating Scale III (motor) at 1-year follow-up.

Dorsomedial Nucleus of the Thalamus

In addition to the CM-Pf/Voi region of the thalamus, there has been a single report of dorsomedial nucleus thalamic implantation and stimulation for a patient with TS. Vernaleken and colleagues[60] reported on a patient who had previously failed GPi stimulation for TS and subsequently underwent thalamic implantation at the dorsomedial nucleus of the thalamus. The patient experienced a 36% reduction in global YGTSS score at 6 months' follow-up. Thalamic stimulation was positively correlated with decreased thalamic dopamine release, and discontinuing stimulation resulted in a dramatic large increase in thalamic dopamine levels. These findings were the first to corroborate surgical intervention with changes in neurotransmitter levels postoperatively, and are in concordance with the dopamine hypothesis of TS, because neuroleptic medications are commonly used to treat and reduce tics.

Target Comparison

Given the heterogeneity in patient demographics, disease characteristics, stimulation parameters, and length of follow-up time, it is difficult to compare clinical outcomes across the various studies to date to determine target efficacy. However, there exist several reports that have independently compared the efficacy of sites of stimulation in the suppression of tics in TS.[14–16,39] The first comparison was made in a prospective, double-blinded, sham controlled trial initially in 1 patient[14] and ultimately 3 patients[16] who underwent bilateral CM-Pf/Voi and anteromedial GPi lead implantation. Patients were randomized to 2-month periods during which either the thalamic leads, pallidal leads, both pallidal and thalamic leads, or no leads were stimulated. Although there was no significant difference in efficacy in their single-patient report, at long-term follow-up with 3 patients anteromedial GPi stimulation resulted in a greater reduction in YGTSS scores (78% vs

45%) with no added benefit with combined stimulation (60%). However, following the randomized stimulation periods, 2 of the patients went on to experience significant reductions in YGTSS scores (74% and 82%) with simultaneous pallidal and thalamic stimulation, suggesting that there may still be some usefulness in a multitarget approach. Although the trial was prospective, randomized, and double blinded, it is difficult to make strong conclusions about the efficacy of each target given the limited stimulation period of each one, because some patients continue to improve after many months following initiation of stimulation.

A single-patient comparison of the anterior limb of the internal capsule versus the thalamus was reported by Shields and colleagues.[15] Following only modest benefit from ALIC stimulation (23% reduction in global YGTSS at 18 months), it was decided to place leads in the CM-PF/Voi thalamus when the hardware failed and required replacement. Following the new placement of leads in the CM-Pf/Voi thalamus the patient experienced a 46% reduction in YGTSS at 3 months.

In addition, Martinez-Fernandez and colleagues[39] described an open-label intragroup comparison of anteromedial GPi versus the posterolateral GPi. The patients who received lead placement in the anteromedial GPi had a mean reduction of global YGTSS score of 38%, whereas those with posterolateral GPi stimulation had a mean reduction of 20%. However, there was 1 patient who initially received posterolateral GPi stimulation with only modest results, and subsequently had anterolateral GPi leads placed. At last follow-up, although he experienced greater tic reduction with anterolateral stimulation (75% motor and 74% phonic tics vs 42% motor and 60% phonic tics), he received equal reductions in YGTSS from the two treatment strategies (19%).

CLINICAL OUTCOMES

Despite more than a decade of experience with the DBS of numerous targets for the treatment of TS, most published reports have been open-label studies, many of them including only a single patient (see **Table 1**). Clinical outcomes have focused primarily on the resolution of tics measured either through the percentage reduction in tic frequency or the reduction in the YGTSS.[55] The success of stimulation at various targets was discussed earlier, but has varied from having no clinical benefit[19,29,38,43] to reducing YGTSS by more than 96% in an individual patient.[16] It is difficult to make any strong conclusions because there have been only a limited number of randomized, double-blinded studies. Welter and colleagues[16] in a prospective double-blinded crossover trial with a sham control showed that the anteromedial GPi had greater benefit at reducing YGTSS than CM-Pf stimulation. However, these assessments were made after 2 months of stimulation at each target. It is unclear what time course of stimulation is needed, and whether this varies from target to target, before maximum clinical benefit is achieved during stimulation.

Ackermans and colleagues[28] published the only other double-blinded, randomized assessment of DBS for TS in a trial including 6 patients targeting the CM-Pf/Voi thalamus. They assessed patients in a double-blind fashion after an On and Off stimulation period, each lasting 3 months. The YGTSS was 37% lower following the On period compared with the Off. The randomized period was followed by an unblinded continuous stimulation period of 6 months, during which the tic symptoms of patients continued to improve. The studies discussed earlier, in addition to the open-label reports, suggest that there is clinical benefit to the DBS of these circuits implicated in the pathophysiology of TS. However, randomized double-blinded studies with longer follow-up are needed to determine which targets are superior.

Although initial outcome measures almost exclusively addressed the reduction in tics, it has become increasingly apparent that the reduction in comorbid psychiatric conditions is also important in overall patient outcome. This conclusion was especially highlighted by Servello and colleagues[23] who reported on 2 patients who, despite achieving adequate tic reduction with thalamic stimulation, remained functionally impaired because of their severe obsessions and compulsions. Comorbid conditions that have been seen to improve following stimulation include OCD, depression, anxiety, self-injurious behavior, aggression/impulsivity, and ADHD.[61] The most commonly reported comorbidity assessed was OCD, as measured by changes in YBOCS. Throughout the series that reported on this secondary outcome, reductions in scores ranged from 23% to 75%.[18,20,22,24,44,47] The largest series (n = 18) reporting on this measure had the most modest outcomes, with a mean 23% reduction in YBOCS at last follow-up.[20] Moreover, not all patients experienced a decrease in YBOCS following DBS, with 22% of the patients experiencing an increase in OCD symptoms, with 1 patient experiencing a 27.5% increase. These findings, and others that fail to show decreases in YBOCS following simulation,[28,31] support the need for randomized, double-blind studies to determine the benefits on the comorbid conditions of TS as well.

COMPLICATIONS

Surgical

A limited number of surgery-related complications have been reported, including intracerebral hematomas associated with electrode placement,[26,30,33] abdominal hematomas associated with generator placement,[20,21] mechanical[15,40] or infectious issues[22,28,35,39,40] requiring hardware replacement or removal, and wound breakdown problems.[20–22] There have been 3 patients who were found to have intracerebral hemorrhages following placement of DBS leads. One was in 27-year-old man who received bilateral leads into the posterolateral GPi and who subsequently experienced bradykinesia of the left hand and was found to have a right pallidal hemorrhage.[33] Another was in a 39-year-old man who had bilateral thalamic leads placed in the CM-Pf nucleus.[30] He was found to have an associated intracranial hemorrhage deep to the left electrode resulting in a transient vertical gaze palsy. Idris and colleagues[26] reported on a 24-year-old man who experienced 2 parenchymal hematomas related to lead placement. He was later found to have low levels of factor XIIIA, which they suggested might be related to decreased levels of tryptophan, which may be inherent to some patients with TS. In addition, there was 1 patient who was found to have an abdominal hematoma following peritoneal generator placement that required evacuation.[20,21]

The rate of hardware infection and wound complications in patients with TS seems to be significantly greater than that in the normal movement disorder population.[62] Eight patients with hardware infections requiring removal or replacement across 5 different clinical series have been reported.[22,28,35,39,40] In addition to infection-related hardware complications, 4 patients across 2 series required hardware replacement after breakage of the lead connectors or wires.[15,40] In addition, 3 patients required wound revisions, 1 of which required the assistance of plastic surgery.[20–22] On account of the frequent incidence of infectious complications and wound breakdowns in the TS DBS population, Servello and colleagues[62] performed an internal retrospective analysis of their complication rates following implantation of DBS systems. They found a significant correlation between infectious events and patients with TS. The incidence of infection in their series of patients undergoing DBS for various movement disorders was 3.7% overall (10 of 272) versus 18% in patients with TS ($P<.0001$). Moreover, the patients with TS had recurrent infections requiring multiple revisions, and ultimate removal of hardware in 5 of the 7 patients.[62] The investigators hypothesized that this relationship may be attributable to the decrease in cellular immunity that has been reported in patients with TS.[63] Moreover, Servello and colleagues[62] found that many of their patients admitted to having compulsions to pick at their surgical wounds. This behavior was corroborated by caregivers, and found to be true in additional patients who denied such compulsions. The combination of decreased immunity and compliance with perioperative precautions may explain the greater incidence of infection-related complications in patients with TS undergoing DBS, and should be considered in the preoperative counseling and considerations before surgery.

Stimulation-related Adverse Effects

It is difficult to ascertain which sites and methods of stimulation will reliably reproduce the various stimulation-associated adverse effects given the vast heterogeneity in stimulation parameters and targets used (see **Table 1**). A review of the literature reveals that most patients report problems with loss of energy, visual disturbances, and sexual problems.[6] A considerable number of patients across multiple studies and target sites complained of decreased energy or depressed mood that interfered with their activities of daily life for up to several months.[12,15,17,28,33,42] In addition to the aforementioned hemorrhage-related vertical gaze palsy,[30] numerous patients complained of stimulation-related visual symptoms including excessive eye blinking,[11] blurring of vision,[20,21] and visual and gaze disturbances.[25,28,31,38] Most of these visual symptoms were transient; however, 1 cohort of patients reported permanent blurred vision and fixation problems despite normal ophthalmologic evaluations.[28] Decreased libido and sexual dysfunction were observed with thalamic stimulation in a limited number of reports; however, these were reported with stimulation at other sites.[12,16,17] Other more rare adverse effects of stimulation include acute psychosis[19]; inability to tolerate stimulation, requiring Off periods[31]; and paradoxic increases in tics.[29,40]

Despite the frequent use of neurocognitive testing before and after DBS implantation, the effects of stimulation on neurocognitive performance are unclear. Bergfeld and colleagues[64] recently reviewed the literature on the cognitive sequelae of DBS in neuropsychiatric conditions, including TS. Across different targets and studies there did not seem to be any significant effects of stimulation on multiple cognitive domains, including working memory, visual memory, visuospatial organization, cognitive inhibition, and psychomotor speed.[16,19,24,25,28,36] Notwithstanding most neutral reports, there were limited incidences of improvements and worsening in certain domains as well. Shahed and colleagues[34] reported an improvement on psychomotor functioning, cognitive flexibility, and visuospatial perception in 1 patient, whereas Kaido and colleagues[25] reported mild cognitive improvement in 1 patient as well. Ackermans and colleagues[13,28] observed a decline in cognitive flexibility in 1 patient and a decrease in verbal memory functioning in another. Overall, there seems to be a limited degree of cognitive sequelae resulting from stimulation the commonly used targets in TS. Future studies with improved, double-blinded follow-up are required to further investigate this issue.

CLINICAL EVALUATION AND PERIOPERATIVE MANAGEMENT

Patient Selection

With increasing evidence toward the efficacy of DBS for TS, and a greater number of patients undergoing DBS for treatment, it is critical to establish guidelines regarding the patient population that should be considered for implantation and stimulation. Multiple guideline articles have been published by field experts.[61,65–68] Initial evaluation should ensure first and foremost that the patient has a diagnosis of TS, fulfilling criteria as outlined by the Diagnostic and Statistical Manual of Mental Disorders, Fourth Edition (DSM-IV).[69] An evaluation by a multidisciplinary team consisting of neurosurgeons, neurologists, and psychiatrists should subsequently take place to determine the risk/benefit ratio of surgery. Although there is no clear consensus as to what minimum age the patient should be before being considered for DBS, the patient should be old enough, or have symptoms severe enough, to suggest a poor chance of spontaneous remission with time.[54,61,66,68] Given the potential for therapeutic efficacy and the potential loss of years of function if not treated, there is an increasing trend toward treating patients earlier if symptoms seem unlikely to abate. Patients should have documented severe tics that significantly impair function as assessed by the YGTSS, with a tic score of greater than 35 out of 50 for a period of 12 months. In addition, patients should have failed 3 different trials of medical therapy that were ineffective despite adequate dosing or poorly tolerated secondary to side effects of medication. Medication regimens should include alpha-agonists, typical and atypical dopamine antagonists, and a benzodiazepine. Furthermore, the patient must have had comorbid neurologic, psychiatric, and psychosocial components of their disease adequately managed for at least 6 months before treatment. Patients who have severe medical, neurologic, psychiatric, or cognitive disorders that may inordinately increase the risk of a failed procedure should be excluded.

Target Selection

There is currently no definitive evidence as to which DBS target has the greatest clinical efficacy with stimulation. Based on the most recent guidelines from the 2 most experienced groups in TS DBS, expert opinion agrees that either the CM-Pf with or without the Voi and the GPi are the targets recommended for stimulation, although some centers may advocate for ALIC/NA as well.[61,68] Within the GPi, there is continued debate as to whether the posterolateral (motor) portion or the anterolateral (limbic) portion provides the most clinical benefit with stimulation.[68] In order to resolve the issues regarding target superiority and clinical efficacy, large multicenter trials with a centralized database to allow interinstitution comparison is necessary. The TS Association recently created an online database to allow the exchange of information regarding past, present, and future clinical data regarding TS DBS (http://dbs.tsa-usa.org/). With the continued collaboration across hospitals and nations, it is hoped that the questions regarding target efficacy and objective clinical outcome for TS DBS will be answered.

SUMMARY

Despite the great progress and promising clinical evidence to date, DBS for TS is still in its infancy. With more than a decade of clinical reports and long-term follow-up, the safety and potential efficacy of DBS for TS have become more convincing. The publication of the most recent guidelines by expert panels in neuromodulation for TS and other psychiatric disorders will allow a more standardized recruitment of patients to enroll in larger multicenter trials. These future clinical studies will help answer many of the questions regarding target superiority and long-term efficacy in the neuromodulation of TS.

REFERENCES

1. Leckman JF, Bloch MH, Scahill L, et al. Tourette syndrome: the self under siege. J Child Neurol 2006;21(8):642–9.
2. Knight T, Steeves T, Day L, et al. Prevalence of tic disorders: a systematic review and meta-analysis. Pediatr Neurol 2012;47(2):77–90.
3. Pappert EJ, Goetz CG, Louis ED, et al. Objective assessments of longitudinal outcome in Gilles de

la Tourette's syndrome. Neurology 2003;61(7): 936–40.
4. Freeman RD, Fast DK, Burd L, et al. An international perspective on Tourette syndrome: selected findings from 3,500 individuals in 22 countries. Dev Med Child Neurol 2000;42(7):436–47.
5. Robertson MM. The Gilles de la Tourette syndrome: the current status. Arch Dis Child Educ Pract Ed 2012;97(5):166–75.
6. Muller-Vahl KR. Surgical treatment of Tourette syndrome. Neurosci Biobehav Rev 2013;37(6): 1178–85.
7. Neimat JS, Patil PG, Lozano AM. Novel surgical therapies for Tourette syndrome. J Child Neurol 2006;21(8):715–8.
8. Hassler R, Dieckmann G. Stereotaxic treatment of tics and inarticulate cries or coprolalia considered as motor obsessional phenomena in Gilles de la Tourette's disease. Rev Neurol 1970;123(2):89–100 [in French].
9. Leckman JF, de Lotbiniere AJ, Marek K, et al. Severe disturbances in speech, swallowing, and gait following stereotactic infrathalamic lesions in Gilles de la Tourette's syndrome. Neurology 1993; 43(5):890–4.
10. Babel TB, Warnke PC, Ostertag CB. Immediate and long term outcome after infrathalamic and thalamic lesioning for intractable Tourette's syndrome. J Neurol Neurosurg Psychiatr 2001;70(5): 666–71.
11. Vandewalle V, van der Linden C, Groenewegen HJ, et al. Stereotactic treatment of Gilles de la Tourette syndrome by high frequency stimulation of thalamus. Lancet 1999;353(9154):724.
12. Visser-Vandewalle V, Temel Y, Boon P, et al. Chronic bilateral thalamic stimulation: a new therapeutic approach in intractable Tourette syndrome. Report of three cases. J Neurosurg 2003;99(6): 1094–100.
13. Ackermans L, Duits A, Temel Y, et al. Long-term outcome of thalamic deep brain stimulation in two patients with Tourette syndrome. J Neurol Neurosurg Psychiatr 2010;81(10):1068–72.
14. Houeto JL, Karachi C, Mallet L, et al. Tourette's syndrome and deep brain stimulation. J Neurol Neurosurg Psychiatr 2005;76(7):992–5.
15. Shields DC, Cheng ML, Flaherty AW, et al. Microelectrode-guided deep brain stimulation for Tourette syndrome: within-subject comparison of different stimulation sites. Stereotact Funct Neurosurg 2008;86(2):87–91.
16. Welter ML, Mallet L, Houeto JL, et al. Internal pallidal and thalamic stimulation in patients with Tourette syndrome. Arch Neurol 2008;65(7):952–7.
17. Ackermans L, Temel Y, Cath D, et al. Deep brain stimulation in Tourette's syndrome: two targets? Mov Disord 2006;21(5):709–13.
18. Bajwa RJ, de Lotbiniere AJ, King RA, et al. Deep brain stimulation in Tourette's syndrome. Mov Disord 2007;22(9):1346–50.
19. Maciunas RJ, Maddux BN, Riley DE, et al. Prospective randomized double-blind trial of bilateral thalamic deep brain stimulation in adults with Tourette syndrome. J Neurosurg 2007;107(5): 1004–14.
20. Porta M, Servello D, Zanaboni C, et al. Deep brain stimulation for treatment of refractory Tourette syndrome: long-term follow-up. Acta Neurochir 2012; 154(11):2029–41.
21. Servello D, Porta M, Sassi M, et al. Deep brain stimulation in 18 patients with severe Gilles de la Tourette syndrome refractory to treatment: the surgery and stimulation. J Neurol Neurosurg Psychiatr 2008;79(2):136–42.
22. Servello D, Sassi M, Brambilla A, et al. Long-term, post-deep brain stimulation management of a series of 36 patients affected with refractory Gilles de la Tourette syndrome. Neuromodulation 2010; 13(3):187–94.
23. Servello D, Sassi M, Brambilla A, et al. De novo and rescue DBS leads for refractory Tourette syndrome patients with severe comorbid OCD: a multiple case report. J Neurol 2009;256(9):1533–9.
24. Porta M, Brambilla A, Cavanna AE, et al. Thalamic deep brain stimulation for treatment-refractory Tourette syndrome: two-year outcome. Neurology 2009;73(17):1375–80.
25. Kaido T, Otsuki T, Kaneko Y, et al. Deep brain stimulation for Tourette syndrome: a prospective pilot study in Japan. Neuromodulation 2011;14(2): 123–8 [discussion: 129].
26. Idris Z, Ghani AR, Mar W, et al. Intracerebral haematomas after deep brain stimulation surgery in a patient with Tourette syndrome and low factor XIIIA activity. J Clin Neurosci 2010;17(10):1343–4.
27. Lee MW, Au-Yeung MM, Hung KN, et al. Deep brain stimulation in a Chinese Tourette's syndrome patient. Hong Kong Med J 2011;17(2):147–50.
28. Ackermans L, Duits A, van der Linden C, et al. Double-blind clinical trial of thalamic stimulation in patients with Tourette syndrome. Brain 2011; 134(Pt 3):832–44.
29. Duits A, Ackermans L, Cath D, et al. Unfavourable outcome of deep brain stimulation in a Tourette patient with severe comorbidity. Eur Child Adolesc Psychiatry 2012;21(9):529–31.
30. Ackermans L, Temel Y, Bauer NJ, et al. Vertical gaze palsy after thalamic stimulation for Tourette syndrome: case report. Neurosurgery 2007;61(5): E1100 [discussion: E1100].
31. Okun MS, Foote KD, Wu SS, et al. A trial of scheduled deep brain stimulation for Tourette syndrome: moving away from continuous deep brain stimulation paradigms. J Neurol 2013;70(1):85–94.

32. Savica R, Stead M, Mack KJ, et al. Deep brain stimulation in Tourette syndrome: a description of 3 patients with excellent outcome. Mayo Clin Proc 2012;87(1):59–62.
33. Diederich NJ, Kalteis K, Stamenkovic M, et al. Efficient internal pallidal stimulation in Gilles de la Tourette syndrome: a case report. Mov Disord 2005; 20(11):1496–9.
34. Shahed J, Poysky J, Kenney C, et al. GPi deep brain stimulation for Tourette syndrome improves tics and psychiatric comorbidities. Neurology 2007;68(2):159–60.
35. Gallagher CL, Garell PC, Montgomery EB Jr. Hemi tics and deep brain stimulation. Neurology 2006; 66(3):E12.
36. Dehning S, Mehrkens JH, Muller N, et al. Therapy-refractory Tourette syndrome: beneficial outcome with globus pallidus internus deep brain stimulation. Mov Disord 2008;23(9):1300–2.
37. Dehning S, Feddersen B, Cerovecki A, et al. Globus pallidus internus-deep brain stimulation in Tourette's syndrome: can clinical symptoms predict response? Mov Disord 2011;26(13):2440–1.
38. Dueck A, Wolters A, Wunsch K, et al. Deep brain stimulation of globus pallidus internus in a 16-year-old boy with severe Tourette syndrome and mental retardation. Neuropediatrics 2009;40(5): 239–42.
39. Martinez-Fernandez R, Zrinzo L, Aviles-Olmos I, et al. Deep brain stimulation for Gilles de la Tourette syndrome: a case series targeting subregions of the globus pallidus internus. Mov Disord 2011; 26(10):1922–30.
40. Cannon E, Silburn P, Coyne T, et al. Deep brain stimulation of anteromedial globus pallidus interna for severe Tourette's syndrome. Am J Psychiatry 2012;169(8):860–6.
41. Piedimonte F, Andreani JC, Piedimonte L, et al. Behavioral and motor improvement after deep brain stimulation of the globus pallidus externus in a case of Tourette's syndrome. Neuromodulation 2013;16(1):55–8 [discussion: 58].
42. Flaherty AW, Williams ZM, Amirnovin R, et al. Deep brain stimulation of the anterior internal capsule for the treatment of Tourette syndrome: technical case report. Neurosurgery 2005;57(Suppl 4):E403.
43. Burdick A, Foote KD, Goodman W, et al. Lack of benefit of accumbens/capsular deep brain stimulation in a patient with both tics and obsessive-compulsive disorder. Neurocase 2010;16(4): 321–30.
44. Kuhn J, Lenartz D, Mai JK, et al. Deep brain stimulation of the nucleus accumbens and the internal capsule in therapeutically refractory Tourette-syndrome. J Neurol 2007;254(7):963–5.
45. Zabek M, Sobstyl M, Koziara H, et al. Deep brain stimulation of the right nucleus accumbens in a patient with Tourette syndrome. Case report. Neurol Neurochir Pol 2008;42(6):554–9.
46. Neuner I, Podoll K, Lenartz D, et al. Deep brain stimulation in the nucleus accumbens for intractable Tourette's syndrome: follow-up report of 36 months. Biol Psychiatry 2009;65(4):e5–6.
47. Martinez-Torres I, Hariz MI, Zrinzo L, et al. Improvement of tics after subthalamic nucleus deep brain stimulation. Neurology 2009;72(20):1787–9.
48. Mink JW. Basal ganglia dysfunction in Tourette's syndrome: a new hypothesis. Pediatr Neurol 2001; 25(3):190–8.
49. Mink JW. Neurobiology of basal ganglia circuits in Tourette syndrome: faulty inhibition of unwanted motor patterns? Adv Neurol 2001;85:113–22.
50. Mink JW. Neurobiology of basal ganglia and Tourette syndrome: basal ganglia circuits and thalamocortical outputs. Adv Neurol 2006;99:89–98.
51. Haber SN, Calzavara R. The cortico-basal ganglia integrative network: the role of the thalamus. Brain Res Bull 2009;78(2–3):69–74.
52. Eckert U, Metzger CD, Buchmann JE, et al. Preferential networks of the mediodorsal nucleus and centromedian-parafascicular complex of the thalamus–a DTI tractography study. Hum Brain Mapp 2012;33(11):2627–37.
53. Sidibe M, Pare JF, Smith Y. Nigral and pallidal inputs to functionally segregated thalamostriatal neurons in the centromedian/parafascicular intralaminar nuclear complex in monkey. J Comp Neurol 2002;447(3):286–99.
54. Ackermans L, Temel Y, Visser-Vandewalle V. Deep brain stimulation in Tourette's syndrome. Neurotherapeutics 2008;5(2):339–44.
55. Leckman JF, Riddle MA, Hardin MT, et al. The Yale Global Tic Severity Scale: initial testing of a clinician-rated scale of tic severity. J Am Acad Child Adolesc Psychiatry 1989;28(4):566–73.
56. Dong S, Zhuang P, Zhang XH, et al. Unilateral deep brain stimulation of the right globus pallidus internus in patients with Tourette's syndrome: two cases with outcomes after 1 year and a brief review of the literature. J Int Med Res 2012;40(5): 2021–8.
57. Vilela Filho O, Ragazzo P, Silva DJ, et al. Bilateral GPe-DBS for Tourette's syndrome. Neurotarget 2008;3(66). Available at: http://www.neurotarget.com/v3n1_GPe-DBS.html.
58. Graybiel AM, Rauch SL. Toward a neurobiology of obsessive-compulsive disorder. Neuron 2000; 28(2):343–7.
59. Nuttin BJ, Gabriels LA, Cosyns PR, et al. Long-term electrical capsular stimulation in patients with obsessive-compulsive disorder. Neurosurgery 2003;52(6):1263–72 [discussion: 1272–4].
60. Vernaleken I, Kuhn J, Lenartz D, et al. Bithalamical deep brain stimulation in Tourette syndrome is

associated with reduction in dopaminergic transmission. Biol Psychiatry 2009;66(10):e15–7.
61. Muller-Vahl KR, Cath DC, Cavanna AE, et al. European clinical guidelines for Tourette syndrome and other tic disorders. Part IV: deep brain stimulation. Eur Child Adolesc Psychiatry 2011;20(4):209–17.
62. Servello D, Sassi M, Gaeta M, et al. Tourette syndrome (TS) bears a higher rate of inflammatory complications at the implanted hardware in deep brain stimulation (DBS). Acta Neurochir 2011;153(3):629–32.
63. Martino D, Dale RC, Gilbert DL, et al. Immunopathogenic mechanisms in Tourette syndrome: a critical review. Mov Disord 2009;24(9):1267–79.
64. Bergfeld IO, Mantione M, Hoogendoorn ML, et al. Cognitive functioning in psychiatric disorders following deep brain stimulation. Brain Stimul 2013;6(4):532–7.
65. Visser-Vandewalle V, Ackermans L, van der Linden C, et al. Deep brain stimulation in Gilles de la Tourette's syndrome. Neurosurgery 2006;58(3):E590.
66. Mink JW, Walkup J, Frey KA, et al. Patient selection and assessment recommendations for deep brain stimulation in Tourette syndrome. Mov Disord 2006;21(11):1831–8.
67. Rabins P, Appleby BS, Brandt J, et al. Scientific and ethical issues related to deep brain stimulation for disorders of mood, behavior, and thought. Arch Gen Psychiatry 2009;66(9):931–7.
68. Cavanna AE, Eddy CM, Mitchell R, et al. An approach to deep brain stimulation for severe treatment-refractory Tourette syndrome: the UK perspective. Br J Neurosurg 2011;25(1):38–44.
69. Association AP. Diagnostic and statistical manual of mental disorders. Text revision (DSM-IVTR). 4th edition. Washington, DC: APA; 2000.

Limbic Neuromodulation

Implications for Addiction, Posttraumatic Stress Disorder, and Memory

Ausaf Bari, MD, PhD[a,*], Tianyi Niu, MD[a],
Jean-Philippe Langevin, MD, PhD[b], Itzhak Fried, MD, PhD[c]

KEYWORDS

- Deep brain stimulation • Addiction • Dementia • Memory • Posttraumatic stress disorder • Alzheimer • Limbic system

KEY POINTS

- The nucleus accumbens is a potential target of deep brain stimulation (DBS) for drug addiction.
- The amygdala is a potential DBS target for posttraumatic stress disorder and anxiety.
- The entorhinal area, hippocampus, and fornix are potential DBS targets for dementia.
- Neuromodulation for neuropsychiatric disorders poses ethical challenges.

INTRODUCTION

The limbic system is involved in some of the most challenging neurobehavioral disorders known to medicine, including disorders of mood and anxiety such as depression and posttraumatic stress disorder (PTSD), substance abuse and dependence, and disorders of cognition and memory such as Alzheimer disease. Advances in surgical neuromodulation of the limbic circuitry underlying these disorders offer a new hope for treatment. This article reviews limbic neuromodulation as it applies to addiction, PTSD, and memory.

THE LIMBIC SYSTEM

The definition of the limbic system has evolved over time, but most investigators would agree that affective processing is a central component of this system. Structures commonly included in the limbic system are the hippocampus, cingulate gyrus, amygdala, septal nuclei, hypothalamus, ventral striatum, ventral tegmentum, and prefrontal cortical regions. A full list of the structures and pathways is given in **Table 1**. The concept of the "greater limbic system" involves the role of memory and affect in orchestrating behavior to ensure the survival of the organism and species. This concept incorporates not only affective processing but also the association between memory, affect, and goal-directed behavior. This definition of the greater limbic system provides a key relationship that can help guide research on neuromodulation for addiction, PTSD, and disorders of memory and cognition.

ADDICTION

Addiction is a major global medical, social, economic, and public health challenge. Approximately 25% of all deaths in Western industrial nations are directly or indirectly attributed to the consumption of addictive substances.[1] Alcohol is the most

[a] Department of Neurosurgery, Geffen School of Medicine, University of California, Los Angeles, Room 18-228 NPI, Box 957039, Los Angeles, CA 90095, USA; [b] Department of Neurosurgery, Greater LA VA Healthcare, Geffen School of Medicine, University of California, Los Angeles, 11301 Wilshire Boulevard 10H2, Los Angeles, CA 90073, USA; [c] Department of Neurosurgery, Geffen School of Medicine, University of California, Los Angeles, 740 Westwood Plaza, Los Angeles, CA 90095, USA
* Corresponding author.
E-mail address: abari@mednet.ucla.edu

Neurosurg Clin N Am 25 (2014) 137–145
http://dx.doi.org/10.1016/j.nec.2013.08.004
1042-3680/14/$ – see front matter

Table 1
Brain nuclei and fiber tracts of the limbic system

Nucleus	Tract
Anterior nucleus of the thalamus	Mammillothalamic tract
Amygdala	Stria terminalis
Cingulate gyrus	Cingulum, internal capsule
Dentate gyrus	—
Entorhinal cortex	—
Habenula	Stria medullaris
Hippocampus	Fornix
Hypothalamus	—
Mammillary bodies	Mammillothalamic tract
Mediodorsal nucleus of the thalamus	Internal capsule
Nucleus accumbens	Medial forebrain bundle
Prefrontal cortex	Internal capsule
Subiculum	—
Septal nuclei	Anterior commissure
Ventral tegmental area	Medial forebrain bundle

frequently abused substance in the world, and in the United States, 1 in 6 patients in community-based practice has a problem with alcohol consumption.[2] Other frequently abused substances include opioids, cocaine, and tobacco products. The cost for treatment of the addiction and, more importantly, from the loss of productivity is invaluable. The National Institute of Drug Abuse has estimated the annual cost of substance use disorders to the United States at over half a trillion dollars. A large body of evidence over the last several decades has shown that several components of the limbic system play a major role in addiction.

The nucleus accumbens (NAc) is one of the principal nuclei involved in the neural circuitry underlying reward and motivation, and is one of the main targets of the mesocorticolimbic reward pathway. A large body of evidence from several species, including humans, has implicated this pathway in reward processing, addiction, and goal-directed behavior.

The NAc is located in the ventral portion of the striatum, and its principal neuronal subtype is the γ-aminobutyric acid (GABA)ergic medium spiny inhibitory neuron. Single-neuron recordings from the NAc during self-administration of drug reinforcement have shown a population of neurons that exhibit increasing firing rates while the animals are working toward receiving a drug reward, and are quiescent immediately after reward acquisition.[3,4] Ablation of the NAc may result in a decrease in reward-seeking behavior, and certain investigators have indicated that this has potential as a treatment for severe intractable drug addiction.

Few studies have investigated the role of ablation of the NAc in humans in drug-seeking behavior. Gao and colleagues[5] performed bilateral ablation of the NAc in 28 patients addicted to various opioids. Although complete remission was reported in only 7 patients, the investigators reported decreased withdrawal symptoms in the remaining patients and concluded that bilateral ablation of the NAc is a safe and effective treatment for opioid addiction. These results were extended to a cohort of 12 patients with alcohol dependence who underwent bilateral NAc ablation. In this study there was also a significant reduction in dependence and craving in the majority of patients.[6]

Although these ablative studies confirm the important role of the NAc in drug-seeking in humans, ablation has the disadvantage of being irreversible and, therefore, potentially damaging to normal reward processing. From this perspective, deep brain stimulation (DBS) carries less risk. However, human studies of DBS of the NAc specifically to evaluate drug-seeking behavior are limited to case reports or case series. These reports suggest that DBS of the NAc decreases craving for nicotine, alcohol, and heroin.[7]

The NAc can be subdivided into two anatomically and functionally distinct regions known as the core and shell. Evidence suggests that the shell may be selectively involved in limbic processing, whereas the core may be considered an interface between limbic and motor networks.[8] Thus, the shell may mediate the desire to use a substance and, through its connectivity with the core, translate this desire into action. One could hypothesize that DBS for addiction should target the shell and not the core, as the latter could produce undesired motor suppression. The role of the core in nonspecific motor response has also been described in animal studies.[9]

Just as the activity of striatal neurons is modulated by dopaminergic input from the substantia nigra pars compacta, analogous input from the ventral tegmental area (VTA) provides dopaminergic modulation of accumbal neurons. This mesoaccumbens pathway, located within the medial forebrain bundle (MFB), has long been known to be a powerful substrate for electrical self-stimulation that mimics addictive drug-seeking behavior.[10,11] Thus, other nuclei and pathways in this reward network such as the VTA, MFB, ventral pallidum, mediodorsal thalamic nucleus, and cortical regions such as the cingulate, prefrontal, and orbitofrontal cortices, are potential targets of DBS for addiction (**Fig. 1**). However, neuromodulation of most of these regions specifically for addiction has not been described in humans with the exception of the accumbens and cingulate gyrus. Inadvertent DBS of the MFB has been shown to cause hypomania.[12] Thus, stimulation of the MFB supports the role of the NAc in goal-directed behavior in humans. Hypomania in MFB stimulation seems to confirm the role of the NAc in goal-directed motor activity in humans.

The cingulate gyrus is another major limbic region with connectivity to the medial prefrontal cortex, mediodorsal thalamus, amygdala, hippocampus, and NAc.[13] Neuromodulation of the cingulate gyrus has been shown to be effective for pain and obsessive-compulsive disorder (OCD).[14] Early clues as to role of this region in addiction came from cingulotomies performed in patients to treat intractable pain. Most of these patients had narcotic dependence that improved following cingulotomy.[15] Since then, several studies have reported successful cingulotomy for narcotic dependence.[16,17] More recently, a Russian group reported the successful use of bilateral cryocingulotomies for the treatment of intractable heroin addiction in 348 patients. Follow-up was reported in 187 of these patients, 62% of whom were found to be completely free of opioid use after 2 years, while another 13% showed partial improvement.[18]

In addition to the NAc and the cingulate gyrus, other nuclei in the limbic reward network that may be potential targets of neuromodulation for drug addiction include the hypothalamus, basolateral amygdala, lateral habenula, substantia innominata, and subthalamic nucleus (STN).[19–24]

Witjas and colleagues[25] reported on 2 patients with a history of addiction who underwent DBS of the STN for the treatment of Parkinson disease. In 1 patient, premorbid excessive alcohol intake was greatly reduced after stimulation was initiated.[1] The STN is divided into motor, associative, and limbic regions. Rouaud and colleagues[26] proposed that high-frequency stimulation of the STN decreases incentive motivation for cocaine while inducing the opposite effect for food.[3,4]

The ventromedial nucleus of the hypothalamus has also been tested as a target for alcohol addiction. Unfortunately, all patients showed side effects including reduction of sexual drive, decreased impulsivity, amnesia, visual disturbances, and vegetative crisis.[5,23] Application of electrical stimulation to the lateral hypothalamus has been shown to potentially lead to weight loss in patients with intractable morbid obesity.[6,27] In obese patients, functional neuroimaging studies have shown that food activates the ventral striatum in the same way that drugs do in patients with substance dependence.[7,28]

The amygdala has also been proposed as a target of DBS for drug addiction, based on evidence showing that inactivation of the basolateral amygdala in rats reduces cue-induced reinstatement of cocaine-seeking and activation of the amygdala during presentation of drug-associated cues.[8,29]

DBS of the lateral habenula at low frequency also results in increasing target activity and increasing self-administration of cocaine, whereas high-frequency stimulation had no effect. Unconventional stimulation alternating between 10 and 100 Hz decreased self-administration of cocaine; however, it also decreased general motivation.[9,30]

DBS for the treatment of addiction is still in its infancy, and is based largely on the studies of neuromodulation in rodent models. This brings us to an interesting and unique limitation and ethical dilemma. Animal models of addiction do not represent the full complexity of the disorder. Furthermore, there are differences in anatomic brain regions between rodents and humans, and many technical aspects of DBS in rodents differ significantly from human clinical parameters. Additional caveats for studying the effects of DBS in animal models include the difficulties in replicating the social and environmental factors associated with different clinical disease states, the multitude of cognitive and physiologic domains that characterize psychiatric disorders, and the differences in structural homology among rodents, nonhuman primates, and humans.[12,31] Because of these neuroanatomic and pathophysiologic differences between rodent models and human patients, Müller and colleagues[7] suggest that it is necessary to carefully continue to study the effects of DBS in severely addicted individuals in addition to the translational studies in animal models.[13] These investigators further state that in their opinion, enough is known to ethically justify continuing to analyze the risk versus benefit of DBS, comparing the enormous medical and socioeconomic burden of the disease with the risks of DBS and its potential to alleviate disease severity and even prevent relapses.[7,14] A recent cost analysis was conducted by Stephen and colleagues[32] to evaluate the cost of DBS in comparison with that of medical treatment of opiate addiction. The study revealed that the threshold success rate, which is defined as the percentage of patients remaining heroin-free after 6 months of treatment, at which DBS

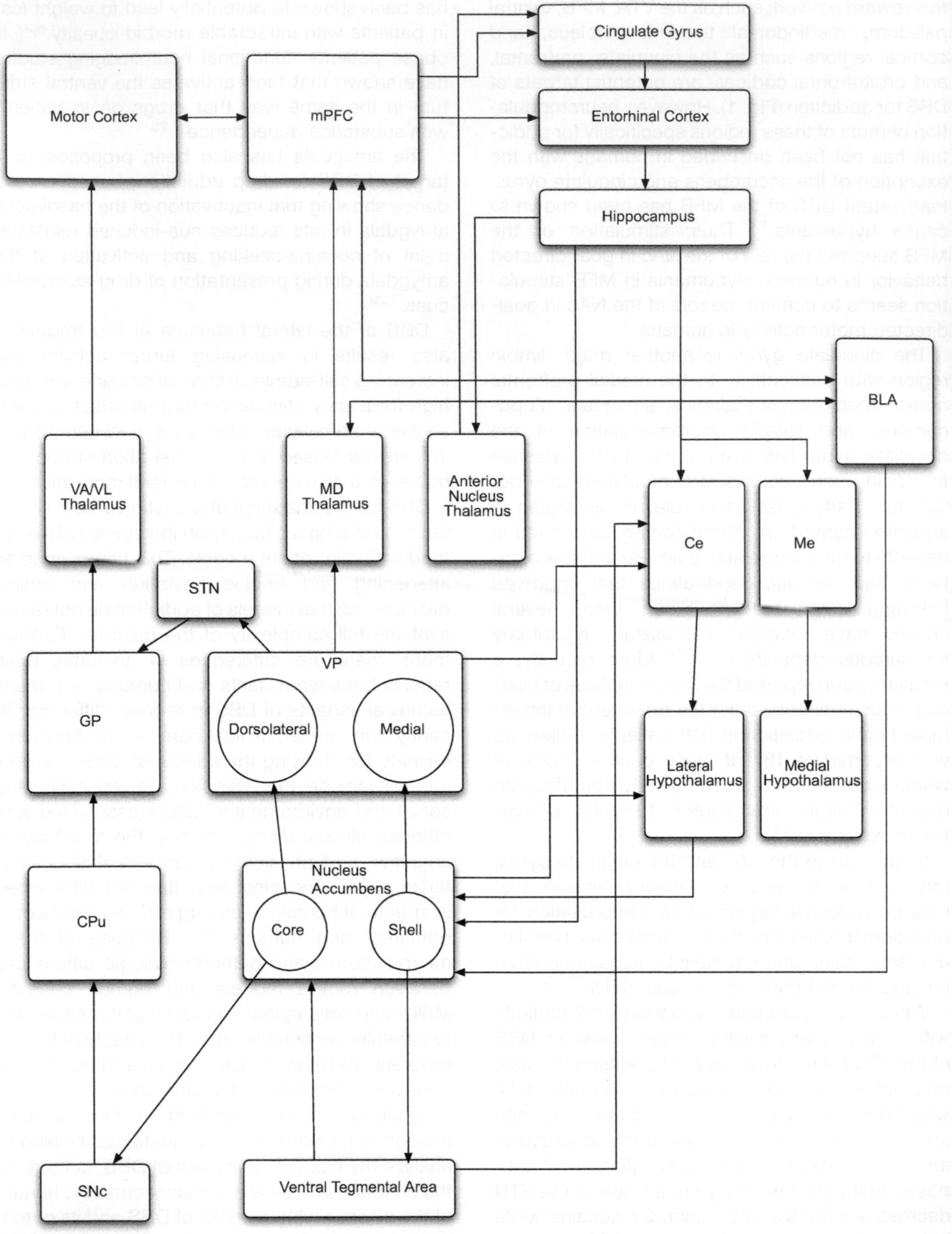

Fig. 1. Nuclei within the limbic system and their connectivity to motor output systems. BLA, basolateral nucleus of amygdala; Ce, central nucleus of amygdala; CPu, caudate-putamen; GP, globus pallidus; MD, mediodorsal nucleus; Me, medial nucleus of amygdala; mPFC, medial prefrontal cortex; SNc, substantia nigra pars compacta; VA/VL, ventral anterior/ventral lateral nuclei. Note that the ventral striatum/nucleus accumbens projects to the motor striatum via its core subdivision. In addition, the hypothalamus has efferents to the brainstem and spinal cord. These pathways provide a route for the limbic system to influence behavioral output.

would be as cost-effective as methadone is estimated at only 49%. This group concluded that a theoretical course of DBS would need a success rate of 36.5% to match the current methadone treatment, but a success rate of 49% to be cost-effective.[15]

It is therefore imperative that DBS for addiction can only be considered when the highest medical ethical standards are applied, given the nature of the conditions that are being treated.[16,17,33] Furthermore, patients should be carefully screened and followed by an interdisciplinary team that includes the neurosurgeon, psychiatrists, neurologists, social workers and support groups, because DBS is an intensive procedure that requires extensive follow-up and careful observation of symptoms and possible side effects. As Luigjes and colleagues[34] point out, DBS should be restricted to chronically addicted, treatment-refractory patients stable enough to comply with an intensive period of treatment and research.[18]

POSTTRAUMATIC STRESS DISORDER

PTSD is an anxiety disorder that develops following a life-threatening or an integrity-threatening traumatic event, and often includes perceptual, cognitive, affective, physiologic, and psychological features. PTSD is characterized by hyperarousal, intrusive vivid reliving of memories, and persistent avoidance of trauma-associated stimuli.[19–24,35] The estimated lifetime prevalence of PTSD in the United States is approximately 6.8%, and the 12-month prevalence is about 3.8%.[36,37] Unfortunately, 30% of patients still suffer from PTSD at least 10 years after the initial trauma despite the best current medical therapy.[38]

Functional neuroimaging studies in veterans indicate that the amygdala may play a critical role in the development of PTSD. In fact, PTSD patients subjected to provocative testing have shown increased activity in the amygdala on functional magnetic resonance imaging or positron emission tomography (PET)/computed tomography.[39–43] The intensity of the amygdala activity seen on imaging also correlates with the severity of PTSD symptoms.[41,44] Of note, veterans with injury to the amygdala never develop PTSD.[45] Koenigs and Grafman[46] showed that 40% of veterans who suffered brain injury in combat develop PTSD unless the amygdala is injured. The amygdala seems to be responsible for the encoding and retrieval of the memories associated with the traumatic events. In this sense, it is responsible for the symptoms and suffering associated with PTSD.

If it is assumed that DBS can functionally reduce the activity of a cerebral target and that activity in the amygdala seems to be responsible for PTSD development, DBS of the amygdala may treat the symptoms of PTSD. Langevin and colleagues[47] tested this hypothesis using a rodent model of PTSD in which rats were given inescapable shock in the presence of an unfamiliar object. The rats then developed a tendency to bury the object when reexposed to it several days later. This behavior mimics the symptoms of PTSD. Ten rats underwent placement of an electrode in the right basolateral nucleus of the amygdala (BLn). The rats were then subjected to a session of inescapable shocks while being exposed to an object. Five rats received high-frequency DBS treatment while the other 5 rats did not. Rats that were treated with BLn DBS spent on average 13-fold less time burying the ball than the control rats, and thus the behavior of treated rats was nearly normalized. More recently, Stidd and colleagues[48] demonstrated that the effects of BLn DBS in this rat model of PTSD were preserved even when DBS was initiated late after the establishment of the PTSD behavior.

Alternative methods of neuromodulation in the treatment of PTSD, such as vagus nerve stimulation (VNS), have also been studied. In VNS, electrical pulses are applied to the vagus nerve in the neck to activate afferents. VNS does not provide direct stimulation to the cortex but acts broadly by activating the parasympathetic nervous system. The Food and Drug Administration approved VNS in 1997 for epilepsy and in 2005 for treatment-resistant depression. George and colleagues[49] performed an open-label study of adjunctive VNS treatment for anxiety, and suggested that this treatment was well tolerated and possibly efficacious in patients with a range of anxiety disorders, including OCD, panic disorder, and PTSD. The group speculated that the effects likely derived from downstream modulation by the vagus nerve afferents on the locus coeruleus, orbitofrontal cortex, insula, hippocampus, and amygdala.[22]

Unfortunately, human investigations of neuromodulation for the treatment of PTSD are limited. There are currently no human studies involving amygdala DBS. A longitudinal study in humans is needed to evaluate the effects of DBS of the amygdala on PTSD.

MEMORY

Alzheimer disease is the most common form of dementia. It is a progressive disease, and currently there is no cure. Pharmacologic agents such as acetylcholinesterase inhibitors and *N*-methyl-D-aspartate receptor antagonists are used to delay the progression, but they are not effective in all patients and carry significant side-effect profiles. Alzheimer disease is usually diagnosed in people older than 65 years. Early onset is less frequent but is also possible. In 2006, there were 26.6 million patients with Alzheimer globally, and the number is expected to reach 1 in 85 by 2050.[5] Therefore, it is imperative to develop a different strategy in Alzheimer treatment. This section reviews the role of limbic neuromodulation in the treatment of dementia.

At the heart of the limbic system since its earliest conceptualization lie the mesial temporal lobe structures and their targets, including the hippocampal formation and fornix. The role of this region in the formation of memory is well established. Abnormalities of these regions have been linked to disorders of cognition and memory such as Alzheimer disease and other forms of dementia. For example, hippocampal atrophy and volume have been used to predict the onset of dementia.[50–52] Other regions with connectivity to the hippocampus and fornix include the mammillary bodies, anterior nucleus of the thalamus, cingulate gyrus, and basal forebrain cholinergic nuclei.

The anterior nucleus of the thalamus (AN) has already been studied as a target of DBS in the treatment of intractable epilepsy. The AN receives afferent fibers from mammillary bodies via the mammillothalamic tract and from the subiculum via the fornix. Efferent fibers from the AN project to the cingulate gyrus. The AN is an integral part of the limbic system that seems to play a role in modulating alertness, and is involved in learning and memory. Oh and colleagues[53] studied DBS of the AN in the treatment of patients with intractable epilepsy, and found that not only did it result in seizure control but was also associated with improvements in both verbal recall and oral information processing. The investigators proposed that the effect on memory could be related to the bilateral activation of a thalamacortical circuit following DBS surgery. These results suggest that DBS of the AN and functionally related regions may be used to enhance memory. Indeed, high-frequency stimulation of the AN in rats has been shown to increase hippocampal neurogenesis and to reverse experimentally suppressed hippocampal neurogenesis. These findings suggest that DBS not only alters neuronal activity but also produces long-term neuronal changes that may potentially enhance memory formation.[54]

High-frequency stimulation to isolated hippocampal slices also increases synaptic plasticity in the CA1 region and results in a 2-fold increase of nonamyloidogenic α-secretase activity, in comparison with controls stimulated at low frequency.[55] DBS treatment has also been shown to facilitate acquisition of object-recognition memory in rats in comparison with the baseline.[55] Stone and colleagues[56] took this idea one step further and showed that stimulation of the entorhinal cortex in rats influences cognitive function via activity-dependent regulation of hippocampal neurogenesis. Acute stimulation of entorhinal cortex transiently promoted proliferation in the dentate gyrus. New cells generated as a consequence of stimulation eventually differentiated into neurons, survived for at least several weeks, and acquired normal dentate granule cell morphology. After maturation, these neurons integrated into hippocampal circuits supporting memory.[56] Another group confirmed this finding by showing that DBS of the fornix in rats reverses the memory-impairing effects of scopolamine when compared with sham.[57] Furthermore, they reported that the fornix is not sensitive to the frequency but rather the current and no side effects on anxiety or general motor activity were encountered.[57]

Human studies have corroborated these results in a single patient who underwent DBS of the hypothalamus for obesity. Hamani and colleagues[58] discovered that DBS in this region surprisingly evoked detailed autobiographical memories. Electroencephalographic source localization in this patient identified activity in mesial temporal lobe structures in response to DBS of the hypothalamus. The investigators hypothesized that they were actually stimulating fibers of the fornix within the hypothalamus, which resulted in activation of mesial temporal lobe structures.[58]

Based on this initial result, the investigators from the previous study conducted a phase I clinical trial of DBS of the fornix/hypothalamus in patients with mild Alzheimer disease, using PET imaging to illustrate an early and striking reversal of the impaired glucose utilization in the temporal and parietal lobes that was maintained after 12 months of continuous stimulation. Stimulation of the fornix/hypothalamus drove neural activity in the memory circuit, including the entorhinal and hippocampal areas, and activated the brain's default mode network. At 6 and 12 months follow-up, evaluations suggested possible improvements and/or slowing in the rate of cognitive decline. In addition, there were no serious adverse events reported.[59]

Fontaine and colleagues[60] also conducted a prospective study in a single patient with Alzheimer disease who underwent bilateral forniceal DBS. Electrodes were placed in the fornix within the hypothalamus bilaterally; at 1-year follow-up, the patient's memory score stabilized in comparison with baseline, with an increased metabolism in the mesial temporal lobes. No complications were reported.

Whereas the aforementioned human studies indirectly stimulated the mesial temporal lobe by purportedly stimulating forniceal fibers in the hypothalamus, Suthana and colleagues[61] studied the effect of direct entorhinal stimulation in patients without dementia. This study involved stimulation of the entorhinal cortex in patients implanted with depth electrodes for the purpose of seizure monitoring. In this study, 7 subjects underwent stimulation of the entorhinal cortex while learning a visuospatial memory task involving reaching locations by using landmarks. The subjects who underwent stimulation during the learning phase reached their target locations more quickly and by shorter routes. Remarkably, this study suggests that direct stimulation of mesial temporal lobe structures may enhance learning and memory in patients without baseline dementia.[61]

Other targets have been tested and studied for possible impact on memory and treatment of dementia. Freund and colleagues[62] reported a single patient with dementia treated with DBS of the nucleus basalis of Meynert (nbM). Stimulation of the nbM resulted in markedly improved cognitive function. Improvement in attention, concentration, alertness, drive, and spontaneity resulted in the patient's renewed enjoyment of former interests and enhanced social communication. While the exact mechanism for the success of nbM DBS in memory improvement remains unknown, many hypotheses have been proposed, including enhancement of the synthesis of nerve growth factor and possible facilitating/resetting of neural oscillation.[63]

Costa and colleagues[64] reported experimental investigations into the effect of low-frequency electrical stimulation (25 Hz) of the pedunculopontine (PPN) area on working memory in patients with Parkinson disease. Patients showed a consistent decrease in response time on both the verbal and visual-object tasks when going from the "Off" to the "On" condition. However, the accuracy score did not significantly differ between the two experimental conditions. Costa proposed that stimulation of the PPN area may facilitate the speed of processing of information in the content of working memory, or the memory system that keeps multiple pieces of information in a place where they can be manipulated.

In conclusion, our understanding of the neural substrates underlying memory is still in its infancy, despite important discoveries over the last few years. DBS as a means to modulate and augment memory and cognition shows promise in the treatment of conditions characterized by cognitive impairment. Learning and recall are highly dynamic processes. Therefore, dynamic neuromodulatory devices and technologies are likely to be required to modulate these functions.[65] The initial goal of neuromodulation in memory is to help patients suffering from cognitive difficulties such as dementia. However, the remote possibility of cognitive enhancement using neuromodulation may raise ethical dilemmas in the future.

SUMMARY

The limbic system lies at the center of some of the most intractable neuropsychiatric disorders such as addiction, PTSD, and dementia. Successful treatment of these disorders has eluded physicians and scientists for decades. Preliminary results show that DBS to specific nuclei within the limbic system may be at least as successful as traditional pharmacologic therapies. In addition, advances in limbic neuromodulation are increasing our understanding of how the limbic system works in healthy people. There remains a mix of healthy skepticism and misunderstanding among the public and physicians outside of neurosurgery regarding the safety and efficacy of DBS for neuropsychiatric disorders. The ethical and legal challenges to the widespread application of this technology offer new opportunities for education and increasing social awareness, and will require the cooperative effort of multidisciplinary treatment teams consisting of neurosurgeons, neurologists, psychiatrists, and other specialties.

REFERENCES

1. McGinnis JM, Foege WH. Actual causes of death in the United States. JAMA 1993;270:2207–12.
2. Xu F, et al. Surveillance for certain health behaviors among States and selected local areas—United States, 2010. MMWR Surveill Summ 2013; 62:1–247.
3. Carelli RM. Nucleus accumbens cell firing during goal-directed behaviors for cocaine vs. 'natural' reinforcement. Physiol Behav 2002;76:379–87.
4. Carelli RM. The nucleus accumbens and reward: neurophysiological investigations in behaving animals. Behav Cogn Neurosci Rev 2002;1:281–96.
5. Gao G, et al. Clinical study for alleviating opiate drug psychological dependence by a method of ablating the nucleus accumbens with stereotactic surgery. Stereotact Funct Neurosurg 2003; 81:96–104.
6. Wu HM, et al. Preliminary findings in ablating the nucleus accumbens using stereotactic surgery for

alleviating psychological dependence on alcohol. Neurosci Lett 2010;473:77–81.
7. Müller UJ, et al. Deep brain stimulation of the nucleus accumbens for the treatment of addiction. Ann N Y Acad Sci 2013;1282:119–28.
8. Zahm DS. Functional-anatomical implications of the nucleus accumbens core and shell subterritories. Ann N Y Acad Sci 1999;877:113–28.
9. Bari AA, Pierce RC. D1-like and D2 dopamine receptor antagonists administered into the shell subregion of the rat nucleus accumbens decrease cocaine, but not food, reinforcement. Neuroscience 2005;135:959–68.
10. Wise RA. Addictive drugs and brain stimulation reward. Annu Rev Neurosci 1996;19:319–40.
11. Olds J, Milner P. Positive reinforcement produced by electrical stimulation of septal area and other regions of rat brain. J Comp Physiol Psychol 1954;47: 419–27.
12. Coenen VA, et al. Medial forebrain bundle stimulation as a pathophysiological mechanism for hypomania in subthalamic nucleus deep brain stimulation for Parkinson's disease. Neurosurgery 2009;64:1106–14 [discussion: 1114–5].
13. Zahm DS. An integrative neuroanatomical perspective on some subcortical substrates of adaptive responding with emphasis on the nucleus accumbens. Neurosci Biobehav Rev 2000;24:85–105.
14. Lipsman N, Neimat JS, Lozano AM. Deep brain stimulation for treatment-refractory obsessive-compulsive disorder: the search for a valid target. Neurosurgery 2007;61:1–11 [discussion: 11–3].
15. Foltz EL, White LE. Pain 'relief' by frontal cingulumotomy. J Neurosurg 1962;19:89–100.
16. Kanaka TS, Balasubramaniam V. Stereotactic cingulumotomy for drug addiction. Appl Neurophysiol 1978;41:86–92.
17. Balasubramaniam V, Kanaka TS, Ramanujam PB. Stereotaxic cingulumotomy for drug addiction. Neurol India 1973;21:63–6.
18. Medvedev SV, Anichkov AD, Poliakov II. Physiological mechanisms of the effectiveness of bilateral stereotactic cingulotomy in treatment of strong psychological dependence in drug addiction. Fiziol Cheloveka 2003;29:117–23 [in Russian].
19. Knight G. Chronic depression and drug addiction treated by stereotactic surgery. Nurs Times 1969; 65:583–6.
20. Müller D, Roeder F, Orthner H. Further results of stereotaxis in the human hypothalamus in sexual deviations. First use of this operation in addiction to drugs. Neurochirurgia (Stuttg) 1973;16:113–26.
21. Langevin JP. The amygdala as a target for behavior surgery. Surg Neurol Int 2011;2:7.
22. Lu L, Wang X, Kosten TR. Stereotactic neurosurgical treatment of drug addiction. Am J Drug Alcohol Abuse 2009;35:391–3.
23. Stelten BM, Noblesse LH, Ackermans L, et al. The neurosurgical treatment of addiction. Neurosurg Focus 2008;25:E5.
24. Pelloux Y, Baunez C. Deep brain stimulation for addiction: why the subthalamic nucleus should be favored. Curr Opin Neurobiol 2013. http://dx.doi.org/10.1016/j.conb.2013.02.016.
25. Witjas T, et al. Addiction in Parkinson's disease: impact of subthalamic nucleus deep brain stimulation. Mov Disord 2005;20:1052–5.
26. Rouaud T, et al. Reducing the desire for cocaine with subthalamic nucleus deep brain stimulation. Proc Natl Acad Sci U S A 2010;107:1196–200.
27. Whiting DM, et al. Lateral hypothalamic area deep brain stimulation for refractory obesity: a pilot study with preliminary data on safety, body weight, and energy metabolism. J Neurosurg 2013;119:56–63.
28. Volkow ND, Wise RA. How can drug addiction help us understand obesity? Nat Neurosci 2005; 8:555–60.
29. Langevin JP. The amygdala as a target for behavior surgery. Surg Neurol Int 2012;3:40–6.
30. Friedman A, et al. Electrical stimulation of the lateral habenula produces enduring inhibitory effect on cocaine seeking behavior. Neuropharmacology 2010;59:452–9.
31. Hamani C, Temel Y. Deep brain stimulation for psychiatric disease: contributions and validity of animal models. Sci Transl Med 2012;4:142.
32. Stephen JH, et al. Deep brain stimulation compared with methadone maintenance for the treatment of heroin dependence: a threshold and cost-effectiveness analysis. Addiction 2012;107: 624–34.
33. Carter A, Hall W. Proposals to trial deep brain stimulation to treat addiction are premature. Addiction 2011;106:235–7.
34. Luigjes J, et al. Deep brain stimulation in addiction: a review of potential brain targets. Mol Psychiatry 2012;17:572–83.
35. Novakovic V, et al. Brain stimulation in posttraumatic stress disorder. Eur J Psychotraumatol 2011;2.
36. Kessler RC, et al. Lifetime prevalence and age-of-onset distributions of DSM-IV disorders in the National Comorbidity Survey Replication. Arch Gen Psychiatry 2005;62:593–602.
37. Kessler RC, Chiu WT, Demler O, et al. Prevalence, severity, and comorbidity of 12-month DSM-IV disorders in the National Comorbidity Survey Replication. Arch Gen Psychiatry 2005;62:617–27.
38. Breslau N. Outcomes of posttraumatic stress disorder. J Clin Psychiatry 2001;62(Suppl 17):55–9.
39. Protopopescu X, et al. Differential time courses and specificity of amygdala activity in posttraumatic stress disorder subjects and normal control subjects. Biol Psychiatry 2005;57:464–73.

40. Semple WE, et al. Higher brain blood flow at amygdala and lower frontal cortex blood flow in PTSD patients with comorbid cocaine and alcohol abuse compared with normals. Psychiatry 2000;63:65–74.
41. Shin LM, et al. Regional cerebral blood flow in the amygdala and medial prefrontal cortex during traumatic imagery in male and female Vietnam veterans with PTSD. Arch Gen Psychiatry 2004;61: 168–76.
42. Shin LM, et al. A functional magnetic resonance imaging study of amygdala and medial prefrontal cortex responses to overtly presented fearful faces in posttraumatic stress disorder. Arch Gen Psychiatry 2005;62:273–81.
43. Etkin A, Wager TD. Functional neuroimaging of anxiety: a meta-analysis of emotional processing in PTSD, social anxiety disorder, and specific phobia. Am J Psychiatry 2007;164:1476–88.
44. Armony JL, Corbo V, Clément MH, et al. Amygdala response in patients with acute PTSD to masked and unmasked emotional facial expressions. Am J Psychiatry 2005;162:1961–3.
45. Koenigs M, et al. Focal brain damage protects against post-traumatic stress disorder in combat veterans. Nat Neurosci 2008;11:232–7.
46. Koenigs M, Grafman J. Posttraumatic stress disorder: the role of medial prefrontal cortex and amygdala. Neuroscientist 2009;15:540–8.
47. Langevin JP, De Salles AA, Kosoyan HP, et al. Deep brain stimulation of the amygdala alleviates post-traumatic stress disorder symptoms in a rat model. J Psychiatr Res 2010;44:1241–5.
48. Stidd DA, Vogelsang K, Krahl SE, et al. Amygdala deep brain stimulation is superior to paroxetine treatment in a rat model of posttraumatic stress disorder. Brain Stimul 2013. http://dx.doi.org/10.1016/j.brs.2013.05.008.
49. George MS, et al. A pilot study of vagus nerve stimulation (VNS) for treatment-resistant anxiety disorders. Brain Stimul 2008;1:112–21.
50. Laakso MP, et al. Hippocampal volumes in Alzheimer's disease, Parkinson's disease with and without dementia, and in vascular dementia: an MRI study. Neurology 1996;46:678–81.
51. Junqué C, et al. Amygdalar and hippocampal MRI volumetric reductions in Parkinson's disease with dementia. Mov Disord 2005;20:540–4.
52. Aybek S, et al. Hippocampal atrophy predicts conversion to dementia after STN-DBS in Parkinson's disease. Parkinsonism Relat Disord 2009;15:521–4.
53. Oh YS, et al. Cognitive improvement after long-term electrical stimulation of bilateral anterior thalamic nucleus in refractory epilepsy patients. Seizure 2012;21:183–7.
54. Toda H, Hamani C, Fawcett AP, et al. The regulation of adult rodent hippocampal neurogenesis by deep brain stimulation. J Neurosurg 2008;108: 132–8.
55. Arrieta-Cruz I, Pavlides C, Pasinetti GM. Deep brain stimulation in midline thalamic region facilitates synaptic transmission and short-term memory in a mouse model of Alzheimer's disease. Transl Neurosci 2010;1:188–94.
56. Stone SS, et al. Stimulation of entorhinal cortex promotes adult neurogenesis and facilitates spatial memory. J Neurosci 2011;31:13469–84.
57. Hescham S, et al. Deep brain stimulation of the forniceal area enhances memory functions in experimental dementia: the role of stimulation parameters. Brain Stimul 2013;6:72–7.
58. Hamani C, et al. Memory enhancement induced by hypothalamic/fornix deep brain stimulation. Ann Neurol 2008;63:119–23.
59. Laxton AW, et al. A phase I trial of deep brain stimulation of memory circuits in Alzheimer's disease. Ann Neurol 2010;68:521–34.
60. Fontaine D, et al. Symptomatic treatment of memory decline in Alzheimer's disease by deep brain stimulation: a feasibility study. J Alzheimers Dis 2013;34:315–23.
61. Suthana N, et al. Memory enhancement and deep-brain stimulation of the entorhinal area. N Engl J Med 2012;366:502–10.
62. Freund HJ, et al. Cognitive functions in a patient with Parkinson-dementia syndrome undergoing deep brain stimulation. Arch Neurol 2009;66:781–5.
63. Hardenacke K, et al. Stimulate or degenerate: deep brain stimulation of the nucleus basalis Meynert in Alzheimer dementia. World Neurosurg 2012. [Epub ahead of print].
64. Costa A, et al. Effects of deep brain stimulation of the pedunculopontine area on working memory tasks in patients with Parkinson's disease. Parkinsonism Relat Disord 2010;16:64–7.
65. Hu R, Eskandar E, Williams Z. Role of deep brain stimulation in modulating memory formation and recall. Neurosurg Focus 2009;27:E3.

Neuromodulation for Eating Disorders: Obesity and Anorexia

Alessandra A. Gorgulho, MD, MSc[a,b,c,*],
Julio L.B. Pereira, MD[a,b], Scott Krahl, PhD[a,d],
Jean-Jacques Lemaire, MD, PhD[e,f],
Antonio De Salles, MD, PhD[a,b,c]

KEYWORDS

• Eating disorders • Neuromodulation • Deep brain stimulation • Hypothalamus

KEY POINTS

- Based on our increasing knowledge of neurophysiology, functional neuroimaging, and previous experience with deep brain stimulation, neuromodulation should help patients with eating disorders.
- The relative low complication rate of deep brain stimulation (DBS) surgery, its reversibility, and the potential success of this approach in morbid obesity and anorexia nervosa is supported by the animal experimental literature and by a limited number of humans submitted to this procedure.
- DBS potentially can play a pivotal role in the management of patients with refractory eating disorder.

INTRODUCTION

Extremes of eating disorders (ED) have come to the attention of neurosurgeons as they have become prevalent in society.[1–4] Therapies available, although largely effective, fail in a substantial number of patients and carry considerable side effects. Morbid obesity and anorexia nervosa (AN) represent important causes of morbidity and mortality among young adults in the developed countries, and this trend is spreading to the developing world.[5] Morbid obesity, in particular, has reached epidemic proportions,[6] affecting disproportionate numbers of children in a worrisome way.[7] AN is also important for its high mortality in young adults, leading also to severe depression, malnourishment, and suicide. The challenges of effectively treating AN are well recognized.[8,9] In this article, important aspects of ED are reviewed in detail, and novel approaches to the treatment of ED are proposed.

MORBID OBESITY

Comorbidity factors such as cardiac disease, high blood pressure, myocardial infarction, metastatic disease, and spine problems that may need neurosurgical intervention directly affect patients with morbid obesity.[10] Deep brain stimulation (DBS), currently used to influence brain function in several neurologic diseases, has the potential also to be used for the treatment of systemic diseases encountered in daily practice, such as morbid obesity.[11,12]

[a] Department of Neurosurgery, David Geffen School of Medicine, University of California, Los Angeles, Los Angeles, CA, USA; [b] Department of Radiation Oncology, David Geffen School of Medicine, University of California, Los Angeles, Los Angeles, CA, USA; [c] HCor Neuroscience, Hospital do Coração, Rua Abilio Soares, 250, Paraiso, São Paulo 05005-000, Brazil; [d] VA Great Los Angeles Healthcare Hospital, 11301 Wilshire Blvd, Los Angeles, CA, USA; [e] Service of Neurosurgery, University Hospital, Clermont-Ferrand, France; [f] EA 7292 (Image-Guided Clinical Neuroscience and Connectomics), Auvergne University, France
* Corresponding author. Department of Neurosurgery, David Geffen School of Medicine, University of California, Los Angeles, 10945 Le Conte Avenue, Suite 2120, Los Angeles, CA 90095.
E-mail addresses: a_gorgulho@yahoo.com; agorgulho@mednet.ucla.edu

Neurosurg Clin N Am 25 (2014) 147–157
http://dx.doi.org/10.1016/j.nec.2013.08.005
1042-3680/14/$ – see front matter

The Problem

The World Health Organization (WHO) estimates that by 2015 the number of overweight people globally will increase to 2.3 billion and that more than 700 million will be obese.[6,7,13] The increasing prevalence of obesity has been reported in the United States, Canada, Australia, Europe, and nonindustrialized countries. It was estimated in 2003 that 66% of American adults were overweight, 32% were obese, and 5% were morbidly or severely obese (body mass index $\geq$40 kg/m^2). Over the last 20 years, the incidence of morbid obesity has doubled.[14] Among adults, obesity is associated with nearly 112,000 excess deaths relative to normal weight. More than 9 million children and adolescents are considered overweight (National Health and Nutrition Examination Survey 2003–2004).[7,15,16] Increasing rates of obesity-related chronic diseases not previously seen in children, such as type 2 diabetes mellitus, have been observed.[10] Morbid obesity has many ramifications on both individual and societal levels. The health risks associated with morbid obesity include hypertension, hyperlipidemia, cardiomyopathy, stroke, diabetes, hypoventilation disorders, increased risk of malignancy,[17] cholelithiasis, degenerative arthritis, gastroesophageal reflux, infertility, and psychosocial impairment.[14,16]

Need for New Obesity Therapies

Present treatments to control morbid obesity include a wide variety of drugs, nutritional and dietetic counseling, and surgical procedures focused on the gastrointestinal tract. Medical weight-reduction programs have rarely achieved long-term success in this population, with nonsurgical options resulting in less than a 1% chance of chronic weight control. Therefore, undesired side effects and failure of long-term control keep morbid obesity as an open field regarding the search for new and more effective therapeutic modalities.

The mortality rate in bariatric surgery is reported to range from 0.1% to 2%.[18–20] Risk factors identified included advanced age, body mass index greater than 50 kg/m^2, and comorbidities. When sustained weight loss is achieved over the long term, epidemiologic studies show a significant reduction in mortality from any cause, particularly deaths from diabetes, cardiovascular events, and cancer.[18–20] Bariatric surgery is the current standard of treatment for morbidly obese patients. However, despite the success as regards decreasing mortality risk, morbidities associated with bariatric surgery are not insignificant. Dumping syndrome can occur in up to 70% of cases submitted to Roux-en-Y gastric bypass,[21] the singular surgery leading to the best results in terms of weight reduction. Other side effects described include nausea and vomiting; deficiency in iron, vitamin B_{12}, folate, copper, calcium, and fat-soluble vitamins; peripheral neuropathy; polyradiculoneuropathy; myelopathy; and encephalopathy.[19,22,23]

Based on all of this evidence, it is of utmost relevance that neurosurgeons make efforts to develop surgical techniques leading to sustained weight loss and lowered morbidity and mortality. As neurosurgeons have direct access to brain centers controlling food intake, it is natural that their expert knowledge of stereotactic techniques should be used to reach these centers and modulate them, using proven effective devices that discretely influence brain function.

Role of Hypothalamic Nuclei in Obesity

The hypothalamus is crucially involved in many physiologic, endocrine, and behavioral processes. Although the human hypothalamus accounts for only 4 cm^3, or 0.3%, of the adult brain volume, it contains the integrative systems critical for all these processes.[24]

Since the early 1940s it was noted that lesions of specific brain areas led to alterations in normal food and water intake. A lesion of the ventromedial hypothalamus (VMH) can cause overeating and obesity,[25,26] whereas a lesion of the lateral hypothalamus can lead to anorexia.[27] Many scientific experiments have demonstrated that high-frequency electrical stimulation of the VMH induces a pronounced bout of eating in previously satiated animals, and that electrical stimulation of the lateral area of the hypothalamus (LHA) causes food-deprived animals to stop eating.[28] Other studies have demonstrated that bilateral electrolytic lesions in the VMH cause rats to become obese, but when bilateral destruction of the extreme lateral portion of the LHA is performed in addition to VMH lesions, the animals lapse into anorexia and adipsia. The effects of LHA ablation are so severe that it can result in death.[29,30] Taken together, the results of these experiments suggest that high-frequency stimulation mimics the results observed with ablation, suggesting a suppressive effect of high-frequency stimulation on these hypothalamic nuclei. In Denmark, 3 human subjects were submitted to ablation of the lateral hypothalamus, 2 of whom received unilateral lesions. Subjects experienced weight loss temporarily.[31]

Integration of the various mechanisms controlling feeding results from the complex interplay of medial and lateral hypothalamic circuits. The VMH acts as a "satiety center," which is the set point for regulation of caloric intake, whereas the LHA acts as a "feeding center."[32] Thus, activation of the VMH or a lesion of the LHA induces primary increases in metabolism rates that precede and parallel the period of food-intake inhibition.[26,33,34] In other words, the modulation of these neural structures results in a tendency toward weight loss by way of a double influence on both sides of the energy balance. One influence favors the utilization of stored molecules (lipolytic effect), accompanied by a second influence that restricts the income of energy in the organism (inhibition of feeding) (**Fig. 1**).[35–37]

Deep Brain Stimulation

DBS is a well-established and safe procedure that has multiple applications. It is currently approved by the Food and Drug Administration for the treatment of Parkinson disease and essential tremor, and has a humanitarian device exemption for dystonia and refractory obsessive-compulsive disorder. DBS is also frequently used off-label as a treatment for chronic pain syndrome, cluster headaches (CH), and, more recently, some other psychiatric conditions.[12] The potential for clinical neurosurgical applications related to the hypothalamic control of fat distribution and body weight has not been fully explored. Recently, new developments on manipulation of central nervous system functions through DBS have taken place in humans, based on exquisite magnetic resonance imaging (MRI) stereotactic targeting.[38] Moreover, therapeutic electrical stimulation of the hypothalamus for CH is an acceptable approach to the treatment of this refractory pain syndrome.[39,40] Patients under hypothalamic stimulation for CH have demonstrated loss of weight.[39,40] The authors' group has also observed such an effect of hypothalamic stimulation on CH; one patient lost more than 20 kg after DBS stimulation and also changed his food preferences.

Implantation of the VMH for the treatment of human obesity has been alluded to in the literature.[41] Recently DBS was applied to the lateral hypothalamus in a trial to decrease food intake, manipulate energy metabolism, and engender weight loss.[2] However, in this small study it was not possible to show it to be an effective treatment for morbidly obese patients.

Hypothalamus and Regulation of Food Intake

The early model of bimodal regulation of food intake by VMH and LHA has now become

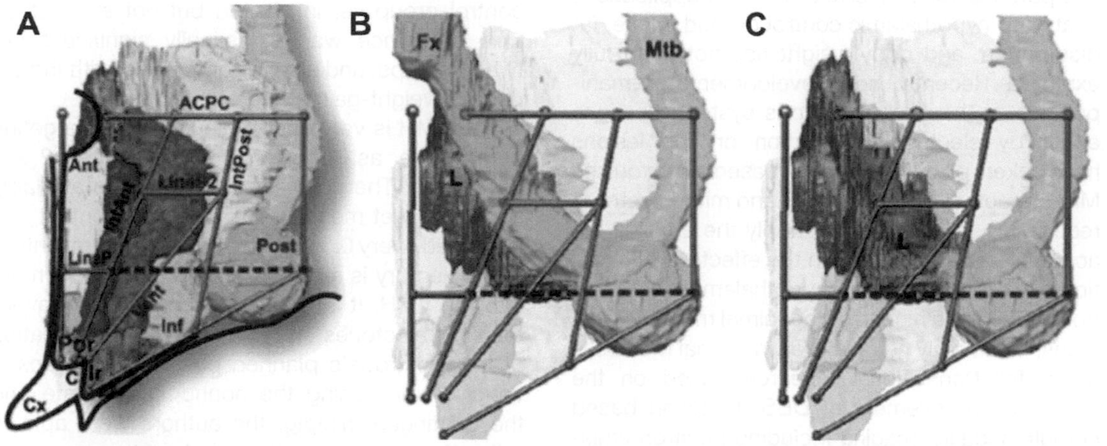

Fig. 1. The hypothalamus is defined posteriorly by the vertical line (Post) placed behind the mammillary body and perpendicular to ACPC, anteriorly by a line (Ant) rising from the preoptic recess (Por) also perpendicular to ACPC, and inferiorly by a line (Inf) from the infundibular recess (Ir) to the posterior point of mammillary body (at the origin of Post). Two intermediate lines, anterior (IntAnt) and posterior (IntPost) go from the dorsal region of the optic chiasma (Cx) to the anterior point of the intermediate third of ACPC, and from the midpoint of Inf to the posterior point of the intermediate third of ACPC. The anterior part (LineP) of the horizontal line (*doted black line*) goes parallel to ACPC (toward the posterior point at the origin of Post). The intermediate horizontal line (LineP2) is parallel to ACPC and origins at the midpoint of the segment of IntAnt between the point where IntAnt crosses LineP and the point where IntAnt crosses ACPC. The ventral line (Vent) goes from "c" to the intersection of LineP2 and IntPost. (*From* Lemaire JJ, Nezzar H, Sakka L, et al. Maps of the adult human hypothalamus. Surg Neurol Int 2013;4:159.)

increasingly refined to include other hypothalamic regions, for example, the arcuate and periventricular nuclei as centers for the regulation of metabolism and modulation of food intake.[22,42–44] The hypothalamus integrates peripheral reward and hormonal afferent signals of satiety and energy reserve, and directs neuroendocrine efferent "arms" to affect energy storage in relation to energy expenditure. Activities of 5 groups of cells in the hypothalamus (the arcuate, paraventricular, ventromedial, and dorsomedial nuclei, and the dorsolateral hypothalamic area) are modulated by anorexigenic peptides (α-MSH, CART peptide, corticotropin-releasing hormone, urocortin III, cholecystokinin, and glucagon-like peptides) and orexigenic peptides (neuropeptide Y, agouti-related peptide, orexins, melanin concentrating hormone, and galanin). Intrahypothalamic neuronal circuits have been identified between these peptidergic neurons, prominently including the arcuate-paraventricular and arcuate-dorsolateral hypothalamic projections. Efferent projections of hypothalamic neurons give rise to projections to autonomic centers in the brainstem and the spinal cord with potential for stimulation or inhibition of peripheral factors related to food intake, energy balance, and ingestion behavior.[21]

Deep Brain Stimulation for the Treatment of Eating Disorders

The potential for clinical neurosurgery applications related to hypothalamic control of food intake, fat distribution, and body weight has not been fully explored. Recently, new developments on manipulation of the central nervous system functions either by electrical stimulation or fine lesions have taken place in humans based on exquisite MRI stereotactic targeting[38,45] and microelectrode recordings.[46] It is timely to apply the body of the accumulated knowledge on the effects of stimulation and lesions of the hypothalamus obtained from rodent and higher-order animal models to humans. This highly studied area in animal models is ready for translational research based on the exquisite improvement of DBS, targeting based in multimodality imaging including positron emission tomography (PET),[47,48] and functional and morphologic MRI with fiber tracking, including the hypothalamus, as presented by the authors' group.[48,49] Coupled with the exquisite imaging available for stereotactic electrode placement, there has been an increasing understanding of stimulation parameters needed to modulate neural networks.[2,50,51] The ultimate goal of developing therapies for humans with morbid obesity is at hand.[2,4,52]

Deep Brain Stimulation of the Hypothalamus

Recently, electrodes were implanted in the posterior hypothalamus for long-term DBS treatment of refractory chronic CH.[39] This therapeutic approach has been based solely on adoption of DBS methods used successfully in the treatment of Parkinson disease, with the assumption that high-frequency DBS would exert similar inhibitory effects on hyperactive posterior hypothalamus functional activity. DBS of the posterior hypothalamus was not evaluated in animal models before the application to humans, although the effects of electrical stimulation of the hypothalamus had been previously explored in different animals, predominantly in nonhuman primates.[53,54]

The authors placed DBS leads in the VMH of free-moving, unrestrained nonhuman primates using human stereotactic methods. This experiment established the feasibility and safety of long-term bilateral VMH DBS as a potential intervention for ED in humans, based on changes of feeding behavior through modulation of VMH activity.[55] The translation research was continued using the VMH target with low-frequency stimulation in swine, a species that fulfills the criteria of a natural model of obesity. The authors have shown that it is possible to modulate the weight of these animals without affecting food intake.[4] Animals implanted and receiving stimulation in the VMH consumed all the food offered ad libitum. Nevertheless, these animals did not gain weight as prominently as the control group (ie, implanted but not stimulated). This difference was statistically significant between groups, and also in comparison with the expected weight-gain curve of this species.

The VMH is very challenging from the targeting perspective, as it measures approximately $2 \times 3 \times 5$ mm.[56] The smallest electrode size available on the market measures 1.5 mm per contact and is spaced every 0.5 mm. Moreover, an intraventricular trajectory is required for electrode placement into the VMH. It is well established that intraventricular trajectories carry a higher risk of deviation of the electrode's planned position.[57] In translational studies using the nonhuman primate and the Göttingen minipig, the authors were able to refine the technique with the help of the armamentarium available to make stereotaxis safe in such a busy region. The proper selection of the stimulation contact showed that chronic electrical stimulation of this area is tolerable and safe from autonomic and behavior perspectives, in both models.[58,59] However, small variations in the technique for targeting may affect the clinical results.[58] Torres and colleagues[59] also studied the impact of different ranges of electrical stimulation in the

VMH using a single electrodes placed through the third ventricle. Their results using low-frequency stimulation in the VMH suggested an increase in metabolic rate, corroborating the authors' findings using the minipig model.

Neuroimaging and Obesity

Recent advances in neuroimaging have allowed in vivo measurement of parameters of the dopaminergic system.[60] A PET study using [^{11}C]raclopride to measure dopamine D_2 receptor availability in the striatum found that obese patients had significantly lower D_2 receptor levels than normal-weight controls.[61] The involvement of the dopaminergic (DA) system in reward and reinforcement has led to the hypothesis that low brain DA activity in obese subjects predisposes them to excessive consumption of food. A better understanding of the role of the DA system in the motivation for food intake will help the development of better therapeutic interventions. In subjects of normal weight, [^{11}C]raclopride PET was also used to demonstrate that extracellular concentrations of dopamine in the dorsal striatum increase in response to the sight and smell of food.[62] Increases in extracellular dopamine were positively correlated with self-reports of hunger and desire for food, suggesting that dopamine release in the dorsal striatum is involved in food motivation in humans.

Another line of evidence implicating the dopaminergic system in the regulation of weight is the problematic side effect observed in antipsychotic therapy. Treatment with antipsychotic medications that principally block the dopamine D_2 receptor causes weight gain.[63] Long-term administration of typical and atypical antipsychotic drugs induces excessive weight gain, which afflicts up to 50% of patients.[64,65] Conversely, treatment of obesity with anorectic drugs has been shown to be successful only in a limited number of studies.[66,67]

The anorectic agents that currently represent the main pharmacologic approach to appetite suppression and resultant weight loss include indirect sympathomimetic action, which potentiates dopamine and/or serotonin neurotransmission, and dopamine receptor agonists.[66,67] Because pharmacologic manipulation of the DA system has been well documented to influence body weight in humans, it may be that in the nondrug context the overall steady-state activity of the DA system also contributes to the motivation and maintenance of an individual's food intake patterns, and is likely associated with corresponding D_1 and D_2 receptor profiles in striatum and hypothalamus. Parkinson disease is a readily available example of imbalance in the DA system that can be modulated by the DBS technique.

Treatment of morbid obesity with functional neurosurgery approaches is at hand. This approach obviates several of the difficulties in operating on the morbidly obese patient, as intracranial anatomy is not affected by obesity. The efficacy of bariatric surgery in the treatment of morbid obesity is well established. A study evaluated how efficient DBS results would need to be to achieve weight loss comparable with that observed after bariatric surgery.[68] However, it is expected that neuromodulation will induce weight loss at a slower pace. The mechanisms involved in the neuromodulation of the hypothalamus are quite different from mechanical modifications achieved with bariatric intervention. Given the low complication rate of DBS surgery and the potential success of this approach in morbid obesity supported by the animal experimental literature, DBS may become a very attractive alternative for morbidly obese patients.

ANOREXIA NERVOSA

AN is defined as refusal to maintain body weight at or above a minimal weight for height, associated with fear of gain in weight and distorted perception of body shape.[69] It is associated with others psychological factors, such perfectionism, anxiety, and humor deregulation. AN is an eating disorder that can be life threatening because of general medical and psychiatric complication, such as depression and suicide. Severe forms of AN are difficult to treat, leading to a high mortality rate.[70,71]

The Problem

The diagnosis of AN is currently based on the DSM-IV-TR (*Diagnostic and Statistical Manual of Mental Disorders* 4th edition, text revision). DSM criteria have changed over time, making it difficult to evaluate in epidemiologic studies. Moreover, self-reported samples are unreliable. Some studies show a lifetime prevalence of anorexia in women to be 0.3% to 2.2%, and 0.3% in men.[5,8,72]

The occurrence of AN has increased over the past 30 years. Adolescent and young adult women are most afflicted with this disease.[70,71] Women in this age group are particularly vulnerable to ED because of the tendency in our culture to idolize skinny phenotypes. Mortality for AN ranges from 6% to 11%, and more than 20% of patients do not derive benefit from current clinical treatment.[8,73]

Need for New Anorexia Therapies

The standard treatment of anorexia involves a multidisciplinary care of nutritional rehabilitation, treatment of clinical complications, and psychotherapy. A review shows that only 50% of AN patients have a good outcome, defined by return to a healthy weight.[70] Anorexia is a chronic disease with a poor outcome (defined as failure to reach a healthy weight) in more than 25% of patients, despite decades of research.[73,74]

Psychiatric surgery has evolved, with several studies showing it to be safe and effective when using DBS.[12] It is important to remember that research in psychiatric neuromodulation must follow universal rules of ethics of clinical research. Any study must be approved by institutional review boards, which are composed of independent psychiatrists corroborating the diagnosis and treatment eligibility.[12,75]

AN remains one of the most challenging psychiatric diseases.[74,76] In this context, new research and advances in neuroimaging, implantable brain stimulation, and stereotactic guidance have offered new hope for neuromodulation in AN. DBS surgery has been proved to be beneficial in improving quality of life in adults with medically refractory psychiatric disorders such as obsessive-compulsive disorders. A phase II to III trial is under way evaluating its impact on refractory major depressive disorders.[77]

Treatment of AN requires an interdisciplinary approach and should include, at minimum, a mental health professional, a medical doctor, and a nutritionist. Many psychiatric comorbidities are associated with AN, and family members need to be included in the treatment. The neurosurgeon should be supported by this highly specialized team when trying to treat AN.

Evidence Supporting Neurosurgery for Anorexia Nervosa

The frontostriatal system plays a key role in thoughts and behavior. Basic research has shown that there are changes in the frontostriatal circuitry during self-regulatory control of food intake in AN.[78,79] Moreover, there are substantial psychological and social aspects associated with AN, and it has been difficult to separate those factors.[74]

Imaging in Anorexia Nervosa

Recently, abnormality of brain connectivity has been suggested to exist in AN patients. Favaro and colleagues[80] showed a specific association with visual spatial difficulties that may explain disturbance in recognition of own body image in AN patients. AN patients who underwent a resting-state functional MRI scan showed increased coactivation in the left parietal cortex, in an area implicated in long-term multimodal spatial memory and representation of the body, even in the absence of visual information. Schulte-Rüther and colleagues[81] showed reduced activation in the middle and anterior temporal cortex and in the medial prefrontal cortex in AN patients. Hypoactivation in the medial prefrontal cortex at admission to hospital was correlated with better clinical outcome at follow-up.

Functional and anatomic brain-imaging studies have showed that forebrain areas are associated with mood, reward, and motivation. Functional abnormality in cortical-limbic-striatal control systems has been associated with anorexia. Marsh and colleagues[82] showed BOLD (blood oxygen level dependent) signal hypoactivation in multiple regions of frontostriatal regions among individuals with ED. Wagner and colleagues[83] reported that women who had recovered from AN showed hypoactivation in the anterior ventral striatum in response to correct answers in a guessing-game task. Friederich and colleagues[84] performed a morphometric analysis of brain regions within cortical-striatal networks in patients suffering from acute AN as well as patients with restored long-term weight ($n = 39$). AN patients showed decreased gray matter volume in the anterior cingulate cortex and supplementary motor area, unrelated to stage of the disease. Other investigators have shown hypometabolism and limbic circuit dysfunction in the subcallosal area. This finding is known to relate to mood disturbance in AN.[79]

The absence of a good animal model to study AN contributes to the limited understanding about the neuropathologic mechanisms leading to the disease. Available rodent models are a result of forced restriction of calorie intake. In humans, there is evidence that genetic factors play a role in AN. Familial studies showed that a female relative with AN is 7 to 20 times more likely to have the disease than females in the general population.

Basic research suggests a role for serotonin pathways in deregulation of appetite and mood. The serotonin pathway is modulated by estrogen, explaining the gender differences. Other studies have tried to show the role of cortisol pathways in the pathogenesis of AN.[85,86] This deregulation is still under debate, and there is no primary pharmacologic approach for AN based on the assumption of disturbance in the cortisol pathways.[86] Trials of DBS in AN may help to elucidate a truly effective treatment, considering that almost 50%

of the patients diagnosed with AN do not reach satisfactory results.[8]

Neurosurgical Indication

Recently, Lipsman and colleagues[87] conducted a literature review on the surgical treatment of refractory AN. The literature search selected 35 patients who underwent a neurosurgical procedure for AN. The first report in the literature was a lobotomy for this disease, performed in 1950. Since then, stereotactic ablation and, more recently, DBS has taken the stage regarding neurosurgical treatment of AN.[1] Surgical procedures for AN have evolved over the last few years. DBS has been progressively studied as a promising option. There is no standard indication for DBS in AN. Small series and case reports suggest a good outcome after DBS surgery (**Table 1**).[3,88] The recent literature on AN has shown that DBS might be useful in select cases with chronic, severe, medically, and behaviorally refractory disease.

Old and New Trends for Anorexia Nervosa

Since 1950, when Drury and colleagues performed the first neurosurgery for AN, the same question prevails: where is the best target? Between 1950 and 1973, the goal was to disconnect white matter tracts connecting frontal cortical structures. Surgery was described as unilateral lower quadrant frontal leucotomy, bilateral lower quadrant frontal leucotomy, or prefrontal lobotomy.

In the medical literature, there are 6 cases reported between 1973 and 2011. The target was the anterior cingulate bilaterally, the rostral cingulate, and lower medial quadrant of the frontal lobes. Radiofrequency lesions were performed. Two patients improved and 1 committed suicide.[90,91] Zamboni and colleagues[92] performed a bilateral dorsomedial thalamotomy in 2 patients, with improvement of the symptoms. Lastly, Barbier and colleagues[93] targeted the anterior capsule bilaterally, and observed normalization of weight within 3 months.

The first trial with 6 patients was reported in 2013. The target was the subcallosal cingulate region. Three of the 6 women gained weight during 9 months of follow-up. There was an improvement in scores measuring mood and anxiety, suggesting a similar mechanism of action on controlling obsession, reported earlier in patients implanted for obsessive-compulsive disorder. AN improved in 4 patients.[3] The series showed a change in cerebral glucose metabolism revealed in PET scans. The investigators compared PET scans at baseline and at 6 months after surgery. There was a significant decrease in glucose metabolism in the subcallosal cingulate area, insula, and medial frontal lobe. DBS led to an increase in glucose metabolism in the parietal lobe.[3] This finding is interesting because this location is related to AN distortion of self body image, according to previous studies.[80,84,94]

The Shangai group's DBS case series was reported in 2013.[90] The target was bilateral DBS of nucleus accumbens. All 4 patients were female. Procedures were performed between 2007 and 2011. All patients had psychiatric comorbidities (3 had obsessive-compulsive disorder and 1 had anxiety disorder). After the procedure there was a 65% increase in weight at 38 months of follow-up. This study showed that DBS might be a valuable option for weight restoration in severe AN. However, it must be emphasized that DBS for AN remains investigational (**Table 2**).[90]

DBS is still an investigational procedure for chronic, intractable, and severe AN.[3,87,90] A large trial of DBS for AN has not yet been carried out. Even an indirect comparison is difficult, as the accumulated number of cases in the literature is still very limited. A recent pilot trial demonstrated the safety of DBS surgery in AN patients. Nevertheless, further investigation is essential to clarify the long-term efficacy and safety of DBS for AN.

Table 1
Studies of deep brain stimulation for anorexia nervosa

Authors,[Ref.] Year	Patients	Target	Outcome
Israël et al,[89] 2010	1	Bilateral DBS of subcallosal cingulate	2-y F/U, good outcome
Wu et al,[90] 2013	4	Bilateral DBS of nucleus accumbens	38-mo F/U, 65% increase in BMI
McLaughlin et al,[77] 2013	1	Bilateral DBS of ventral caudate/striatum	Partial improvement
Lipsman et al,[3] 2013	6	Bilateral DBS of subcallosal cingulate	9-mo F/U, 3 of 6 had increase in BMI

Abbreviations: BMI, body mass index; DBS, deep brain stimulation; F/U, follow-up.

Table 2
Clinical trials on DBS for anorexia nervosa (ClinicalTrials.gov)

Chief Investigator, Hospital	Start	Title	Status
Wei Liu, Ruijin Hospital, Shanghai	August 30, 2012	Deep brain stimulation and capsulotomy for the treatment of refractory anorexia nervosa	Recruitment of participants
Andres M. Lozano, University Health Network, Toronto	November 15, 2011	Deep brain stimulation for the treatment of refractory anorexia nervosa	Recruitment of participants

SUMMARY

Based on our increasing knowledge of neurophysiology, functional neuroimaging, and previous experience with DBS, neuromodulation should help patients with ED. The relative low complication rate of DBS surgery, its reversibility, and the potential success of this approach in morbid obesity and AN are supported by the animal experimental literature and by limited data from humans submitted to this procedure. DBS potentially can play a pivotal role in the management of patients with refractory eating disorder.

REFERENCES

1. Sun B, Liu W. Stereotactic surgery for eating disorders. Surg Neurol Int 2013;4:164.
2. Whiting DM, Tomycz ND, Bailes J, et al. Lateral hypothalamic area deep brain stimulation for refractory obesity: a pilot study with preliminary data on safety, body weight, and energy metabolism. J Neurosurg 2013;119:56–63.
3. Lipsman N, Woodside DB, Giacobbe P, et al. Subcallosal cingulate deep brain stimulation for treatment-refractory anorexia nervosa: a phase 1 pilot trial. Lancet 2013;381:1361–70.
4. Melega WP, Lacan G, Gorgulho AA, et al. Hypothalamic deep brain stimulation reduces weight gain in an obesity-animal model. PLoS One 2012;7(1):e306–72.
5. Hoek HW, Van Hoeken D. Review of the prevalence and incidence of eating disorders. Int J Eat Disord 2003;34(4):383–96.
6. Obesity: preventing and managing the global epidemic. World Health Organ Tech Rep Ser 2000;894:i–xii, 1-253.
7. Wang Y, Lobstein T. Worldwide trends in childhood overweight and obesity. Int J Pediatr Obes 2006;1:11–25.
8. Keski-Rahkonen A, Hoek HW, Susser ES, et al. Epidemiology and course of anorexia nervosa in the community. Am J Psychiatry 2007;164:1259–65.
9. Wilson GT, Shafran R. Eating disorders guidelines from NICE. Lancet 2005;365:79–81.
10. Mokdad AH, Serdula MK, Dietz WH. The continuing epidemic of obesity in the United States. JAMA 2000;284(13):1650–1.
11. Kalia SK, Sankar T, Lozano AM. Deep brain stimulation for Parkinson's disease and other movement disorders. Curr Opin Neurol 2013;26:374–80.
12. Lipsman N, Ellis M, Lozano AM. Current and future indications for deep brain stimulation in pediatric populations. Neurosurg Focus 2010;29:E2.
13. Prentice AM. The emerging epidemic of obesity in developing countries. Int J Epidemiol 2006;35(1):93–9.
14. Tessier DJ, Eagon JC. Surgical management of morbid obesity. Curr Probl Surg 2008;45(2):68–137.
15. Kelishadi R. Childhood overweight, obesity, and the metabolic syndrome in developing countries. Epidemiol Rev 2007;29(1):62–76.
16. Rosamond W, Flegal K, Furie K, et al, American Heart Association Statistics Committee and Stroke Statistics Subcommittee. Heart disease and stroke statistics—2008 update: a report from the American Heart Association Statistics Committee and Stroke Statistics Subcommittee. Circulation 2008;117(4):e25.
17. Reeves GK, Pirie K, Beral V, et al. Cancer incidence and mortality in relation to body mass index in the Million Women Study: cohort study. BMJ 2007;335(7630):1134.
18. DeMaria EJ. Bariatric surgery for morbid obesity. N Engl J Med 2007;356:2176–83.
19. Flum DR, Salem L, Elrod JA, et al. Early mortality among Medicare beneficiaries undergoing bariatric surgical procedures. JAMA 2005;294:1903–8.
20. McMahon MM, Sarr MG, Clark MM, et al. Clinical management after bariatric surgery: value of a multidisciplinary approach. Mayo Clin Proc 2006;81:S34–45.
21. Rayner DV, Trayhurn P. Regulation of leptin production: sympathetic nervous system interactions. J Mol Med 2001;79:8–20.

22. Elmquist JK, Elias CF, Saper CB. From lesions to leptin: hypothalamic control of food intake and body weight. Neuron 1999;22:221–32.
23. Higa KD, Boone KB, Ho T, et al. Laparoscopic Roux en Y gastric bypass for morbid obesity: technique and preliminary results of our first 400 patients. Arch Surg 2000;135:1029–33.
24. Hofman MA, Swaab DF. The human hypothalamus: comparative morphometry and photoperiodic influences. Prog Brain Res 1992;93:133–47.
25. Niijima A, Rohner-Jeanrenaud F. Role of ventromedial hypothalamus on sympathetic efferents of brown adipose tissue. Am J Physiol 1984;242: 650–4.
26. Monda M, Sullo A, De Luca V, et al. Acute lesions of the ventromedial hypothalamus reduce sympathetic activation and thermogenic changes induced by PGE 1. J Physiol 1997;91: 285–90.
27. De Luca B, Monda M, Pellicano MP, et al. Cortical control of thermogenesis induced by lateral hypothalamic lesion and overeating. Am J Physiol 1987;253:R626–33.
28. Brown FD, Fessler RG, Rachlin JR, et al. Changes in food intake with electrical stimulation of the ventromedial hypothalamus in dogs. J Neurosurg 1984;60:1253–7.
29. Anand BK, Brobeck JR. Hypothalamic control of food intake in rats and cats. Yale J Biol Med 1951;24(2):123–40.
30. Hetherington AW, Ranson SW. The relation of various hypothalamic lesions to adiposity in the rat. J Comp Neurol 1942;76:475–99.
31. Quaade F, Veernet K, Larsson S. Stereotaxic stimulation and electrocoagulation of the lateral hypothalamus in obese humans. Acta Neurochir (Wien) 1974;30:111–7.
32. Carmel PW. Surgical syndromes of the hypothalamus. Clin Neurosurg 1980;27:133–59.
33. O'Brien PE, Dixon JB, Laurie C. Treatment of mild to moderate obesity with laparoscopic adjustable gastric banding or an intensive medical program randomized trial. Ann Intern Med 2006;144(9): 625–33.
34. Raftopoulos Y, Gatti GG, Luketich JD. Advanced age and sex as predictors of adverse outcomes following gastric bypass surgery. JSLS 2005;9(3): 272–6.
35. Ruffin MP, Nicolaidis S. Electrical stimulation of the ventromedial hypothalamus enhances both fat utilization and metabolic rate that precede and parallel the inhibition of feeding behavior. Brain Res 1999; 846(1):23–9.
36. Tokunaga K, Matsuzawa Y, Fujioka S, et al. PVN-lesioned obese rats maintain ambulatory activity and its circadian rhythm. Brain Res Bull 1991; 26(3):393–6.
37. Vilberg TR, Keesey RE. Reduced energy expenditure after ventromedial hypothalamic lesions in female rats. Am J Physiol 1984;27:183–8.
38. De Salles AA, Frighetto L, Behnke E, et al. Functional neurosurgery in the MRI environment. Minim Invasive Neurosurg 2004;47:284–9.
39. Franzini A, Ferroli P, Leone M. Hypothalamic deep brain stimulation for the treatment of chronic cluster headaches: a series report. Neuromodulation 2004;7(1):1–8.
40. Franzini A, Leone M, Messina G, et al. Neuromodulation in treatment of refractory headaches. Neurol Sci 2008;29(Suppl 1):S65–8.
41. Hamani C, McAndrews MP, Cohn M, et al. Memory enhancement induced by hypothalamic/ fornix deep brain stimulation. Ann Neurol 2008; 63:119–23.
42. Keen-Rhinehart E, Kalra SP, Kalra PS. AAV-mediated leptin receptor installation improves energy balance and the reproductive status of obese female Koletsky rats. Peptides 2005;26(12):2567–78.
43. Meguid MM, Fetissov SO, Varma M, et al. Hypothalamic dopamine and serotonin in the regulation of food intake. Nutrition 2000;16(10):843–57.
44. Shiraishi T, Oomura Y, Sasaki K, et al. Effects of leptin and orexin-A on food intake and feeding related hypothalamic neurons. Physiol Behav 2000; 71(3–4):251–61.
45. Anzal Y, Lufkin R, Salles AD. Radiofrequency ablation of brain tumours using MR guidance. Minim Invasive Ther Allied Tech 1996;5(3):232–42.
46. Lozano AM, Hutchison WD, Tasker RR. Microelectrode recordings define the ventral posteromedial pallidotomy target. Stereotact Funct Neurosurg 1998;71:153–63.
47. Lemaire JJ, Nezzar H, Sakka L, et al. Maps of the adult human hypothalamus. Surg Neurol Int 2013; 4(Suppl 3):S156–63.
48. Lemaire JJ, Frew AJ, McArthur D, et al. White matter connectivity of human hypothalamus. Brain Res 2011;1371:43–64.
49. Sedrak M, Gorgulho A, Frew A, et al. The role of modern imaging modalities on deep brain stimulation targeting for mental illness. Acta Neurochir Suppl 2008;101:3–7.
50. Hashimoto T, Elder CM, Vitek JL. A template subtraction method for stimulus artifact removal in high-frequency deep brain stimulation. J Neurosci Methods 2002;113:181–6.
51. Barkhoudarian G, Klochkov T, Sedrak M, et al. A role of diffusion tensor imaging in movement disorder surgery. Acta Neurochir (Wien) 2010;152: 2089–95.
52. Halpern CH, Attiah M, Bale TL. Deep brain stimulation for the treatment of binge eating: mechanisms and preclinical models. Animal Models of Eating Disorders 2013;74:193–200.

53. Takaki A, Aou S, Oomura Y. Feeding suppression elicited by electrical and chemical stimulations of monkey hypothalamus. Am J Physiol 1992;262: 586–94.
54. Aou S, Takaki A, Karádi Z, et al. Functional heterogeneity of the monkey lateral hypothalamus in the control of feeding. Brain Res Bull 1991;27:451–5.
55. Laćan G, De Salles A, Gorgulho AA, et al. Modulation of food intake following deep brain stimulation of the ventromedial hypothalamus in the vervet monkey. J Neurosurg 2008;108:336–42.
56. Schaltenbrand G, Warren W. Atlas for stereotaxy of the human brain. Stuttgart (Germany): Thieme; 1977.
57. Zrinzo L, van Hulzen AL, Gorgulho AA, et al. Avoiding the ventricle: a simple step to improve accuracy of anatomical targeting during deep brain stimulation. J Neurosurg 2009;110:1283–90.
58. Ettrup KS, Sorensen JC, Rodell A, et al. Hypothalamic deep brain stimulation influences autonomic and limbic circuitry involved in the regulation of aggression and cardiocerebrovascular control in the Göttingen minipig. Stereotact Funct Neurosurg 2012;90:281–91.
59. Torres N, Chabardes S, Piallat B, et al. Body fat and body weight reduction following hypothalamic deep brain stimulation in monkeys: an intraventricular approach. Int J Obes 2012;1:1–8.
60. Tataranni PA, DelParigi A. Functional neuroimaging: a new generation of human brain studies in obesity research. Obes Rev 2003;4(4):229–38.
61. Wang GJ, Volkow ND, Logan J, et al. Brain dopamine and obesity. Lancet 2001;357:354–7.
62. Volkow ND, Wang GJ, Fowler JS, et al. "Nonhedonic" food motivation in humans involves dopamine in the dorsal striatum and methylphenidate amplifies this effect. Synapse 2002;44(3):175–80.
63. Korner J, Aronne LJ. The emerging science of body weight regulation and its impact on obesity treatment. J Clin Invest 2003;111(5):565–70.
64. Allison DB, Mentore JL, Heo M. Antipsychotic-induced weight gain: a comprehensive research synthesis. Am J Psychiatry 1999;156:1686–96.
65. Weiden PJ, Mackell JA, McDonnell DD. Obesity as a risk factor for antipsychotic noncompliance. Schizophr Res 2004;66(1):51–7.
66. Haddock CK, Poston WS, Dill PL, et al. Pharmacotherapy for obesity: a quantitative analysis of four decades of published randomized clinical trials. Int J Obes Relat Metab Disord 2002;26(2):262–73.
67. Doknic M, Pekic S, Zarkovic M. Dopaminergic tone and obesity: an insight from prolactinomas treated with bromocriptine. Eur J Endocrinol 2002;147:77–84.
68. Halpern CH, Wolf JA, Bale TL, et al. Deep brain stimulation in the treatment of obesity. A review. J Neurosurg 2008;109:625–34.
69. American Psychological Association. Diagnostic and Statistical Manual of Mental Disorders. 4th edition. Washington, D.C.: American Psychological Association; 1994. In Press.
70. Steinhausen HC. The outcome of anorexia nervosa in the 20th century. Am J Psychiatry 2002;159:1284–93.
71. Korndörfer SR, Lucas AR, Suman VJ, et al. Long-term survival of patients with anorexia nervosa: a population-based study in Rochester, Minn. Mayo Clin Proc 2003;78:278–84.
72. Hudson JI, Hiripi E, Pope HG, et al. The prevalence and correlates of eating disorders in the National Comorbidity Survey Replication. Biol Psychiatry 2007;61:348–58.
73. Strober M, Freeman R, Morrell W. The long-term course of severe anorexia nervosa in adolescents: survival analysis of recovery, relapse, and outcome predictors over 10-15 years in a prospective study. Int J Eat Disord 1997;22:339–60.
74. Sylvester CJ, Forman SF. Clinical practice guidelines for treating restrictive eating disorder patients during medical hospitalization. Curr Opin Pediatr 2008;20:390–7.
75. Pisapia JM, Halpern CH, Muller UJ, et al. Ethical considerations in deep brain stimulation for the treatment of addiction and overeating associated with obesity. AJOB Neuroscience 2013;4(2):35–46.
76. Morris J, Twaddle S. Anorexia nervosa. BMJ 2007; 334:894–8.
77. McLaughlin NC, Didie ER, Machado AG, et al. Improvements in anorexia symptoms after deep brain stimulation for intractable obsessive-compulsive disorders. Biol Psychiatry 2013;73:e29–31.
78. Mair RG, Onos KD, Hembrook JR. Cognitive activation by central thalamic stimulation: the Yerkes-Dodson Law revisited. Dose Response 2011;9: 313–31.
79. Weiner MW, Veitch DP, Aisen PS, et al. The Alzheimer's disease neuroimaging initiative: a review of papers published since its inception. Alzheimers Dement 2012;8:S1–68.
80. Favaro A, Santonastaso P, Manara R, et al. Disruption of visuospatial and somatosensory functional connectivity in anorexia nervosa. Biol Psychiatry 2012;72:864–70.
81. Schulte-Rüther M, Mainz V, Fink GR, et al. Theory of mind and the brain in anorexia nervosa: relation to treatment outcome. J Am Acad Child Adolesc Psychiatry 2012;51:832–41.e11.
82. Marsh R, Maia TV, Peterson BS. Functional disturbances within frontostriatal circuits across multiple childhood psychopathologies. Am J Psychiatry 2009;166(6):664–74.
83. Wagner A, Aizenstein H, Venkatraman VK, et al. Altered reward processing in women recovered from anorexia nervosa. Am J Psychiatry 2007; 164:1842–9.

84. Friederich HC, Walther S, Bendszus M, et al. Grey matter abnormalities within cortico-limbic-striatal circuits in acute and weight-restored anorexia nervosa patients. Neuroimage 2012;59:1106–13.
85. Connan F, Lightman SL, Landau S, et al. An investigation of hypothalamic-pituitary-adrenal axis hyperactivity in anorexia nervosa: the role of CRH and AVP. J Psychiatr Res 2007;41:131–43.
86. Klein DA, Walsh BT. Eating disorders: clinical features and pathophysiology. Physiol Behav 2004; 81:359–74.
87. Lipsman N, Woodside DB, Giacobbe P, et al. Neurosurgical treatment of anorexia nervosa: review of the literature from leucotomy to deep brain stimulation. Eur Eat Disord Rev 2013. [Epub ahead of print].
88. Treasure J, Schmidt U. DBS for treatment-refractory anorexia nervosa. Lancet 2013;381:1338–9.
89. Israël M, Steiger H, Kolivakis T, et al. Deep brain stimulation in the subgenual cingulate cortex for an intractable eating disorder. Biol Psychiatry 2010;67(9):e53–4.
90. Wu H, Van Dyck-Lippens PJ, Santegoeds R, et al. Deep-Brain Stimulation for Anorexia Nervosa. World Neurosurg 2013;80(3–4):1–10.
91. Kelly D, Mitchell-Heggs N. Stereotactic limbic leucotomy—a follow-up study of thirty patients. Postgrad Med J 1973;49:865–82.
92. Zamboni R, Larach V, Poblete M. Dorsomedial thalamotomy as a treatment for terminal anorexia: a report of two cases. Acta Neurochir Suppl (Wien) 1993;58:34–5.
93. Barbier J, Gabriëls L, Van Laere K, et al. Successful anterior capsulotomy in comorbid anorexia nervosa and obsessive-compulsive disorder: case report. Neurosurgery 2011;69(3): E745–51.
94. Luyten L, Welkenhuysen M, van Kuyck K, et al. The effects of electrical stimulation or an electrolytic lesion in the mediodorsal thalamus of the rat on survival, body weight, food intake and running activity in the activity-based anorexia model. Brain Res Bull 2009;79:116–22.

Techniques in Neuromodulation

Image-Guided Deep Brain Stimulation

Rafael A. Vega, MD, PhD[a], Kathryn L. Holloway, MD[b], Paul S. Larson, MD[c,*]

KEYWORDS

- Deep brain stimulation • Functional neurosurgery • Movement disorders • Stereotactic surgery
- Target localization • Intraoperative imaging • Magnetic resonance imaging
- Computed tomography

KEY POINTS

- The clinical efficacy of deep brain stimulation (DBS) is highly dependent on accurate lead placement; traditional stereotactic techniques have an average accuracy of 2 to 3 mm.
- Intraoperative computed tomography can be used during DBS surgery with minimal disruption, and provides an effective means to confirm lead placement with a high degree of accuracy; however, it cannot visualize DBS targets directly and thus depends on fusion with preoperative magnetic resonance imaging (MRI).
- Intraoperative MRI allows DBS surgery to be done under general anesthesia using real-time anatomic targeting and can account for intraoperative brain shift, but usually requires significant changes in implantation techniques.
- The merits of purely anatomic targeting versus physiologic targeting are still under debate.

INTRODUCTION

Deep brain stimulation (DBS) has been advantageous to patients with medically intractable movement disorders and severe psychiatric illness.[1–3] The efficacy of DBS depends on the accurate placement of the leads at the targeted locations.[4–6] Knowledge of the anatomic position of the DBS electrode in the brain is essential in quality control, selection of the stimulation parameters, and ultimately for the success of the therapy. Various types of imaging modalities have been used for intraoperative targeting. Both computed tomography (CT) and magnetic resonance imaging (MRI) have been successfully integrated into the workflow of DBS surgery by a variety of groups. Several examples of these techniques and a discussion of their relative merits are discussed herein.

INTRAOPERATIVE CT-GUIDED DBS

There are 2 types of intraoperative CT available: fan-beam CT (FBCT), which is the same technology used for diagnostic imaging in radiology suites, and flat-panel cone-beam CT (CBCT), which typically is portable and increasingly common in the operating room (OR) environment. A small portable FBCT device (Ceretom; NeuroLogica Corp, Danvers, MA) is commercially available, and its utility in DBS surgery has recently been reported.[7,8] Its small bore makes it difficult to use during the procedure itself,

[a] Department of Neurosurgery, Virginia Commonwealth University, 417 North 11th Street, PO Box 980631, Richmond, VA 23298, USA; [b] Department of Neurosurgery, Parkinson's Disease Research, Education, and Clinical Care Center at the McGuire VAMC, Virginia Commonwealth University, 417 North 11th Street, PO Box 980631, Richmond, VA 23298, USA; [c] Department of Neurological Surgery, University of California, San Francisco, 505 Parnassus Avenue, Box 0112, San Francisco, CA 94143-0112, USA
* Corresponding author.
E-mail address: larsonp@neurosurg.ucsf.edu

Neurosurg Clin N Am 25 (2014) 159–172
http://dx.doi.org/10.1016/j.nec.2013.08.008
1042-3680/14/$ – see front matter Published by Elsevier Inc.

but it can be used to obtain the registration scan and to check final lead position before leaving the OR. In Richmond, the authors have studied the utility of a commercially available CBCT (O-arm; Medtronic Inc, Minneapolis, MN), which has a field of view large enough to image the whole head and a ring aperture large enough to be used repetitively throughout the procedure to check microelectrode tracks during physiologic recording. However, it has inferior soft-tissue resolution. The results of the authors' experience using the O-arm are presented, as well as others' experience with the Ceretom, as examples of well-studied CT-guided DBS.

O-Arm–Guided DBS with Physiologic Testing

Procedure overview

The philosophy of the Richmond program is to maximize any information that improves targeting while improving patient comfort during the surgery. Thus the authors' procedure combines anatomic imaging and physiologic testing. Intraoperative imaging with the O-arm allows for correction of the average 2-mm targeting error seen with frame and frameless stereotaxy.[9–12] Physiologic testing provides adjustment for interpatient variability in physiology and symptomatology. Both microelectrode recording (MER) and intraoperative Unified Parkinson's Disease Rating Scale (UPDRS) testing are useful in this regard. A determined effort is made to assure that the awake portion of the procedure is as comfortable as possible for the patient. Use of the frameless device provides comfortable head and neck support, and allows the patient to adjust head and body position during the surgery. The patient is sedated for infiltration of local anesthetic and drilling. Attachment of the anterior cervical portion of the head rest provides safety during arousal from sedation and can be removed once the patient is awake. The incorporation of the O-arm into the procedure provides the opportunity to incorporate the fiducials within the sedated portion of the procedure and to obtain the registration scan in situ, which further improves patient comfort. O-arm images can be obtained in standard mode to minimize the radiation dose (0.6 mSv), or in enhanced mode to enhance soft-tissue contrast (2.2 mSv), which has radiation dosing similar to that of a regular CT scan (~2–4 mSv) (**Fig. 1**).[10] The authors have determined that enhanced-mode imaging provides slightly better accuracy for fiducial localization than nonenhanced images (0.61 vs 0.70, $P = .04$); therefore, the enhanced mode is used for the registration scan standard mode is used for subsequent scans. MRI and CT images are obtained preoperatively, and the target is selected on the volumetric T1-weighted and T2-weighted images. The burr-hole entry site is chosen to optimize the maximum number of contacts within the

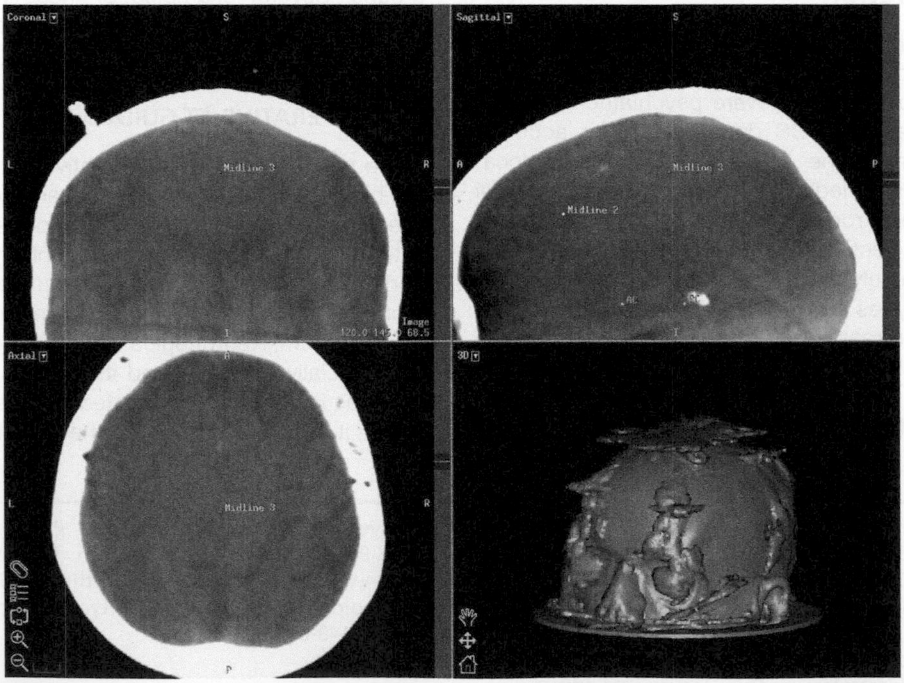

Fig. 1. Example of image obtained by the O-arm in enhanced mode, which increases the soft-tissue contrast thus providing sulcal anatomy and increased accuracy for intraoperative localization of fiducial markers.

target region and to minimize approximation to the internal capsule. The planned trajectory is reviewed on T1-weighted images to avoid transgression of cortical veins, sulci, or ventricles, and is adjusted accordingly.

A radiolucent head holder is used to minimize artifacts on the O-arm scans, and the radiolucent Medtronic Nexframe head support or collar is attached to the bed so that the vertical profile of the apparatus is minimized (**Fig. 2**). The O-arm is then positioned with the base at the patient's shoulders and neck. Three O-arm positions are created at this point, and saved. The ring is positioned with the head in the center of the ring for imaging. The park position should optimize surgical access, and an intermediate position is chosen to allow transition between scan and park positions without collision with the bed or cranial devices. The entire top of the head is prepped and a clear hip drape is adhered to the patient's head. The sedated patient is then injected with local anesthesia, and 6 bone fiducials are placed through 3-mm incisions created with the Colorado tip (**Fig. 3**A). The planned burr-hole entry sites are approximated by measuring distance from the coronal and sagittal sutures on the images and the patient's head. The location is marked with fiducials taped to the scalp (**Fig. 3**B). An enhanced-mode O-arm image is then obtained, transferred to the stealth station, and chosen as the reference scan. The preoperative images are then merged to the reference scan. The imaged locations of the taped fiducials are compared with the planned trajectories, and any deviation is corrected by altering the planned incision site and marking the skull with a fiducial or drill (**Fig. 3**C). The centers of the implanted fiducials are then marked on the images while the burr hole is created (**Fig. 4**). The Stimloc base and Nexframe base are secured over the burr hole, and the patient is registered into stereotactic space. The dura is then opened and sealed with gelfoam and fibrin glue. The tower is assembled and aligned to the target (**Fig. 5**). One or more cannulas are then introduced through the microelectrode drive so that they extend to a point that is 10 mm above the planned target to allow for physiologic testing. MER and test stimulation is carried out (**Fig. 6**). Once the microcannulas have reached the target depth, a standard-mode O-arm scan is obtained, transferred, and merged with the existing scans. The imaged position of the electrode is compared with the planned trajectory (**Fig. 7**).

The physiologic data are then interpreted in light of the position of the electrodes on the scan. A subsequent track can be created, or the DBS lead can replace one of the microelectrodes. Imaging of the DBS lead after placement assures the surgeon that its position is acceptable. Because nothing has been disassembled for the scan it is easy to adjust the lead if desired, and surprises are rare if the corresponding microelectrode track has been imaged. This scan does not currently have the soft-tissue resolution to rule out a small bleed.

Outcomes

The O-arm serves 2 purposes during surgery: (1) to serve as the registration scan (this allows the fiducial placement to be incorporated in the sedated portion of the procedure without having to leave the OR for a scan), and (2) to detect the location of the microelectrode track or lead to allow for intraoperative adjustment. To realize these goals, the authors first assessed whether the O-arm introduces a measurement error that is greater than diagnostic CT. Measurement error is the error introduced by the measuring tool rather than a true real

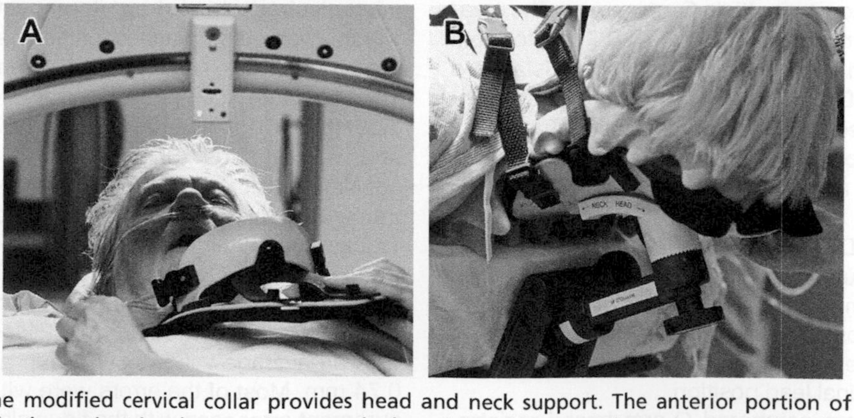

Fig. 2. (*A*) The modified cervical collar provides head and neck support. The anterior portion of the collar is attached while the patient is asleep, and removed when the patient is awake and cooperative. (*B*) The headrest is attached to the bed with a radiolucent Mayfield, minimizing its vertical profile for the ease of imaging.

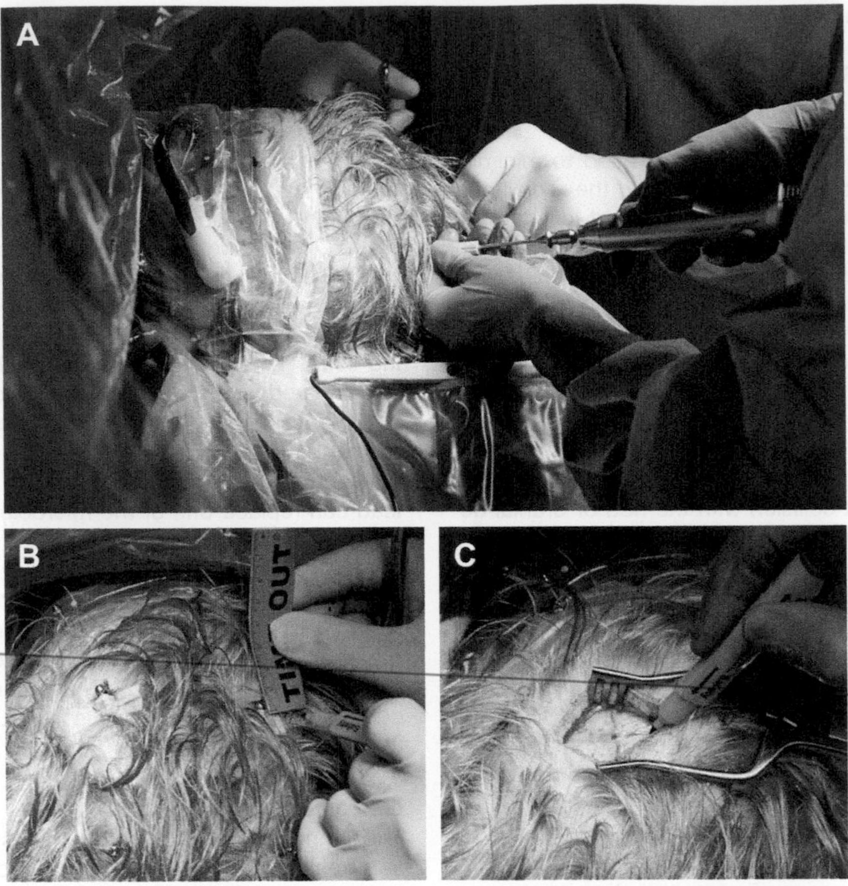

Fig. 3. (*A*) Placement of 5 to 6 bone fiducials under sedation. (*B*) Fiducials are taped to the scalp to mark the approximate location of the burr-hole sites. (*C*) Any deviation of the approximate burr-hole sites from the planned trajectory is corrected, and the true location is marked on the skull with a pilot hole.

world discrepancy in object locations. When 2 images are properly merged with each other, the expected result is that fixed objects will appear at exactly the same location on both scans; however, some error is expected and can be measured. The locations of fiducials and DBS leads were compared across multiple O-arm scans. The measurement error of the O-arm was 0.7 mm for both fiducials and leads.[10] A similar error (0.78 [standard deviation (SD) 0.38]) was found with repeated imaging of fixed leads using diagnostic CT imaging, and in comparing final lead position on an O-arm image and a CT image (0.72 mm [SD 0.38]).[10] This error is considerably smaller than the 1.65-mm (SD 0.19) discrepancy found by Shahlaie and colleagues[11] and the 1.52-mm (SD 1.78) error found by Smith and Bakay.[13] This difference in accuracy is most likely due the use of a postoperative MRI in these other studies as the standard for the location of final lead position.

The authors compared O-arm–based registration accuracy with diagnostic CT-based registration. The accuracy of final lead position was 2.04 mm (SD 0.80) in procedures with registration based on an O-arm image, which was not significantly different from CT-based registration: 2.16 mm (SD 0.92).[10]

The O-arm was used to assess the deviation of a microelectrode track from its expected location, which was the planned initial target.[10] The mean first track error was 2.12 mm (SD 1.04). The absolute component errors were lateral 1.09 (SD 0.78), anteroposterior 1.07 (SD 0.66), and vertical 1.09 (SD 1.03). This deviation is consistent with the authors' previous work on frame and frameless stereotactic accuracy.[9,14] Tracks subsequent to the first track are placed through the BenGun device in a presumed parallel path to the first. In fact, the error of these parallel tracks ranged from 0.21 to 3.04 mm, with an average value of 1.12 mm and an SD of 0.74 mm. Most of the errors were within the measurement error seen with the fiducials and stationary implants. However, 7 of 33 (22%) errors were

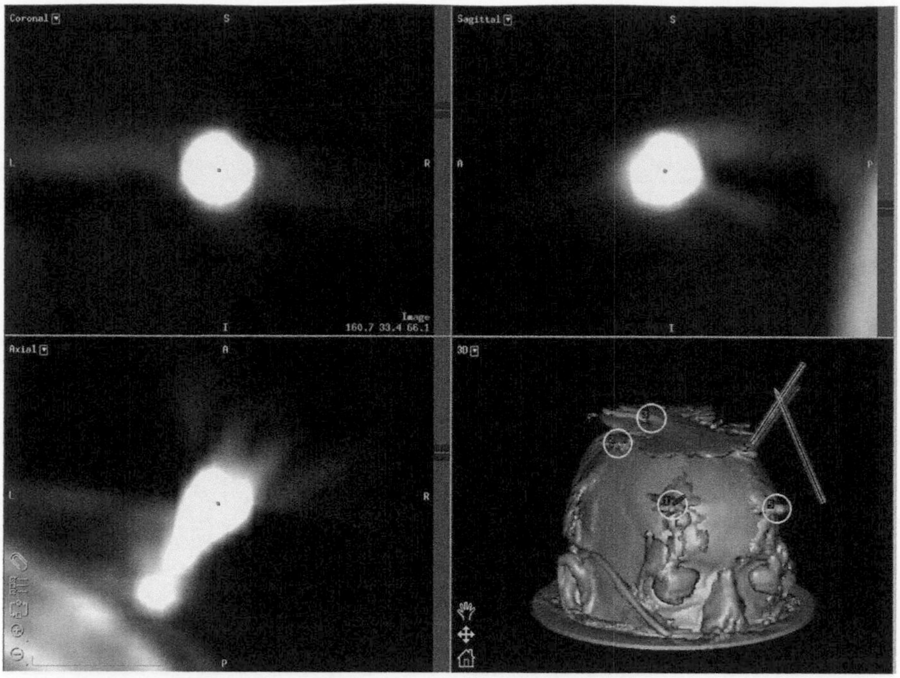

Fig. 4. The centers of the fiducials are selected on the enhanced-mode scan for registration.

greater than 1.8 mm, which is the largest error seen with stationary objects. There was a significant tendency for the tracks to be more medial and superior than intended. Changes in trajectory in the preferred direction tended to travel beyond the targeted area (overshoot), whereas those that moved in the opposite direction tended to fall short of the intended target (undershoot). The authors were thus able to demonstrate that the O-arm was able to detect the initial targeting error of the stereotactic system as well as the 22% skewed tracks through the BenGun.[10]

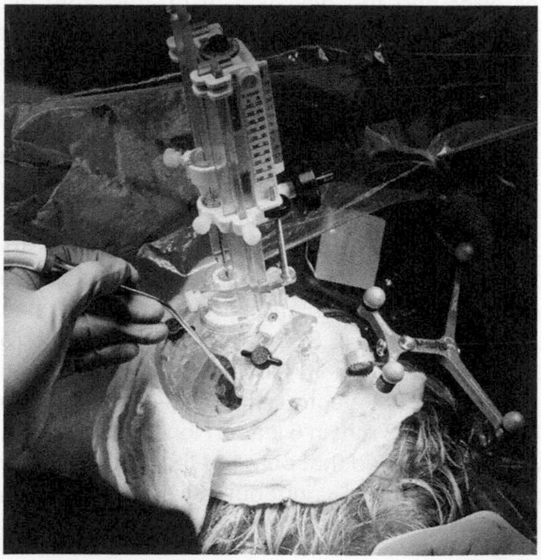

Fig. 5. The Nexframe tower is aligned to the target and the drive is mounted over the burr hole. The cannulas are introduced to the brain, and microelectrodes or the DBS lead are inserted.

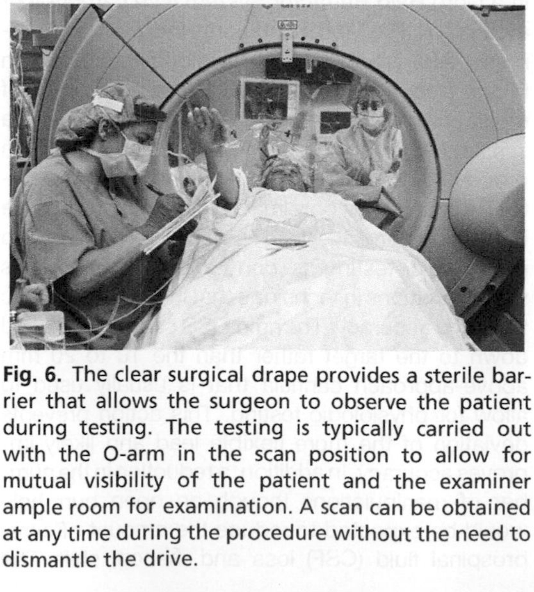

Fig. 6. The clear surgical drape provides a sterile barrier that allows the surgeon to observe the patient during testing. The testing is typically carried out with the O-arm in the scan position to allow for mutual visibility of the patient and the examiner ample room for examination. A scan can be obtained at any time during the procedure without the need to dismantle the drive.

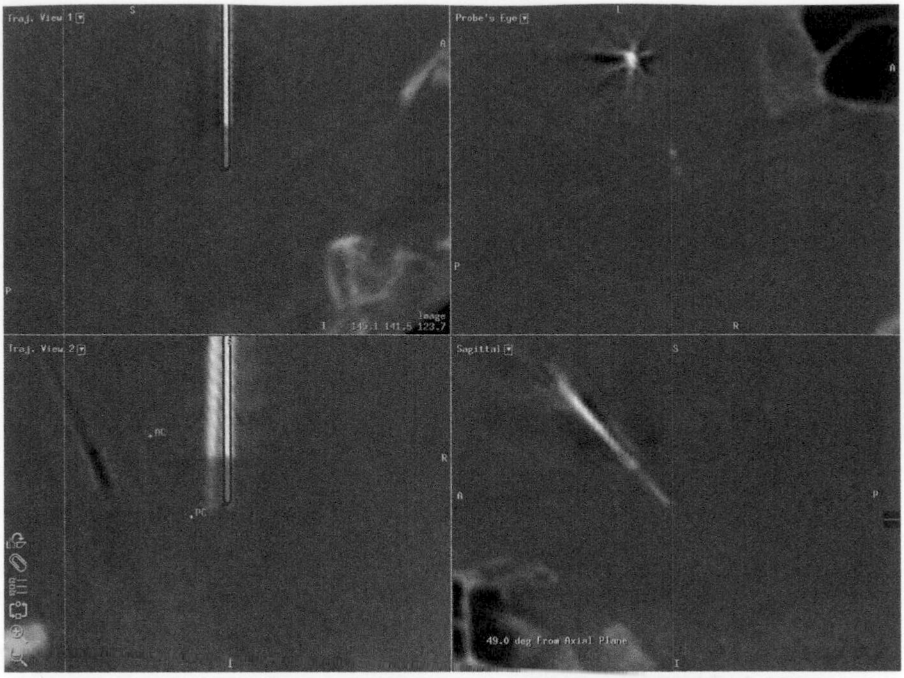

Fig. 7. An O-arm image obtained with 2 microelectrodes and a contralateral DBS in the brain.

Ceretom-Guided DBS Without Physiologic Testing

DBS electrode placement using intraoperative CT without MER has recently been explored.[7] In this study, the investigators enrolled 66 patients to target common areas of interest in movement disorders (ie, globus pallidus internus [GPi], ventral intermediate nucleus, and subthalamic nucleus [STN]). The target is planned using preoperative MRI images. The patient is intubated, and the head is secured in a Doro Halo Retractor System with carbon-fiber extensions (Pro Med Instruments Inc, Freiburg, Germany). After placement of bone fiducials, a Ceretom image is obtained. This image serves as the basis of registration and alignment of the Nexframe, in a similar fashion to the previously described O-arm procedure. Because of the small bore of the Ceretom, the patient is only imaged again after the drive is removed and the lead is secured in place. No physiologic testing is conducted, which allows some variations in technique that increase anatomic targeting accuracy. The rigid DBS cannula is placed down to the target rather than the 10 to 20 mm above-approach cannula that is usually used to allow for physiologic testing. This action prevents deviation of the more flexible lead and likely improves accuracy. In addition, a reduction in the number of manipulations though an open burr hole would be expected to reduce the amount of cerebrospinal fluid (CSF) loss and, hence, shift. The amount of intracranial air affects the accuracy of targeting on the second side.[10,15–17] Furthermore, rigid head fixation and intubation during imaging eliminates respiratory motion. Examining the patient with the same scanner in the same position may also increase accuracy.

Postimplantation CT scans were merged with the registration CT and MR to calculate both vector error and the deviation of off-trajectory distances. Two measures were used to assess the accuracy of electrode placement, which includes vector error and deviation off the trajectory. Vector error was defined as the distance between the position of the center of the target DBS electrode contact and the intended target location. Deviation from the trajectory was defined as the perpendicular distance from the target electrode to the planned trajectory. The mean overall vector error was 1.59 ± 1.11 mm and the deviation off trajectory was 1.24 ± 0.87 mm.[7] The trajectory error exceeded 2 mm in 14 leads and exceeded 3 mm in 3 leads. The vector error exceeded 2 mm in 19 leads and 3 mm in 6 leads. Nonetheless, the investigators noted that only 1 of the 119 electrodes placed required intraoperative replacement because of a vector error of greater than 3 mm.[7]

INTERVENTIONAL MRI-GUIDED DBS

MRI has been the preferred method for most brain-imaging needs since shortly after its commercial introduction in the 1980s. Functional neurosurgeons prefer it primarily for its superior tissue resolution, particularly in differentiating gray matter versus white matter, and the ability to visualize larger blood vessels both on the surface and in the parenchyma. Despite this, some surgeons have been reluctant to rely on MRI as the primary means of targeting and stereotactic registration for several reasons, the most common of which are the potential for motion artifact and image distortion. Individual MRI scans can take upward of 10 minutes or more to obtain, depending on the sequences acquired. In the case of DBS placement, whereby the patients frequently suffer from tremor or other involuntary movements, this can lead to motion artifact that significantly degrades image quality. Second, and more subtle, is the fact that all MR images suffer from small distortions caused by inhomogeneity in the static magnetic field, nonlinearity in the gradient fields, and variable magnetic susceptibility in various regions of the brain. Inherent MR image distortion varies from scanner to scanner and depends on several factors, including field strength and the relative position of the anatomy being imaged to the isocenter of the bore. Some surgeons have devised techniques to overcome these issues, including performing MRI under general anesthesia to eliminate motion artifact.[18]

MRI was not incorporated into the neurosurgical OR until the mid-1990s, when the first widespread use of intraoperative MRI was described.[19] At that time the primary use of this technology was in open craniotomy for tumor resection, but burr-hole–based brain biopsies were also performed using a simple targeting paradigm built into the scanner software.[20] It was not until 2004 that a technique for electrode placement using purely MRI guidance was developed in San Francisco. This method was crude but effective, using a commercially available skull-mounted aiming device (Nexframe) and standard scanner software running on a 1.5-T Philips Intera MRI console (Philips, Best, the Netherlands). The application accuracy of DBS electrode placement using this first-generation technique was assessed in several ways. The average radial error, defined as the 2-dimensional linear difference between intended and actual placement in the axial plane used for targeting, was found to be 1.2 $\pm$ 0.65 mm. The average tip error, defined as the 3-dimensional vector difference between intended and actual placement of the lead tip, was 2.18 $\pm$ 0.92 mm, which was superior to the average tip error seen using a stereotactic frame, previously shown to be 3.06 $\pm$ 1.41 mm.[21] The interventional MRI technique also provided shorter average procedure times (225 minutes for bilateral, 215 minutes for unilateral), fewer brain penetrations (87% of placements with 1 pass, and never more than 2 passes), and improved patient tolerance.[21] However, this first-generation method depended heavily on an imaging scientist who was intimately familiar with the imaging software, MR physics, and the surgical requirements of DBS implantation. These factors hindered widespread adoption of this technique until a second-generation system was developed and approved by the Food and Drug Administration in 2010.[22,23]

Procedure Overview

The current methodology consists of a skull-mounted aiming device (SmartFrame; MRI Interventions, Irvine, CA) that works in collaboration with a software environment (ClearPoint; MRI Interventions). This system can stream MR images in real time from any 1.5-T or 3-T scanner, and guide the surgical team through the implantation procedure. The procedure is referred to as "interventional" MRI (iMRI) as opposed to "intraoperative" MRI DBS placement, which is meant to reflect the fact that the procedure can take place with any 1.5-T or 3-T scanner regardless of whether it is located in an operating suite or the radiology department (in San Francisco, surgery is performed in the radiology department on a diagnostic 1.5-T scanner).

In brief, the patient is placed under general anesthesia and positioned on the MR gantry in the supine position. The technique uses real-time targeting and imaging for placement, so there is no preprocedure imaging or planning required. A stereotactic frame is not needed, and no registration steps are involved because there is no dependence on images acquired before the day of surgery. This method marks a departure from traditional stereotactic techniques, whereby targeting is performed on "historical" images and some sort of registration step (as well as an image fusion step) is needed to align the placement device with the intended target. Likewise, because the target can be identified throughout the implantation process in real time, physiologic mapping is not necessary.

The patient is moved all the way through the bore of the scanner until the head is protruding from the far end. The head is prepped and draped with a sterile, accordion-style drape that establishes a sterile field in the distal half of the bore and the distal face of the scanner (**Fig. 8**). A series of elastic tensioners attach to both ends of the magnet and work together to allow the patient to be moved between isocenter and the bore edge

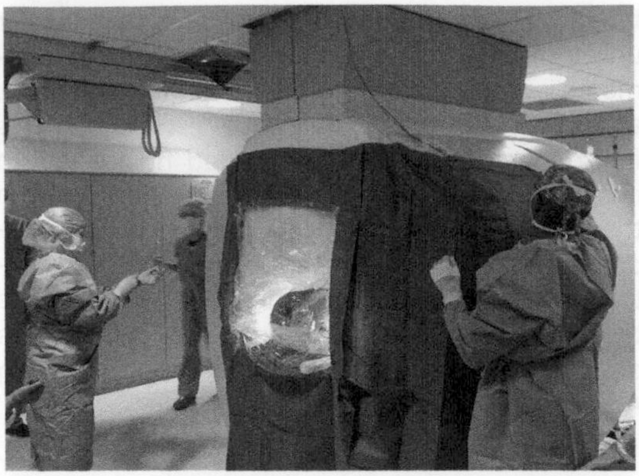

Fig. 8. A custom sterile drape being placed on a 1.5-T diagnostic MRI scanner in the radiology department. The drape adheres to the top of the patient's head, establishing a sterile field in the distal half of the bore and the end of the scanner. The drape wraps partially around one side of the scanner to allow the sterile back table to be positioned close to the sterile field.

without pulling the drape off the head. One or 2 marking grids comprising of MR-visible markers are placed in the anticipated entry region (usually just anterior to the coronal suture), and initial scans are obtained to plan the entry point and trajectory to the target region. The software then shows the surgeon where to make the skin incision and burr hole relative to the marking grids (**Fig. 9**). Skin incision, retraction, burr-hole formation, and all other steps of the procedure are performed with MRI-compatible instrumentation. These instruments are made of a variety of materials including nonferromagnetic metals (titanium, low-grade stainless steel), carbon fiber, ceramic, and plastic (**Fig. 10**). Once the burr hole is created, the dura is opened as early as possible to allow CSF egress and intracranial air entry to occur. In a standard DBS case, surgeons typically take steps to prevent these events to minimize inaccuracies caused by brain shift; in the iMRI technique, targeting is not performed until after dural opening, so it is advantageous to allow any brain shift to occur early in the procedure. The ability to target after dural opening, and on images that are not historical but truly reflect the brain position at the time of surgery, is one of the major advantages of this technique.

The SmartFrame is mounted to the skull around the burr hole and the patient is moved to isocenter (the geographic center of the MRI bore, and the area where MR images are most optimal). The SmartFrame has 4 degrees of freedom; angular pitch and roll movements, which allow for gross aiming, and linear X and Y movements, which allow for fine adjustments. It is designed with a narrow profile to allow bilateral simultaneous

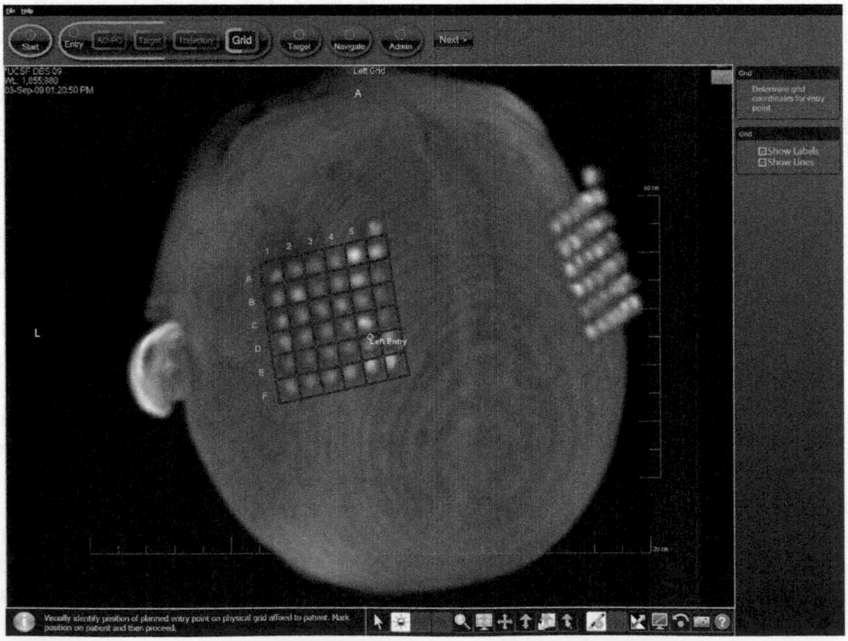

Fig. 9. Screenshot of the ClearPoint software showing the marking grids. The surgeon determines the desired trajectory to the target on coronal and sagittal images, and the software shows the surgeon where to center the skin incision and burr hole relative to the marking grid. A piercing tool is used to mark the skin and skull in this location, and the marking grid is then removed.

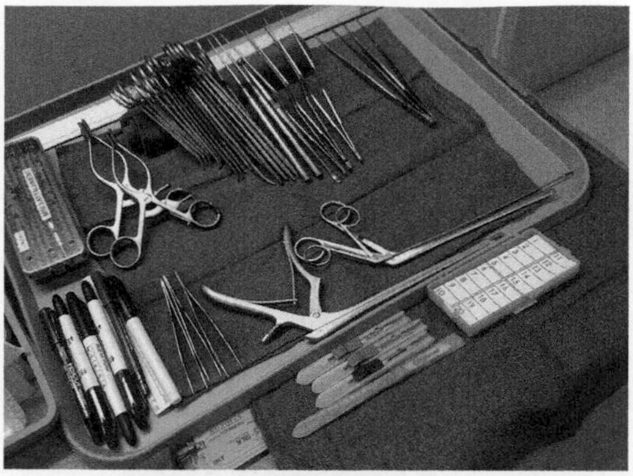

Fig. 10. The main instrument tray on the sterile back table during an interventional MRI procedure. The instruments are made of titanium. The scalpels are standard disposable safety scalpels with blades made of stainless steel with metal of relatively low grade, and their mass is small enough that they are safe to use in the MRI scanner.

placement, and is controlled with a simple cable remote that can be comfortably operated by the surgeon when the patient is at isocenter. The ClearPoint software instructs the MRI technologist to obtain selected MR scans in specific planes through the SmartFrame to allow the surgeon to align the device to the intended target (**Fig. 11**). A plastic-coated ceramic stylet with a surrounding peel-away sheath is then advanced to the target, with serial images acquired at the discretion of the surgeon to monitor the accuracy of placement in real time (**Fig. 12**). Ceramic is used because it provides the smallest, clearest artifact on MR images, which is vital for determining the accuracy of placement. Once proper placement of the stylet is verified, it is removed and the DBS lead is placed down the peel-away sheath to the target. The surgeon may choose to image again at this step to double-check the depth of the DBS electrode if the procedure is being done in a 1.5-T scanner. If a 3-T scanner is being used, any imaging done after the lead is placed would technically be against the DBS-lead manufacturer's current safety labeling, but imaging at this step is optional.

Outcomes

Using the ClearPoint system, clinically acceptable placement can be obtained with a single brain penetration in 98% of cases, with an average application accuracy of 0.6 to 0.8 mm.[23,24] The authors' group in San Francisco has reported preoperative and 6- to 9-month postoperative UPDRS scores in subsets of iMRI-implanted patients using the first-generation technique and subsequently the ClearPoint system. To avoid potential difficulties in interpreting scores obtained from unilaterally implanted patients, only bilaterally stimulated patients were included in this analysis. With the old Nexframe-based technique, the UPDRS III motor scores in the on-stimulation, off-medication state improved by 60% with an average 9 months' follow up.[21] Using the ClearPoint system, bilaterally stimulated patients improved by an average UPDRS III of 49.5%.[24] These motoric improvements are comparable with those in other DBS trials using frame-based, physiologically guided techniques.[3,25] Moreover, in more than 200 consecutive electrodes placed using iMRI, only 1 patient has required lead repositioning for suboptimal clinical outcome. This patient was implanted using the first-generation Nexframe-based method with a particularly narrow and medially positioned STN. This subject had clinical improvement but less than expected, with capsular effects at the upper end of therapeutic amplitudes. He had further improvement with medial lead repositioning.[21] There have been no lead repositions thus far in the authors' series of an initial 101 ClearPoint implantations.[23]

DISCUSSION

Merits and Disadvantages of Intraoperative Imaging

Precise neurosurgical targeting relies on stereotactic principles, initially established by Clarke and Horsley in 1908.[26–28] Stereotaxy provides accurate localization of intracranial targets by ascertaining their triplanar coordinates with reference to a fixed point, thus providing access to surgical targets deep within the brain in a minimally invasive fashion. Functional neurosurgery involves the precise surgical targeting of anatomic structures to modulate neurologic function, such as abnormal movements. As such, accuracy and precision of electrode placement is of great importance.

Stereotactic placement of DBS leads has an average accuracy of 2 to 3 mm, but the range is from 0 to 6 mm.[9,29–32] Because of this wide range in accuracy, intraoperative physiology is usually required to better refine the intended target. However, it is unclear as to how much of the physiologic adjustment is actually a means to compensate for stereotactic error versus physiologic variability. In addition, there are a small but persistent number of times when the physiologic data are conflicting or confusing. All of this results in additional penetrations of the brain, increasing the surgical risk and the operating time, with resultant patient fatigue and loss of cooperation. In addition, the final location of the DBS lead(s) is

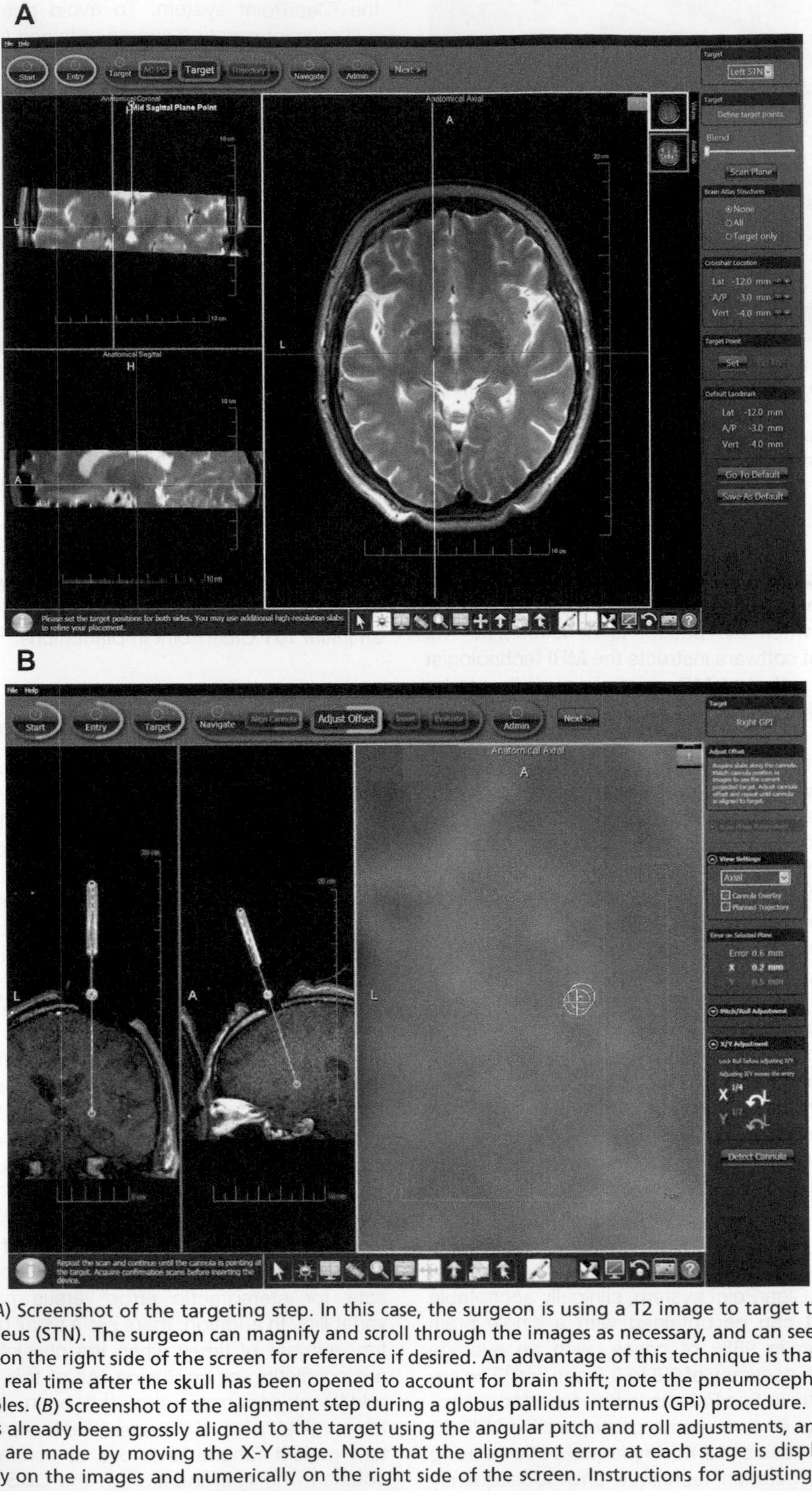

Fig. 11. (*A*) Screenshot of the targeting step. In this case, the surgeon is using a T2 image to target the subthalamic nucleus (STN). The surgeon can magnify and scroll through the images as necessary, and can see AC-PC coordinates on the right side of the screen for reference if desired. An advantage of this technique is that targeting is done in real time after the skull has been opened to account for brain shift; note the pneumocephalus at the frontal poles. (*B*) Screenshot of the alignment step during a globus pallidus internus (GPi) procedure. The SmartFrame has already been grossly aligned to the target using the angular pitch and roll adjustments, and final adjustments are made by moving the X-Y stage. Note that the alignment error at each stage is displayed both graphically on the images and numerically on the right side of the screen. Instructions for adjusting the knobs on the SmartFrame are also provided.

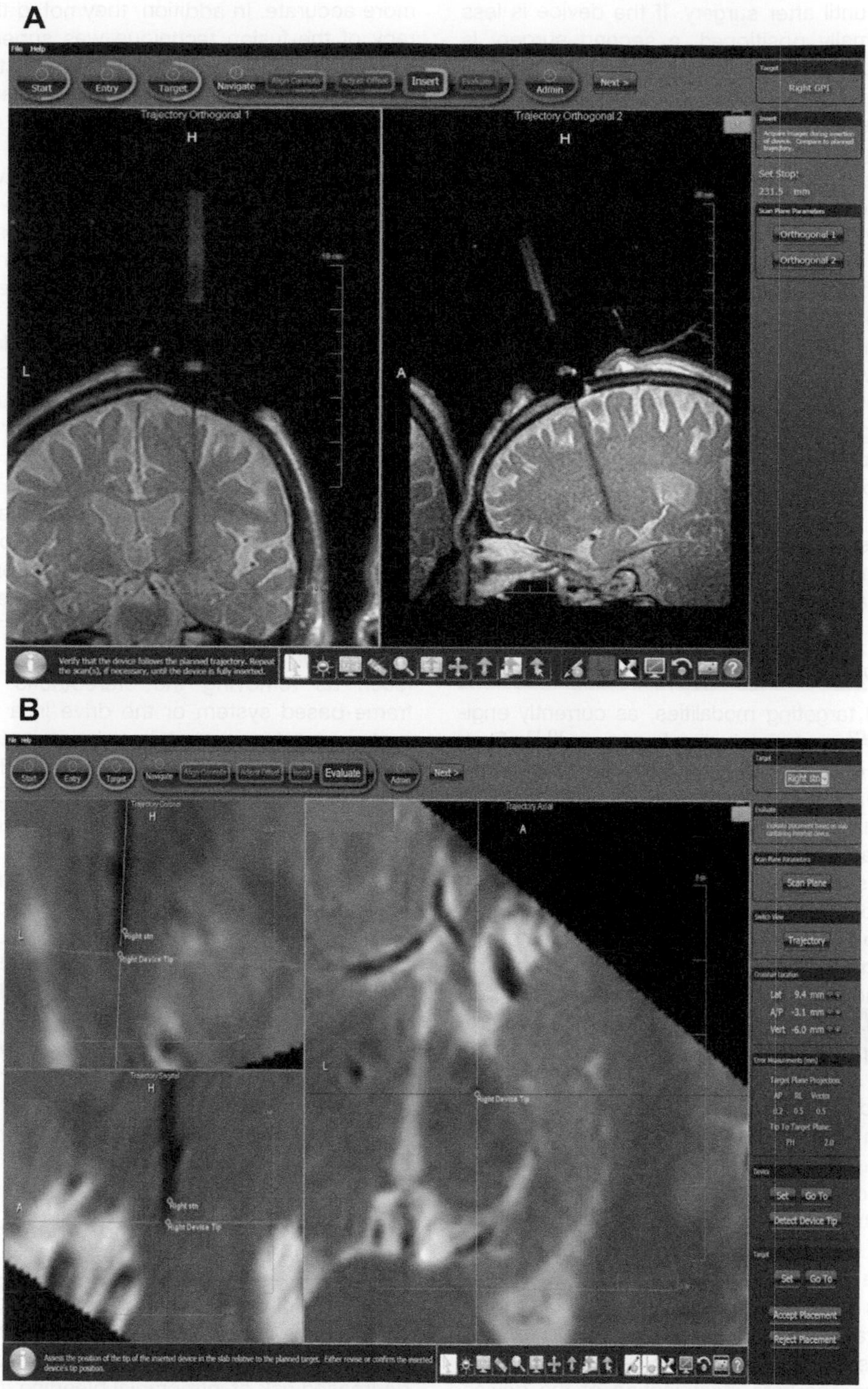

Fig. 12. (*A*) Ceramic stylet being advanced to the target during a GPi procedure. Relatively low-resolution images are obtained at this step to detect any gross deviation or hemorrhage. (*B*) Evaluation of stylet placement during an STN procedure using higher-resolution T2 images. The placement error in this case is 0.2 mm in the anteroposterior direction and 0.5 mm in the right-left direction (as seen on the right side of the screen). Note that the authors' practice is to intentionally place the stylet 2 mm deeper in STN cases to place the desired contact on the DBS lead in the target region.

unknown until after surgery. If the device is less than optimally positioned, a second surgery is often required for correction. The true incidence of DBS leads that require reoperation for repositioning is estimated at 1% to 12.7%.[33–36] Lead repositioning of as small an increment as 2 mm is routinely associated with a change in intraoperative efficacy. This finding has been confirmed by reoperative case series in which repositioning of the DBS was associated with an improved outcome.[4–6,37]

It is clear that methods for the detection and correction of stereotactic targeting error during surgery, with a minimum of brain penetrations, can be beneficial. In addition, the use of intraoperative imaging to provide registration of a stereotactic frame or bone fiducials can improve patient comfort and save time, or in some cases eliminate the need for fiducial registration, and even physiologic mapping, altogether. Both CT-guided and MRI-guided techniques demonstrate excellent accuracy.[7,10,22]

Merits and Disadvantages of Types of Imaging

CT-based targeting modalities, as currently engineered, have several disadvantages.[10,11] First, although excellent for visualizing bone and implanted hardware, the contrast for soft tissue is poor. Therefore, images obtained from approaches such as an O-arm or Ceretom cannot readily be used as "stand-alone" images, but must rather be used in conjunction with fusion to preoperative MR images to accurately localize the DBS electrodes. This method carries the risk of introducing error from intraoperative brain shift and the fusion process itself.[16,32] Second, intraoperative use of CT results in exposure to ionizing radiation, a potential risk factor for subsequent neoplasia.[38,39] Although the radiation dose can be minimized, there is a resultant decline in soft-tissue resolution. Third, there is a mean 0.7-mm (range 0–1.8 mm) measurement error associated with CT imaging, which creates some uncertainty as to true lead position.

On the other hand, CT has several advantages that make it desirable for use in the OR. CT images have high geometric accuracy because of the line-of-sight ray-optic acquisition. The CT artifact of the lead is smaller than the MRI artifact, which allows more accurate identification of the device. Yoshida and colleagues[40] compared localization of DBS contacts as assessed by MRI or postoperative CT fused to the preoperative CT and MRI. Individual contacts were found to be more clearly visualized on the CT, and the distal contact was deviated anteriorly and inferiorly on the MRI. The investigators concluded that the CT method was more accurate. In addition, they noted that accuracy of the fusion technique was superior when the reference scan to which the postoperative scan was merged was a CT rather than an MRI scan. Papavassiliou and colleagues[41] evaluated DBS lead location in 8 cases, using both CT and MRI, and found differences between the techniques ranging anywhere from −2.4 mm to +2.6 mm. In addition, mobile scanners such as the O-arm and Ceretom are becoming more commonplace, and these devices cause the least disruption in the normal workflow of the DBS procedure. In some cases, frame or frameless registration can be done using an intraoperative CT performed immediately before starting the procedure, therefore streamlining the registration and planning process on the day of surgery. Standard surgical instruments and microelectrode recording equipment can be used, and in the case of the larger-bore O-arm, the scanner can accommodate any stereotactic frame and micropositioner currently in use with room to spare. The Ceretom has a much smaller bore (just over 12 inches [30.5 cm]), so some changes in the workflow (such as removing the stereotactic arc in a frame-based system or the drive in a frameless system) must be undertaken during imaging.

Unlike CT, MRI offers superior tissue discrimination and good visualization of targets such as the STN and the GPi. However, its introduction into the surgical procedure necessitates numerous and dramatic changes to the normal DBS workflow. For mobile magnets such as the IMRIS (IMRIS, Minnetonka, MN), standard surgical instruments can be used during the procedure but must be removed from the surgical field for imaging. Microelectrode recording and physiologic confirmation techniques can be used when utilizing a mobile MRI. For fixed magnets, nonferrous and MRI-compatible instrumentation must be used, and microelectrode recording with currently available systems is not feasible.

Merits and Disadvantages of Anatomic Versus Physiologic Targeting

Placement of DBS leads under general anesthesia provides the benefits of increased patient comfort, increased anatomic accuracy, and, potentially, decreased risk of intracranial bleeding. Clearly the quality and type of anatomic imaging becomes paramount with this approach. Anatomic guidance cannot be based on poorly visualized anatomy. Although many groups believe that physiologic mapping should still be the standard method used in the traditional OR, there is also a rational argument that purely anatomic targeting (provided it is done with real-time imaging such as MRI that allows direct visualization) is appropriate for certain targets. These targets include "mature" targets such as the STN and globus pallidus, which are visible on MRI, have well-characterized internal and surrounding anatomy, and have a rich literature describing lead locations within them that are associated with good clinical outcomes. Also included may be some novel targets for experimental therapies whereby the physiology of the target is not well characterized and, therefore, not clinically helpful in guiding surgical placement.

The question still remains as to whether anatomic targeting is equivalent to physiologically based target identification in long-term outcome studies. The authors' experience with the O-arm has shown that, at times, one still has to move away from the anatomic target, as demonstrated by an image of the electrode in the planned target, based on the physiologic response of the patient. The large bore of the O-arm allows the patient to be awake for physiologic testing and repeat imaging if the surgeon prefers this method. Nonetheless, a purely anatomic approach can be accomplished, with excellent anatomic accuracy, using general anesthesia and CT or MR imaging.

SUMMARY

The use of CBCT-guided and FBCT-guided imaging modalities during DBS has been able to provide accurate intraoperative confirmation of lead placement relative to preoperative imaging and planning, and CBCT can be performed at any point during the surgery. Intraoperative CT images must be computationally fused to the preoperative MRI to provide adequate visualization of the target structures and measurement of lead location. Similarly, interventional MRI-guided DBS has been shown to provide a high degree of accuracy using real-time imaging with purely anatomic targeting and placement under general anesthesia. This technique requires a significant technical departure from traditional DBS surgery, and the merits of anatomic targeting versus physiologically based targeting are still under debate. Nevertheless, intraoperative imaging during DBS surgery with both CT and MRI provide the surgeon with useful data that can potentially improve patient outcomes, and these techniques will likely become a mainstay of surgical technique for years to come.

REFERENCES

1. Weaver FM, Follett K, Stern M, et al. Bilateral deep brain stimulation vs best medical therapy for patients with advanced Parkinson disease: a randomized controlled trial. JAMA 2009;301(1):63–73.
2. Holtzheimer PE, Mayberg HS. Deep brain stimulation for psychiatric disorders. Annu Rev Neurosci 2011;34(1):289–307.
3. Follett KA, Weaver FM, Stern M, et al. Pallidal versus subthalamic deep-brain stimulation for Parkinson's disease. N Engl J Med 2010;362(22):2077–91.
4. Anheim M, Batir A, Fraix V, et al. Improvement in Parkinson disease by subthalamic nucleus stimulation based on electrode placement: effects of reimplantation. Arch Neurol 2008;65(5):612–6.
5. Ellis TM, Foote KD, Fernandez HH, et al. Reoperation for suboptimal outcomes after deep brain stimulation surgery. Neurosurgery 2008;63(4): 754–61.
6. Richardson RM, Ostrem JL, Starr PA. Surgical repositioning of misplaced subthalamic electrodes in Parkinson's disease: location of effective and ineffective leads. Stereotact Funct Neurosurg 2009; 87(5):297–303.
7. Burchiel KJ, McCartney S, Lee A, et al. Accuracy of deep brain stimulation electrode placement using intraoperative computed tomography without microelectrode recording. J Neurosurg 2013;119(2):301–6.
8. Rumboldt Z, Huda W, All JW. Review of portable CT with assessment of a dedicated head CT Scanner. AJNR Am J Neuroradiol 2009;30(9):1630–6.
9. Kelman C, Ramakrishnan V, Davies A, et al. Analysis of stereotactic accuracy of the Cosman-Robert-Wells frame and Nexframe frameless systems in deep brain stimulation surgery. Stereotact Funct Neurosurg 2010;88(5):288–95.
10. Holloway K, Docef A. A quantitative assessment of the accuracy and reliability of O-arm images for deep brain stimulation surgery. Neurosurgery 2013;72:47–57.
11. Shahlaie K, Larson PS, Starr PA. Intraoperative computed tomography for deep brain stimulation surgery: technique and accuracy assessment. Neurosurgery 2011;68:114–24.
12. Starr PA, Vitek JL, DeLong M, et al. Magnetic resonance imaging-based stereotactic localization of the globus pallidus and subthalamic nucleus. Neurosurgery 1999;44(2):303–13.
13. Smith AP, Bakay RA. Frameless deep brain stimulation using intraoperative O-arm technology. J Neurosurg 2011;115(2):301–9.
14. Holloway KL, Gaede SE, Starr PA, et al. Frameless stereotaxy using bone fiducial markers for deep brain stimulation. J Neurosurg 2005;103(3): 404–13.
15. Azmi H, Machado A, Deogaonkar M, et al. Intracranial air correlates with preoperative cerebral atrophy and stereotactic error during bilateral STN DBS surgery for Parkinson's disease. Stereotact Funct Neurosurg 2011;89(4):246–52.

16. Slotty PJ, Kamp MA, Wille C, et al. The impact of brain shift in deep brain stimulation surgery: observation and obviation. Acta Neurochir (Wien) 2012; 154(11):2063–8.
17. Miyagi Y, Shima F, Sasaki T. Brain shift: an error factor during implantation of deep brain stimulation electrodes. J Neurosurg 2007;107(5):989–97.
18. Thani NB, Bala A, Lind CR. Accuracy of magnetic resonance imaging-directed frame-based stereotaxis. Neurosurgery 2012;70(1 Suppl Operative): 114–23 [discussion: 123–4].
19. Black PM, Moriarty T, Alexander E 3rd, et al. Development and implementation of intraoperative magnetic resonance imaging and its neurosurgical applications. Neurosurgery 1997;41(4):831–42 [discussion: 842–35].
20. Moriarty TM, Quinones-Hinojosa A, Larson PS, et al. Frameless stereotactic neurosurgery using intraoperative magnetic resonance imaging: stereotactic brain biopsy. Neurosurgery 2000;47(5):1138–45 [discussion: 1145–6].
21. Starr PA, Martin AJ, Ostrem JL, et al. Subthalamic nucleus deep brain stimulator placement using high-field interventional magnetic resonance imaging and a skull-mounted aiming device: technique and application accuracy. J Neurosurg 2010; 112(3):479–90.
22. Larson PS, Starr PA, Bates G, et al. An optimized system for interventional magnetic resonance imaging-guided stereotactic surgery: preliminary evaluation of targeting accuracy. Neurosurgery 2012;70(1 Suppl Operative):95–103 [discussion: 103].
23. Larson P, Starr PA, Ostrem JL, et al. 203 application accuracy of a second generation interventional MRI stereotactic platform: initial experience in 101 DBS electrode implantations. Neurosurgery 2013; 60(Suppl 1):187.
24. Ostrem JL, Galifianakis NB, Markun LC, et al. Clinical outcomes of PD patients having bilateral STN DBS using high-field interventional MR-imaging for lead placement. Clin Neurol Neurosurg 2013; 115(6):708–12.
25. Krack P, Batir A, Van Blercom N, et al. Five-year follow-up of bilateral stimulation of the subthalamic nucleus in advanced Parkinson's disease. N Engl J Med 2003;349(20):1925–34.
26. Compston A. The structure and functions of the cerebellum examined by a new method. By Sir Victor Horsley, FRS, FRCS and R.H. Clarke, MA, MB. Brain 1908: 31; 45-124. Brain 2007;130(6):1449–52.
27. Horsley V, Clarke RH. The structure and functions of the cerebellum examined by a new method. Brain 1908;31(1):45–124.
28. Zrinzo L. The role of imaging in the surgical treatment of movement disorders. Neuroimaging Clin N Am 2010;20(1):125–40.
29. Starr PA, Christine CW, Theodosopoulos PV, et al. Implantation of deep brain stimulators into subthalamic nucleus: technical approach and magnetic imaging-verified electrode locations. J Neurosurg 2002;97(2):370–87.
30. Hamid NA, Mitchell RD, Mocroft P, et al. Targeting the subthalamic nucleus for deep brain stimulation: technical approach and fusion of pre- and postoperative MR images to define accuracy of lead placement. J Neurol Neurosurg Psychiatry 2005;76(3): 409–14.
31. Fitzpatrick JM, Konrad PE, Nickele C, et al. Accuracy of customized miniature stereotactic platforms. Stereotact Funct Neurosurg 2005;83(1): 25–31.
32. Khan MF, Mewes K, Gross RE, et al. Assessment of brain shift related to deep brain stimulation surgery. Stereotact Funct Neurosurg 2008;86(1): 44–53.
33. Blomstedt P, Hariz MI. Hardware-related complications of deep brain stimulation: a ten year experience. Acta Neurochir (Wien) 2005;147(10): 1061–4.
34. Doshi PK. Long-term surgical and hardware-related complications of deep brain stimulation. Stereotact Funct Neurosurg 2011;89(2):89–95.
35. Hu X, Jiang X, Zhou X, et al. Avoidance and management of surgical and hardware-related complications of deep brain stimulation. Stereotact Funct Neurosurg 2010;88(5):296–303.
36. Hamani C, Lozano AM. Hardware-related complications of deep brain stimulation: a review of the published literature. Stereotact Funct Neurosurg 2006; 84(5–6):248–51.
37. Okun MS, Tagliati M, Pourfar M, et al. Management of referred deep brain stimulation failures: a retrospective analysis from 2 movement disorders centers. Arch Neurol 2005;62(8):1250–5.
38. Berrington de González A, Mahesh M, Kim KP, et al. Projected cancer risks from computed tomographic scans performed in the united states in 2007. Arch Intern Med 2009;169(22):2071–7.
39. Smith-Bindman R, Lipson J, Marcus R, et al. Radiation dose associated with common computed tomography examinations and the associated lifetime attributable risk of cancer. Arch Intern Med 2009;169(22):2078–86.
40. Yoshida F, Miyagi Y, Morioka T, et al. Assessment of contact location in subthalamic stimulation for Parkinson's disease by co-registration of computed tomography images. Stereotact Funct Neurosurg 2008;86(3):162–6.
41. Papavassiliou E, Rau G, Heath S, et al. Thalamic deep brain stimulation for essential tremor: relation of lead location to outcome. Neurosurgery 2004; 54(5):1120–30.

Advanced Neuroimaging Techniques for Central Neuromodulation

Angela Downes, MD[a,*], Nader Pouratian, MD, PhD[b]

KEYWORDS

• Brain mapping • Deep brain stimulation (DBS) • fMRI • DTI • 7 T MRI • Functional imaging

KEY POINTS

- The world of modern neuroimaging has seen rapid advances in capability and efficiency, made possible by the ongoing accumulation of discoveries in computational and basic science research.
- Because of the successes of this field, structural and functional image techniques have become the preferred means of evaluating and framing information collected about the function, in vivo, of the human brain.
- Applying these methods to the clinical field of neurosurgery can confer a measure of certainty to surgical undertakings on our patients' brains.
- We must move away from earlier eras when clinical observations were linked with data derived from basic neuroanatomy or animal models, which have resulted in conflicts, competing hypotheses, and incomplete knowledge about the mechanism of deep brain stimulation and the diseases it is used to treat.
- Familiarity with the new perspectives provided by advanced imaging techniques can help achieve a deeper understanding of neurologic and psychiatric disorders and refine both medical and neuromodulatory therapies.

INTRODUCTION

Deep brain stimulation (DBS) has become standard in the treatment paradigm of medically refractory movement disorders. Its efficacy has been proved not only for Parkinson disease (PD) but also for essential tremor and dystonia.[1–5] The remarkable effects produced by DBS on quality of life and motor function as well as its reversibility, and personalization of stimulation, have encouraged exploration of DBS as a treatment of other neurologic conditions such as psychiatric disorders, Alzheimer disease, chronic pain, refractory epilepsy, obesity, and addiction.[6–12]

Contemporary central neuromodulation has continually evolved from the foundation created by stereotactic neurosurgery for lesioning in the mid-twentieth century.[13] Techniques developed during that time, such as ventriculographic guidance and Talairach proportions, were considered the gold standard until the mid-1990s, when the advent of multimodality imaging such as computed tomography (CT) and magnetic resonance imaging (MRI) afforded millimetric precision, and obviated painful and variable contrast ventriculography.[14] This was the birth of direct targeting, which is one of 3 means of target identification and verification used in current practice. The

Financial Support: None.
[a] Department of Neurosurgery, Morsani College of Medicine, University of South Florida, 2 Tampa General Circle, 7th Floor, Tampa, FL 33606, USA; [b] Department of Neurosurgery, David Geffen School of Medicine, University of California, Los Angeles, 10945 Le Conte Avenue, Suite 2120, Los Angeles, CA 90095, USA
* Corresponding author.
E-mail address: adownes@mednet.ucla.edu

Neurosurg Clin N Am 25 (2014) 173–185
http://dx.doi.org/10.1016/j.nec.2013.08.012
1042-3680/14/$ – see front matter

second means of target verification is indirect targeting, in which each subcortical target has standardized atlas-based coordinates relative to the anterior commissure (AC) and posterior commissure (PC). The most commonly used systems are the Talairach coordinate system published in 1988 from the analysis of 1 brain and the stereotactic atlas developed in 1977 by Schaltenbrand and Wahren, which consists of photographs of microscopic sections of 2 cadaveric brains sliced with reference to the AC-PC planes.[15,16] After optimizing direct and indirect modalities, verification of the target occurs with microelectrode recording (MER), a technique described in 1961 by Albe-Fessard and colleagues,[17] and intraoperative stimulation testing.

Many studies over the past several decades have focused on validating the data used in the creation of such print atlases, and suggesting methods to improve, modify, and integrate both structural and functional data to facilitate multimodal mapping, as was the intention of Schaltenbrand and colleagues.[15,18,19] Although such population-based atlases have their place in the anatomic identification of targets and surrounding structures, they are useful only for a subset of patients, and inadequately address the well-documented problem of interindividual structure and functional variability of subcortical targets.[20–25] Advances in MRI technology and availability have helped to expose these differences. A study published in 2009 looking at the variability of subthalamic nucleus (STN) in patients with PD found that the MRI-derived position, size, and shape for the STN was statistically different compared with the Schaltenbrand and Wahren atlas coordinates.[25] These individual differences have been highlighted in many studies over the past decade.[26–29] Richter and colleagues[27] compared the position of STN borders on MRI with the atlases of Talairach and Tournoux and Schaltenbrand and Wahren and found that the lateral border on MRI was 3.1 mm more medial than predicted, and the position of the anterior border was 7.8 cm more posterior on MRI than was shown in the atlases. These positional differences are clinically significant because they are of a similar order of magnitude to the nucleus itself. The clinical impact of these differences is highlighted in the 2008 study by Patel and colleagues,[26] who reported that targeting STN based on atlas-based coordinates results in failure to identify the nucleus in 55% of initial MER passes.

The challenge of targeting is even more significant when trying to target certain subregions of the STN. An anteromedially placed electrode within the STN has been attributed to the emotional and cognitive side effects often seen with this target.[30,31] The optimal position for efficacy in PD is reported to be in the lateral anterodorsal portion of the STN.[32] Other reports describing efficacy have provided conflicting information as to the optimal location of stimulating electrodes within a scalable atlas of the STN.[33] Adding to the difficulty in optimal electrode placement within the STN is the limitation of standard 1.5-T MRI to reliably identify the nucleus, because its borders can often blend into the substantia nigra (SN).[27]

Such variability is even more profound in context of inconsistencies caused by aging, disease, sex, and handedness. In addition to these factors, there are potential influences of variances introduced by neurologic and psychiatric diseases such as depression, psychosis, and dementia, which are particularly relevant to the population of patients with DBS.[34–38] The presence of ventricular enlargement is commonly observed in such neurodegenerative and psychiatric conditions. The individual structural and functional variations in cortical and subcortical structures underscore the limitations of the existing anatomic atlases used in DBS targeting. Advances in neuroimaging modalities can provide a patient-specific solution for the lack of comprehensive targeting strategies.[20–22,24]

NEUROIMAGING TECHNIQUES

The gold standard for present-day DBS surgery remains a combination of indirect and direct targeting and MER. In keeping the techniques of the past, the long-standing controversy remains that has surrounded the imprecision of stereotactic surgery since its inception.[19,39] Although these techniques are certainly valid and account for the success of this therapy to date, they are limited in their ability to provide patient-specific details of subcortical targets, thus representing a potential limitation of current therapeutic strategies and thereby compromising, in part, the goal of DBS surgery: to provide excellent clinical outcomes with the lowest stimulation power required. Advances in neuroimaging techniques have already revolutionized the practice of medicine and are vital to the modernization of central neuromodulation by providing personalized target identification, segmentation of target subregions for network modulation, and understanding the mechanism of DBS and the diseases it treats. These advances include improvements in structural imaging capabilities with ultrahigh field (7-T) MRI for improved resolution and contrast for direct targeting, diffusion tensor imaging (DTI) to characterize and reconstruct white matter tracts surrounding subcortical nuclei, novel applications of and functional imaging such as functional MRI (fMRI), single-photon emission CT, and positron emission tomography (PET) which have shed light on the role of brain function and neuroplasticity in disease states. Contributing further to these advances are developments in postprocessing software, including segmentation techniques such as voxel-based morphometry to delineate numerous millimeter-sized regions of interest (ROI) in the brain, tractography analysis such as probabilistic tractography, and registration tools to enable accurate comparison of images over time and across groups of patients. Furthermore, improvements in acquisition time have made these scans more tolerable to patients, yielding better data quality and quantity. Taken together, these techniques represent an accumulation of technical advances that promise to revolutionize the current practice of central neuromodulation.

Structural Imaging

Ultrahigh field strength MRI

The success of DBS depends on the accurate and precise delivery of the stimulating electrodes to the target. The limitations of atlas-based indirect targeting have led some to conclude that MRI-based direct targeting is a more robust method of optimal target identification, because it considers interpersonal variations in subcortical anatomy.[25–27] However, conventional 1.5-T MRI methods are limited by their lower resolution and tissue contrast to discriminate divisions between nuclei in the thalamus, the divisions between the lateral and medial segments of the internal segment of the globus pallidus (GPi), and differentiate the anterior portion of the STN from the SN, all of which have clinical implications for the success of the surgery.[30] Motion artifact and factors affecting MRI quality such as voxel size and volume averaging are also believed to jeopardize the quality of these images for use in stereotactic surgery.[25,27,40]

Recent advances in the development of ultra-high field strength MRI scanners such as 3 T and 7 T have led to their increased usefulness in neuroscience applications. The advantages of a higher magnetic field are enhanced signal-to-noise ratio (SNR) and the use of certain sequences that are optimal at higher strength fields. The resultant images from 7-T MRI are high resolution, with markedly enhanced tissue contrast, which allow for better edge representation between gray and white matter structures, and even within gray matter.[41,42] Furthermore, the availability of susceptibility-weighted imaging (SWI) (both at 3 T and 7 T), in addition to the standard T1-weighted and T2-weighted images, results in an unprecedented level of anatomic detail. SWI was originally developed to better visualize venous anatomy from magnetic resonance (MR) venograms.[30] SWI provides a higher level of tissue contrast relative to T1-weighted and T2-weighted images, and at 7 T has been used to delineate in vivo the internal thalamic nuclei, including the anterior and medial aspect of the pulvinar and the boundary of the ventral caudal nucleus of the thalamus (Vc).[43]

However, there is concern that the powerful 7-T MR images have an increased susceptibility to geometric distortions, which renders them impractical for clinical applications. Increased susceptibility for geometric distortions can lead to scaling, skew, and volume change of the image data when transforming a high field image onto true patient coordinates such as a CT scan.[41] Quantitative analysis of the integrity of 7-T MRI compared with 1.5-T MRI showed that distortion was more evident in peripheral parts of the brain rather than regions targeted for DBS such as the STN, ventrointermediate (VIM) nucleus, or GPi.[41] Nonetheless, given the fact that approximately 46% of patients with suboptimal outcomes after DBS are found to have improperly placed electrodes, advances in structural imaging like 7-T MRI have great potential to improve target visualization and presurgical planning.[44] However, the major limitation at this time is the limited availability of such high-strength magnets in common clinical practice.

Diffusion imaging

Target visualization can be improved not only by making the target itself more evident (by increasing signal-to-noise) but also by emphasizing the surrounding and internal structures (effectively increasing contrast-to-noise). Diffusion-weighted imaging is an MRI modality that was developed in the 1980s, and most commonly used in the early detection of cerebral ischemia. However, the usefulness of diffusion-weighted imaging also extends to investigating brain microstructure and anatomy in vivo. Diffusion imaging is based on the principle of the diffusion of water molecules. The degree to which different tissues restrict the directional diffusion of water range from equal restriction in all directions such as in cerebrospinal fluid (CSF) (isotropic diffusion), to strong unequal restriction in white matter, and weak unequal restriction in gray matter, referred to as strong and weak anisotropic diffusion, respectively. For example, strong anisotropic diffusion means that the water in white matter diffuses strongly in the direction of the white matter tracts. Diffusion parameters can be modeled as a tensor at each voxel (ie, DTI) and are most often quantified with respect to fractional anisotropy (FA) and mean diffusivity (MD). FA is a measure of the directional diffusion of water, and the tissue or ROI is given a score of 0 to 1. The relative unity of the FA signal reflects the level of fiber tract organization and orientation within a region; the tightly organized regions of the corpus callosum show a high FA (1), and the areas with no directionality (eg, CSF) has an FA of 0. Tissue with intermediate characteristics of gray and white matter has an intermediate FA signal.[45] A low FA signal in white matter is reflective of damage to underlying axons or myelin. MD is a quantitative measure of the average displacement of water molecules at a given time and is highest in tissues without restrictions to diffusion (eg, CSF), and lowest in dense tissues with a high level of water diffusion restriction (eg, nuclei with multiple crossing white matter fibers). MD reflects general tissue density. FA and MD have a similar origin, but represent different tissue characteristics and can be used to infer different neural structural pathologies when correlated to an extrinsic clinical outcome measure.

Studies of the relationship between FA age-related cognitive decline have shown the usefulness of FA as a surrogate marker for structural changes that occur with age-related cognitive decline.[45] Grieve and colleagues[45] found that relative to increased age, FA decreased in a linear fashion in the frontal, temporal, and parietal lobes. This low FA signal was correlated with poorer cognitive performance in executive functions. On the opposite end of the spectrum, high FA in the left temporoparietal white matter connecting Broca and Wernicke areas has been positively correlated with improved reading performance in children[46] and improved executive function in adults.[47] Studies using FA and MD values have also been conducted to better understand PD pathology. For example, Zheng and colleagues[48] used this technology to perform an in-depth analysis of the relationship between the degree of structural white matter changes and the degree of neurocognitive impairments specific to PD. Cognitive deficits seen in PD span many domains, including language, attention, memory, and visuospatial abilities; however, the most common is impairment in executive functions, including planning, initiating, and monitoring goal-directed behavior.[49] The results of the analysis by Zheng and colleagues showed that an increase in FA signal in distinct white matter regions correlated with a better outcome on measures of cognitive performance tested, including executive function, attention, memory, and language. On the other hand, high MD values, reflecting white matter density, were negatively correlated with performance. This study shows the usefulness of FA and MD as unique and direct imaging correlates of intrinsic structural changes as they relate to extrinsic clinical outcome measures and may be a useful data source for diagnosis, management, and guiding therapy.

Diffusion tractography Diffusion tractography represents another application and derivation of DTI that can be used to visualize white matter tracts. Diffusion tractography can improve personalization of DBS surgery by enhancing our knowledge of the neural networks involved, and thus help to better target treatments. Images of white matter tracts can be generated by essentially drawing lines connecting adjacent voxels with similar anisotropy and direction.[50] The result is a representation of white matter tracts that correspond well to classic neuroanatomy and have a high degree of interobserver and intraobserver reliability.[50,51] Sedrak and colleagues[52] used tractography to explore large fiber tracts connecting structures relevant to psychiatric disorders and identified reciprocal connections such as medial prefrontal cortex (mPFC) and subgenual anterior cingulate area. This study characterizes the DBS targets used in depression such as the subgenual anterior cingulate cortex (sgACC) and the anterior limb of the internal capsule by their white matter connections to other territories. Diffusion tractography has been used to show the connectivity patterns of these targets and how they are interrelated within the neural network activated in depression.[53]

Although diffusion-based imaging is a potentially powerful technique for visualizing white matter tracts, one must have an appreciation for potential sources of errors during image acquisition, processing, and postprocessing. Like other MR-based imaging techniques, diffusion imaging and the various derivative algorithms are subject to motion artifact from active patient movements and even from cardiac pulsations. They are also susceptible to artifacts at the air-bone interface, and CSF signal contamination, which can artificially lower the FA signal.[50] Furthermore, the resolution at which these images are acquired is lower than that used for standard T1-weighted and T2-weighted images. Because of this poor spatial resolution (~2 mm isotropic voxel), voxels are likely to contain multiple crossing, diverging, or converging white matter tracts, limiting the ability to detect and track small fiber bundles. These conditions may be in part mitigated by the use of higher field strength MRI (7 T) or by decreasing the voxel size used in image acquisition.[54]

Connectivity-based segmentation Although DTI can be used to define internal anatomy of subcortical targets,[55] such diffusion tensor-based maps can be difficult to interpret. One approach to addressing these limitations has been an adaptation of another postprocessing algorithm known as probabilistic tractography to segment or partition subcortical targets based on variable patterns of connectivity of the voxels within the ROI. Bypassing the linear restrictions of conventional streamline DTI, probabilistic tractography quantifies the probability that 2 points (voxels) are anatomically connected based on their degree of anisotropy.[50] Targeting this technique to a specific ROI in the brain (eg, the thalamus), via a process known as seeding, results in a visual depiction of the cortical regions with which each voxel in the ROI has the highest probability of connectivity and grouping similar voxels together. This visual depiction is known as a connectivity-based segmentation map. This approach was first described in 2003 by Behrens and colleagues[56] as a valid and reliable tool for visualizing cortical connectivity of functionally distinct thalamic subregions, which correspond to thalamic nuclei or nuclear groups, as seen in **Fig. 1**. This approach of thalamic segmentation has been shown to correspond well to invasive tracer studies of thalamic connectivity in nonhuman primate studies.[56]

Because of the lack of distinct nuclear borders and considerable anatomic and functional variability across individuals, the thalamus has been a particularly popular ROI for assessment with probabilistic tractography. Dysregulation in corticostriatal-thalamocortical networks has been cited as a putative cause of neuropsychiatric disorders,[39] and functional imaging has shown thalamic activation in various sensory,[57] motor,[58,59] and cognitive/associative[60–64] tasks. The thalamus is also an important target for central neuromodulation, having been targeted for tremor, pain, epilepsy, Tourette syndrome, and other diseases. Johansen-Berg and colleagues[65] have spearheaded the validation of probabilistic tractography as a feasible means of parcellating the thalamus into functionally relevant subgroups in vivo. Using 11 healthy individuals, these investigators quantitatively defined the anatomic

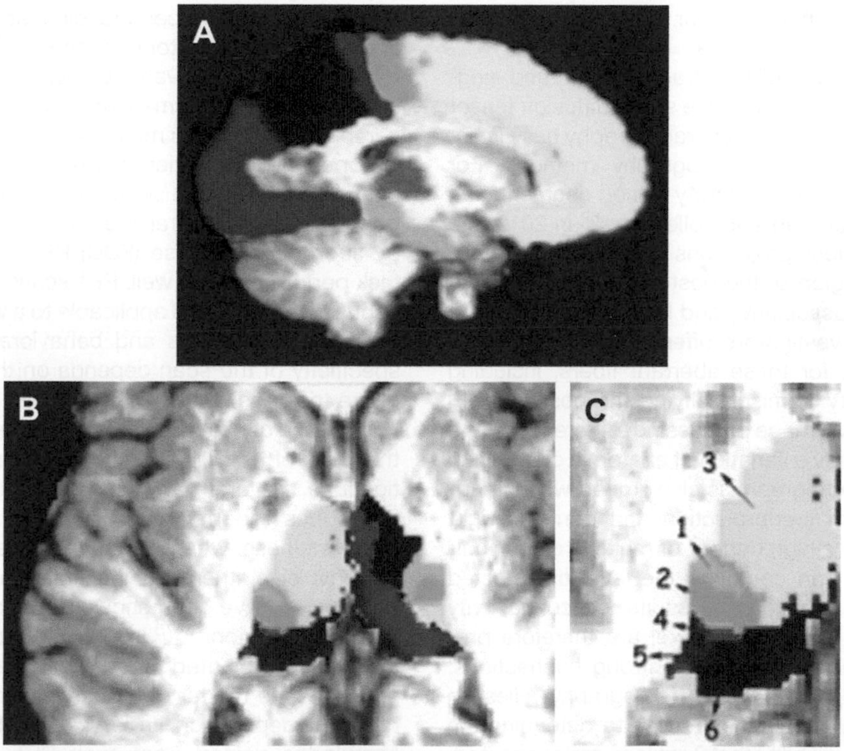

Fig. 1. Connectivity-based thalamic segmentation. Using the methods for probabilistic tractography, the thalamus is segmented based on connectivity with 6 predefined cortical targets. (*A*) Cortical target masks are created for each patient. (*B*) Probabilistic tractography defines each thalamic voxel connecting with the predefined cortical masks. (*C*) Voxels are grouped together based on the region with which they have the highest probability of connection, resulting in a segmentation map corresponding to known thalamic nuclear organization. (1) Precentral gyrus; (2) postcentral gyrus; (3) prefrontal cortex; (4) parietal lobe; (5) occipital lobe; (6) temporal lobe.

variation of thalamic segmentation between individuals and used this information to generate a probabilistic thalamic atlas. This atlas was used as a baseline to further compare tractographic thalamic subregions with previous histologically defined nuclei from cadaveric studies. These investigators also showed the correlation of their probabilistic thalamic atlas to nuclear regions previously implicated in functional activations of motor and memory tasks. For example, the region corresponding to the mediodorsal nucleus had the highest connectivity to prefrontal cortex.

Probabilistic tractography has also been successfully applied to the parcellation of the SN, subgenual cingulate cortex, parietal cortex, and most recently the STN and basal ganglia, to show their distinct patterns of connectivity and functional subregions not otherwise visible by conventional MRI techniques.[54,66–68] The study of anatomic connectivity of the white matter of the anterior cingulate cortex by Johansen-Berg and colleagues[67] found the highest number of strong connections from the subgenual cingulate cortex to targets in frontal, limbic, and visceromotor regions, which supports the use of this target in DBS modulation of the dysfunctional corticolimbic network for treatment-resistant depression.

Because probabilistic tractography and segmentation are based on the same diffusion tensor source data, probabilistic tractography has similar limitations to other tractography methods. For example, in the connectivity-based segmentation of STN by Lambert and colleagues[69] in 2012, the location of fiber projections to the GPi from the motor subregion of the posterior STN was found to be in the associative and limbic portions of the STN. The investigators offered several potential explanations for these aberrant fibers, including the possibility of misclassifying the posterior GPi during manual image processing, differences in atlases, or simply a variation of anatomic distribution of fibers. Tractography is also limited when imaging areas with fiber projections that contain a right angle turn or a high density of multiple crossing fibers, which can confound the level of detected anisotropic diffusion.[70] Results of connectivity analysis for a particular voxel are therefore presented in terms of weak or strong connections. Furthermore, probabilistic tractography relies on this connectivity signal strength to determine the degree of probability that 2 regions are connected. Thus, any general cause of MRI artifact such as patient motion, cardiac pulsations, and target ROI size can result in some regions falling lower than the threshold.[65] Nonetheless, this imaging modality has provided a level of structural and functional detail that is unprecedented and has the potential to be used in the clinical setting.

Functional Imaging

Functional imaging is a means by which we can observe the underlying patterns of neuronal activity through the surrogate use of hemodynamic and metabolic changes. The value of structural imaging techniques such as probabilistic tractography lies in the ability to localize functionally relevant subcortical targets in the human brain. Functional imaging such as fMRI and PET studies have shed light on the neural networks that exist in health and the pathology that alters them in disease states. It is within the context of functional localization that we can begin to improve the personalization of current targets and identify new targets for central neuromodulation. fMRI and PET studies exploit the fact that DBS, at therapeutic stimulation levels, alters cerebral blood flow and glucose metabolism at predictable locations throughout the brain.[71]

PET

PET imaging has a variety of functions, including, depending on the tracer used, detecting regional cerebral blood flow, cerebral glucose metabolism, and dopamine receptor occupancy.[72] Radioactive tracers labeled with various positron emitting isotopes serve different measurements. For example, cerebral blood flow is measured after injecting ^{15}O isotope while the patient performs a task, and the control blood flow is subtracted from that during performance. Cerebral metabolism is measured by fluorodeoxyglucose (FDG)-PET uptake during task performance as well. PET scans are advantageous in that they are applicable to a wide range of functional paradigms and behavioral tasks. The specificity of the scan depends on the specificity of the task design and methodology.

The ease of use for behavioral studies promoted the use of PET imaging in psychiatric investigations. Several early studies by Mayberg and colleagues reported activation of the sgACC in acute sadness, whereas antidepressant and electroconvulsive therapies for treatment-resistant depression have been shown to decrease activation of this region.[73–75] In 2005, Mayberg and colleagues[76] implanted stimulation leads into the sgACC white matter of 6 patients with treatment-resistant depression, in large part driven by the knowledge gained from such PET studies. The study included preprocedure and postprocedure PET scans, which showed a baseline finding of increased sgACC blood flow consistent with past studies in depressed patients. In addition, abnormally decreased blood flow was noted in the dorsolateral prefrontal cortex (DLPFC), premotor, and dorsal anterior cingulate and anterior insula regions. Reversal of these baseline imaging abnormalities was sustained at 3 and 6 months in the 3 patients who had long-term clinical response to stimulation: cerebral blood flow decreased in the sgACC region, whereas it increased in DLPFC, dorsal anterior cingulate, posterior cingulate, and premotor and parietal cortices. Furthermore, treatment responders had a decrease in sgACC CBF that was less than that of control individuals. This study exemplifies the usefulness of PET imaging as a means to qualitatively represent the regional conformation of pathologically activated networks and quantitatively define treatment response when compared with control levels.

Resting-state FDG-PET imaging of glucose metabolism has also been used to investigate the systems-level changes that occur in PD: specific regional metabolic networks have been uncovered with respect to signs and symptoms, disease progression, and treatment response. For example, the PD-related metabolic covariance pattern has been found to correlate with clinical rating scales for akinesia and rigidity. This pattern consists of increased glucose metabolism in the thalamus, globus pallidus, pons, and primary motor cortex and decreased metabolism in the lateral premotor and posterior parietal areas.[77] In 2011, Mure and colleagues[78] obtained FDG-PET images in patients with PD with VIM nucleus DBS both on and off stimulation to identify a novel metabolic network correlating with PD tremor and consisting of increased activity in the cerebellum/dorsal pons and primary motor cortex. This pattern was evident in patients with tremor-dominant PD, and DBS in the VIM nucleus or STN resulted in significantly decreased metabolism in these regions. Such studies using PET imaging to visualize the metabolic differences between signs and symptoms have substantiated previous evidence that tremor differs in pathophysiology from other manifestations of PD such as akinesia and rigidity.[77,79]

Although PET is a powerful tool and resource, PET is limited by a relatively low spatial resolution (4 mm) compared with MRI (2 mm), and partial volume effects, which cause signal to spill over into adjacent areas. This image artifact is particularly evident with small ROIs. Moreover, the relative ease of using fMRI compared with PET (ie, common availability and lack of need of an exogenous contrast agent) have in many instances supplanted the use of PET. Still, PET provides a safe avenue for imaging function and metabolism in patients after implant with neuromodulation devices.

fMRI

fMRI is well recognized in the neurosurgical practice as a potentially powerful imaging technique for mapping brain function. Brain function maps are based on detection of hemodynamic changes that are coupled to regionally specific functional brain activity. fMRI takes advantage of the inherently different magnetic properties of oxyhemoglobin versus deoxyhemoglobin as an intrinsic contrast agent to detect such hemodynamic changes and is therefore most often referred to as blood oxygen level-dependent (BOLD) fMRI. Localized increases in neuronal activity result in a cascade of events that increases local cerebral blood flow and perfusion, thereby increasing the relative proportion of local level of oxyhemoglobin and therefore effectively shortening T2* signal in the area of interest (**Fig. 2**).[72] In most cases, BOLD responses are measured in response to specific stimuli, although more innovative approaches have been described (see discussion of pain literature) and there is an increasing interest in resting-state fMRI BOLD imaging (see later discussion).

Advantages over PET imaging include higher spatial resolution (usually ~2 mm voxels, although the hemodynamic responses that are being detected may inherently have poorer resolution than that), increased SNRs, shortened acquisition times, and no requirement for exogenous contrast agents. Higher field strengths can improve these parameters even more.[80,81] Because fMRI does not depend on radiation or the injection of radioactive tracers, it also enables repeated investigations in a single subject in 1 session or over time, and can be used in children, unlike PET.[72] Although US Food and Drug Administration regulations on specific absorption rate prevent fMRI in routine clinical practice, fMRI has been used in some patients with implanted DBS electrodes.[57] Having evaluated fMRI for both safety and efficacy for detecting cortical areas of activation during thalamic DBS stimulation, Rezai and colleagues reported no adverse events from fMRI performed in 86 patients with thalamic electrodes. Furthermore, their study used fMRI to identify cortical and subcortical patterns of lateral thalamic DBS-coupled activation of various parts of the somatosensory pathway. In the Vc nucleus of the thalamus, stimulation activated the primary somatosensory cortex, whereas periventricular gray matter stimulation resulted in cingulate cortex activation. These areas correspond to the known neuroanatomic pathways of pain perception, and to patient reporting of stimulation-induced parasthesias in most cases.

The potential contributions of fMRI research to neuromodulation are exemplified brain mapping

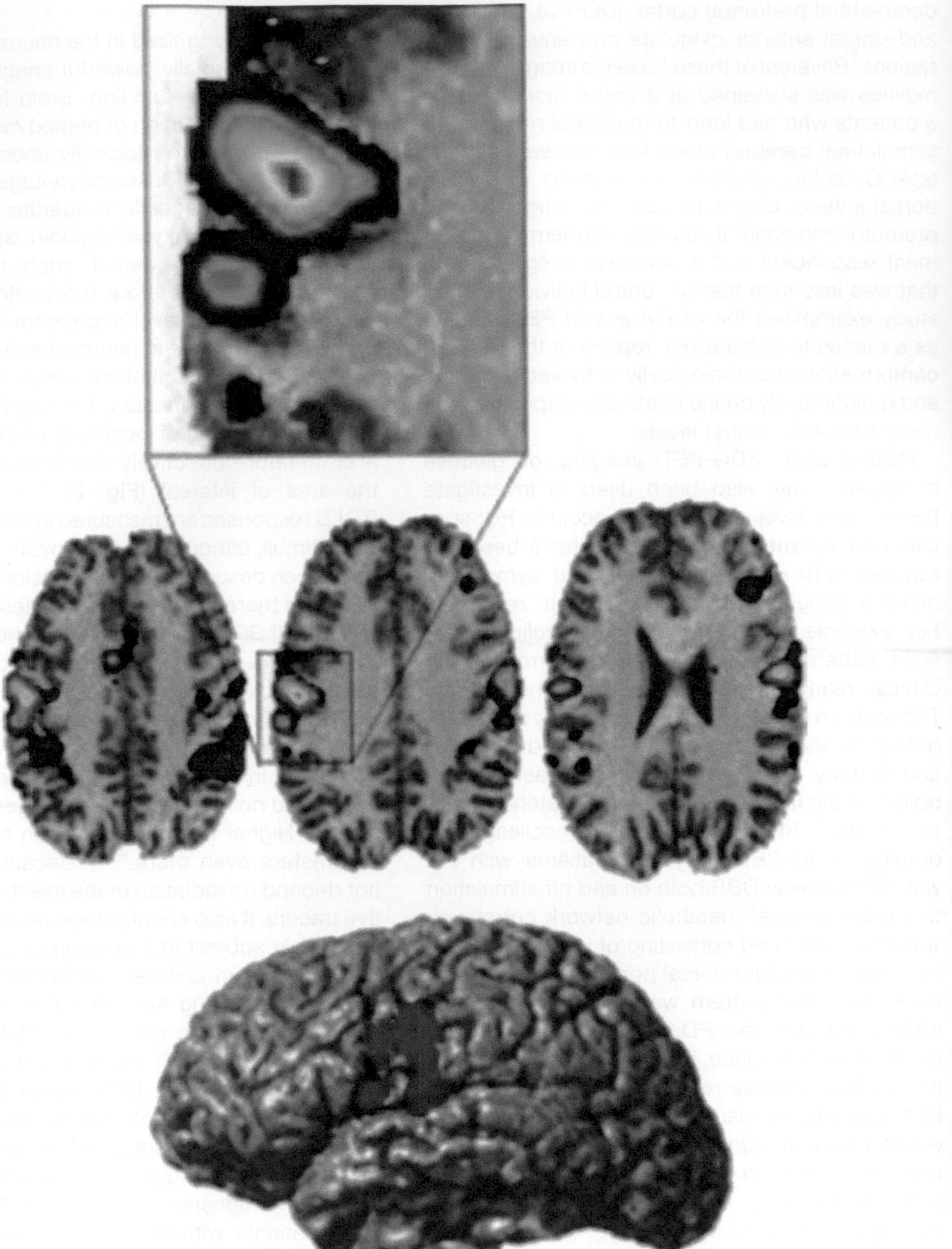

Fig. 2. fMRI motor map. fMRI color-coded map generated during voluntary motor movement showing task-related activation of primary motor cortex (M1), premotor area (PMA), and supplementary motor area (SMA) during tongue movement.

work in the chronic pain literature. In contrast to classic detection of stimulus-related responses in the brain, Baliki and colleagues[82] developed a novel study design using fMRI to evaluate the brain circuitry involved in chronic pain processing. These investigators used an event-related paradigm that recorded fMRI signals continuously, and patients reported real-time pain levels while lying in the scanner. Using this approach, the investigators identified patterns of brain activity related to spontaneous pain of chronic back pain sufferers and to distinguish this from responses to acute nociceptive (thermal) stimuli. Although spontaneous chronic pain correlated with activation of the mPFC and rostral anterior cingulate cortex (rACC), thermal pain activated traditionally accepted pain areas of insula, posterior thalamus, and sensory cortex. The mPFC and rACC are involved in emotional processing and self-referential negative emotional states (ie, suffering).[82]

BOLD fluctuations can also be detected in the resting state based on the intrinsic functional organization of the brain.[83,84] Analysis of resting-state BOLD fMRI fluctuations reveals very low frequency (<0.1 Hz) correlated activity across brain regions, such that several distinct functional networks can be identified. These resting-state functional networks correlate with various task-related and behavior-related neural network activation and behavioral states and provide a biomarker of functional network level connectivity.[84] Many basic science studies have begun to delineate aberrations in resting-state functional networks, or functional connectivity, across disease states. In 2011, Baliki and colleagues[85] used resting-state fMRI to further identify the mechanisms of pain perception and the impact of chronic pain on resting-state brain networks. These investigators found that patients with chronic pain showed a shift toward higher-frequency activations in the resting-state brain network regions, including mPFC, posterior cingulate cortex, and left and right lateral parietal cortices compared with healthy controls. The significance of these fMRI data is that chronic pain generates a change in functional connectivity of regions involved in pain reception and processing. Furthermore, increased high-frequency oscillations perhaps reflect ongoing neural activation or excitability in the areas previously shown to be related to suffering or salience of the pain experience. Thus, fMRI is a powerful tool capable of providing structural and functional information that reflects the process of neuroplasticity during chronic disease. In addition, it offers a new perspective on how we view the brain changes associated with chronic pain and other neuropsychiatric diseases, and the role of neuroplasticity in disease states in general.

FUTURE DIRECTIONS

With the increasing number of indications, and our expanding knowledge of brain structure and function, we are impelled to modernize our techniques and step away from the traditional standardized atlas-based methods. Limitations of indirect targeting have surrounded stereotactic surgery since its inception.[39] Neuroimaging has already been established in neurosurgery in various capacities, including the use of preoperative DTI to visualize critical structures before tumor resections and fMRI to predict the potential for postoperative memory problems in temporal lobectomy.[72] The goals of further integrating advanced neuroimaging into DBS surgery and central neuromodulation in general are similar: to personalize targets, maximize efficiency, and minimize and predict side effects.

The past decade has seen an explosion of advanced neuroimaging techniques to understand the somatotopic organization, psychological function, and temporal relationship of neural networks, both in health and in disease. These techniques have proved reproducible, but few have been clinically validated. Pouratian and colleagues[23] reported in 2011 a probabilistic connectivity-based approach for thalamic segmentation on an individual level. They retrospectively applied this technology to patients who had undergone VIM nucleus DBS for essential tremor, and were able to identify the most efficacious thalamic region electrode placement in each individual patient based on tractography data independent of AC and PC measurements. Furthermore, they found this highly efficacious location was highly variable across individuals relative to AC-PC measurements. Although this was a retrospective study, it underscores the enormous potential impact of using this imaging modality to accurately identify the most efficacious electrode position on an individual basis that produces the best functional outcomes and requires the lowest power.

Precision is tantamount to accuracy for surgical efficiency and avoidance of side effects. Visualizing the white matter tracts at each target with diffusion tensor tractography can help predict side effects, as shown by Barkhoudarian and colleagues.[86] These investigators used 12-direction diffusion tensor tractography for a detailed analysis of white matter tracts around the electrodes placed in STN, GPi, and VIM nucleus. Both low-voltage and high-voltage ROI analyses were performed at each target, which takes into account the theory that higher-voltage stimulation recruits a larger volume of surrounding tissue. The investigators found a variety of tract projections and orientations around each target. Fiber tracts of internal capsule and corona radiata were located medially to GPi, laterally to VIM nucleus, and within STN. Low-voltage analysis revealed that both STN and VIM nucleus had projections to the motor and premotor cortices. High-voltage analysis of STN showed tracts extending to the prefrontal, parietal, inferior occipitofrontal, and frontal eye fields. GPi had a broad range of fiber types even at low voltage, including projections to motor, prefrontal, sensory, and parietal cortices. High voltage of GPi included the cerebellum and frontal eye fields as well. The more diverse fiber tracts around the STN and GPi possibly explains the various side effects that occur with stimulation of these regions, including conjugate eye deviation, sensory disturbances, and psychological changes. This study shows how diffusion tractography can be a practical and accessible adjunctive method of analyzing DBS targets on an individual level to optimize the preoperative targeting process and improve surgical efficiency. Integrating the structural and functional data provided by these clinically validated methods can take into account a significant amount of intersubject variability and offer a clearly improved alternative to traditional methods of direct and indirect targeting.

In trying to optimize the surgical treatments, we must not overlook the importance of improving our knowledge of the diseases that we are treating. In vivo functional imaging performed in human individuals has been integral to improving our understanding of both normal resting brain function and disease states. In the psychiatric domain, both PET and fMRI have been critical to the development of modern views of the pathophysiology of dysregulated networks in disease states and have promoted the use of DBS as a treatment option for network modulation.[39] Chronic pain is another condition that has been redefined by fMRI. For example, Baliki and colleagues[82] confirmed that patients with chronic pain have a spatiotemporally different neural mechanism for the pain experience compared with normal controls. Activation of the mPFC and rACC during spontaneous episodes of chronic back pain were contrasted with the nociceptive regions of the insula, secondary somatosensory cortex, and posterior thalamus. In addition, these investigators found that the overactivation of mPFC inhibits the function of the DLPFC, which is also notably thinner in patients with chronic pain versus healthy patients.[87] These findings show the pathologic role of neuroplasticity in reorganizing neural networks. Sustained activity in the regions of mPFC and rACC are strongly implicated in the depressive state and negative self-referential emotions and accounts for the suffering experienced by patients with chronic pain. This work provides a new perspective and insight into chronic pain as a disease of the brain, regardless of the site of injury within the body. The study by Baliki and colleagues substantiates the findings in depression studies that the rACC and mPFC are primary targets for the idea of suffering and can potentially be modulated with DBS to disrupt this ongoing neural excitability and reset the dysrhythmia within the network, thus ameliorating not the intensity of the pain, but how the patient responds to it.

SUMMARY

Modern neuroimaging has seen rapid advances in capability and efficiency, made possible by the ongoing accumulation of discoveries in computational and basic science research. Because of the successes of this field, structural and functional image techniques have become the preferred means of evaluating and framing information collected about the function, in vivo, of the human brain. Applying these methods to the clinical field of neurosurgery can confer a measure of certainty to surgical undertakings on our patients' brains. We must move away from earlier eras when clinical observations were linked with data derived from basic neuroanatomy or animal models, which have resulted in conflicts, competing hypotheses, and incomplete knowledge about the mechanism of DBS and the diseases it is used to treat. Familiarity with the new perspectives provided by advanced imaging techniques can help achieve a deeper understanding of neurologic and psychiatric disorders and refine both medical and neuromodulatory therapies.

REFERENCES

1. Panov F, Gologorsky Y, Connors G, et al. Deep brain stimulation in DYT1 dystonia: a 10-year experience. Neurosurgery 2013;73(1):86–93.
2. Vidailhet M, Vercueil L, Houeto JL, et al. Bilateral deep-brain stimulation of the globus pallidus in primary generalized dystonia. N Engl J Med 2005; 352(5):459–67.
3. Marks W, Bailey L, Reed M, et al. Pallidal stimulation in children: comparison between cerebral palsy and DYT1 dystonia. J Child Neurol 2013; 28(7):840–8.
4. Okun MS. Deep-brain stimulation for Parkinson's disease. N Engl J Med 2012;367(16):1529–38.
5. Tasker RR, PENN RD. Deep brain stimulation is preferable to thalamotomy for tremor suppression. Commentary. Surg Neurol 1998;49(2):145–54 Elsevier.
6. Lyketsos CG, Targum SD, Pendergrass JC, et al. Deep brain stimulation: a novel strategy for treating Alzheimer's disease. Innov Clin Neurosci 2012; 9(11–12):10–7.
7. Deep brain stimulation for the treatment of Alzheimer's disease–tabular view. 2013. p. 1–3. Available at: ClinicalTrials.gov.
8. Hauptman JS, DeSalles A, Espinoza R, et al. Potential surgical targets for deep brain stimulation in

treatment-resistant depression. Neurosurg Focus 2008;25(1):E3.
9. Taghva AS, Malone DA, Rezai AR. Deep brain stimulation for treatment-resistant depression. World Neurosurg 2012. [Epub ahead of print].
10. Mallet L, Polosan M, Jaafari N, et al. Subthalamic nucleus stimulation in severe obsessive-compulsive disorder. N Engl J Med 2008;359(20):2121–34.
11. Coffey RJ, Lozano AM. Neurostimulation for chronic noncancer pain: an evaluation of the clinical evidence and recommendations for future trial designs. J Neurosurg 2006;105(2):175–89.
12. Hamani C, Schwalb JM, Rezai AR, et al. Deep brain stimulation for chronic neuropathic pain: long-term outcome and the incidence of insertional effect. Pain 2006;125(1–2):188–96.
13. Gildenberg PL. Evolution of neuromodulation. Stereotact Funct Neurosurg 2005;83(2–3):71–9.
14. Kall BA, Goerss SJ, Kelly PJ. A new multimodality correlative imaging technique for VOP/VIM (VL) thalamotomy procedures. Stereotact Funct Neurosurg 1992;58(1–4):45–51.
15. Schaltenbrand G, Wahren W, Hassler RG. Schaltenbrand: atlas for stereotaxy of the human. Thieme. 1977.
16. Talairach J, Tournoux P. Co-planar stereotaxic atlas of the human brain. 3-dimensional proportional system: an approach to cerebral imaging. 1988.
17. Albe-Fessard D, Arfel G, Guiot G, et al. Albe-Fessard: identification et délimitation précise. Google Scholar. CR Acad Sci (Paris). 1961.
18. Niemann K, Naujokat C, Pohl G, et al. Verification of the Schaltenbrand and Wahren stereotactic atlas. Acta Neurochir (Wien) 1994;129(1–2):72–81.
19. Yelnik J, Damier P, Bejjani BP, et al. Functional mapping of the human globus pallidus: contrasting effect of stimulation in the internal and external pallidum in Parkinson's disease. Neuroscience 2000; 101(1):77–87.
20. Littlechild P, Varma TR, Eldridge PR, et al. Variability in position of the subthalamic nucleus targeted by magnetic resonance imaging and microelectrode recordings as compared to atlas co-ordinates. Stereotact Funct Neurosurg 2003; 80(1–4):82–7.
21. Nowinski WL, Belov D, Thirunavuukarasuu A, et al. A probabilistic functional atlas of the VIM nucleus constructed from pre-, intra- and postoperative electrophysiological and neuroimaging data acquired during the surgical treatment of Parkinson's disease patients. Stereotact Funct Neurosurg 2005;83(5–6):190–6.
22. Nowinski WL, Belov D, Pollak P, et al. A probabilistic functional atlas of the human subthalamic nucleus. Neuroinformatics 2004;2(4): 381–98.
23. Pouratian N, Zheng Z, Bari AA, et al. Multi-institutional evaluation of deep brain stimulation targeting using probabilistic connectivity-based thalamic segmentation. J Neurosurg 2011;115(5):995–1004.
24. Pouratian N, Bookheimer SY. The reliability of neuroanatomy as a predictor of eloquence: a review. Neurosurg Focus 2010;28(2):E3.
25. Daniluk S, G Davies K, Ellias SA, et al. Assessment of the variability in the anatomical position and size of the subthalamic nucleus among patients with advanced Parkinson's disease using magnetic resonance imaging. Acta Neurochir (Wien) 2009; 152(2):201–10.
26. Patel NK, Khan S, Gill SS. Comparison of atlas- and magnetic-resonance-imaging-based stereotactic targeting of the subthalamic nucleus in the surgical treatment of Parkinson's disease. Stereotact Funct Neurosurg 2008;86(3):153–61.
27. Richter EO, Hoque T, Halliday W, et al. Determining the position and size of the subthalamic nucleus based on magnetic resonance imaging results in patients with advanced Parkinson disease. J Neurosurg 2004;100(3):541–6.
28. Schlaier J, Schoedel P, Lange M, et al. Reliability of atlas-derived coordinates in deep brain stimulation. Acta Neurochir (Wien) 2005;147(11):1175–80 [discussion: 1180].
29. Starr PA, Christine CW, Theodosopoulos PV, et al. Implantation of deep brain stimulators into the subthalamic nucleus: technical approach and magnetic resonance imaging-verified lead locations. J Neurosurg 2002;97(2):370–87.
30. Abosch A, Yacoub E, Ugurbil K, et al. An assessment of current brain targets for deep brain stimulation surgery with susceptibility-weighted imaging at 7 tesla. Neurosurgery 2010;67(6):1745–56 [discussion: 1756].
31. Sudhyadhom A, Bova FJ, Foote KD, et al. Limbic, associative, and motor territories within the targets for deep brain stimulation: potential clinical implications. Curr Neurol Neurosci Rep 2007; 7(4):278–89.
32. Saint-Cyr JA, Hoque T, Pereira LC, et al. Localization of clinically effective stimulating electrodes in the human subthalamic nucleus on magnetic resonance imaging. J Neurosurg 2002;97(5): 1152–66.
33. Yelnik J, Damier P, Demeret S, et al. Localization of stimulating electrodes in patients with Parkinson disease by using a three-dimensional atlas-magnetic resonance imaging coregistration method. J Neurosurg 2003;99(1):89–99.
34. Annett M. Parallels between asymmetries of planum temporale and of hand skill. Neuropsychologia 1992;30(11):951–62.
35. Ballmaier M, Sowell ER, Thompson PM, et al. Mapping brain size and cortical gray matter changes in

elderly depression. Biol Psychiatry 2004;55(4):382–9.
36. Im K, Lee JM, Lee J, et al. Gender difference analysis of cortical thickness in healthy young adults with surface-based methods. Neuroimage 2006;31(1):31–8.
37. Narr KL, Bilder RM, Luders E, et al. Asymmetries of cortical shape: effects of handedness, sex and schizophrenia. Neuroimage 2007;34(3):939–48.
38. Thompson PM, Hayashi KM, de Zubicaray GI, et al. Mapping hippocampal and ventricular change in Alzheimer disease. Neuroimage 2004;22(4):1754–66.
39. McIntyre CC, Hahn PJ. Network perspectives on the mechanisms of deep brain stimulation. Neurobiol Dis 2010;38(3):329–37.
40. Guehl D, Edwards R, Cuny E, et al. Statistical determination of the optimal subthalamic nucleus stimulation site in patients with Parkinson disease. J Neurosurg 2007;106(1):101–10.
41. Duchin Y, Abosch A, Yacoub E, et al. Feasibility of using ultra-high field (7 T) MRI for clinical surgical targeting. PLoS One 2012;7(5):e37328.
42. Cho ZH, Min HK, Oh SH, et al. Direct visualization of deep brain stimulation targets in Parkinson disease with the use of 7-tesla magnetic resonance imaging. J Neurosurg 2010;113(3):639–47.
43. Duyn JH, van Gelderen P, Li TQ, et al. High-field MRI of brain cortical substructure based on signal phase. Proc Natl Acad Sci U S A 2007;104(28):11796–801.
44. Okun MS, Tagliati M, Pourfar M, et al. Management of referred deep brain stimulation failures: a retrospective analysis from 2 movement disorders centers. Arch Neurol 2005;62(8):1250–5.
45. Grieve SM, Williams LM, Paul RH, et al. Cognitive aging, executive function, and fractional anisotropy: a diffusion tensor MR imaging study. AJNR Am J Neuroradiol 2007;28(2):226–35.
46. Deutsch GK, Dougherty RF, Bammer R, et al. Children's reading performance is correlated with white matter structure measured by diffusion tensor imaging. Cortex 2005;41(3):354–63.
47. Madden DJ, Whiting WL, Huettel SA, et al. Diffusion tensor imaging of adult age differences in cerebral white matter: relation to response time. Neuroimage 2004;21(3):1174–81.
48. Zheng Z, Shemmassian S, Wijekoon C, et al. DTI correlates of distinct cognitive impairments in Parkinson's disease. Hum Brain Mapp 2013. [Epub ahead of print].
49. McKinlay A, Grace RC, Dalrymple-Alford JC, et al. Characteristics of executive function impairment in Parkinson's disease patients without dementia. J Int Neuropsychol Soc 2010;16(2):268–77.
50. Nucifora PG, Verma R, Lee SK, et al. Diffusion-tensor MR imaging and tractography: exploring brain microstructure and connectivity. Radiology 2007;245(2):367–84.
51. Ciccarelli O, Parker GJ, Toosy AT, et al. From diffusion tractography to quantitative white matter tract measures: a reproducibility study. Neuroimage 2003;18(2):348–59.
52. Sedrak M, Gorgulho A, De Salles AF, et al. The role of modern imaging modalities on deep brain stimulation targeting for mental illness. Acta Neurochir Suppl 2008;101:3–7.
53. Gutman DA, Holtzheimer PE, Behrens TE, et al. A tractography analysis of two deep brain stimulation white matter targets for depression. Biol Psychiatry 2009;65(4):276–82.
54. Lenglet C, Abosch A, Yacoub E, et al. Comprehensive in vivo mapping of the human basal ganglia and thalamic connectome in individuals using 7 T MRI. PLoS One 2012;7(1):e29153.
55. Sedrak M, Gorgulho A, Frew A, et al. Diffusion tensor imaging and colored fractional anisotropy mapping of the ventralis intermedius nucleus of the thalamus. Neurosurgery 2011;69(5):1124–9 [discussion: 1129–30].
56. Behrens TE, Johansen-Berg H, Woolrich MW, et al. Non-invasive mapping of connections between human thalamus and cortex using diffusion imaging. Nat Neurosci 2003;6(7):750–7.
57. Rezai AR, Lozano AM, Crawley AP, et al. Thalamic stimulation and functional magnetic resonance imaging: localization of cortical and subcortical activation with implanted electrodes: technical note. J Neurosurg 1999;90(3):583–90.
58. Samuel M, Ceballos-Baumann AO, Blin J, et al. Evidence for lateral premotor and parietal overactivity in Parkinson's disease during sequential and bimanual movements. A PET study. Brain 1997;120(Pt 6):963–76.
59. Krams M, Rushworth M, Deiber MP. The preparation, execution and suppression of copied movements in the human brain. Exp Brain Res 1998;120(3):386–98.
60. Kober H, Barrett LF, Joseph J, et al. Functional grouping and cortical-subcortical interactions in emotion: a meta-analysis of neuroimaging studies. Neuroimage 2008;42(2):998–1031.
61. Baker SC, Rogers RD, Owen AM, et al. Neural systems engaged by planning: a PET study of the tower of London task. Neuropsychologia 1996;34(6):515–26.
62. LaBar KS, Gitelman DR, Parrish TB, et al. Neuroanatomic overlap of working memory and spatial attention networks: a functional MRI comparison within subjects. Neuroimage 1999;10(6):695–704.
63. Davis KD, Kwan CL, Crawley AP. Functional MRI study of thalamic and cortical activations evoked by cutaneous heat, cold, and tactile stimuli. J Neurophysiol 1998;80(3):1533–46.

64. Dove A, Pollmann S, Schubert T, et al. Prefrontal cortex activation in task switching: an event-related fMRI study. Brain Res Cogn Brain Res 2000;9(1):103–9.
65. Johansen-Berg H. Functional-anatomical validation and individual variation of diffusion tractography-based segmentation of the human thalamus. Cereb Cortex 2004;15(1):31–9.
66. Menke RA, Jbabdi S, Miller KL, et al. Connectivity-based segmentation of the substantia nigra in human and its implications in Parkinson's disease. Neuroimage 2010;52(4):1175–80.
67. Johansen-Berg H, Gutman DA, Behrens TE, et al. Anatomical connectivity of the subgenual cingulate region targeted with deep brain stimulation for treatment-resistant depression. Cereb Cortex 2008;18(6):1374–83.
68. Rushworth MF, Behrens TE, Johansen-Berg H. Connection patterns distinguish 3 regions of human parietal cortex. Cereb Cortex 2006;16(10):1418–30.
69. Lambert C, Zrinzo L, Nagy Z, et al. Confirmation of functional zones within the human subthalamic nucleus: patterns of connectivity and sub-parcellation using diffusion weighted imaging. Neuroimage 2012;60(1):83–94.
70. Behrens T, Berg HJ, Jbabdi S, et al. Probabilistic diffusion tractography with multiple fibre orientations: what can we gain? Neuroimage 2007;34(1):144–55.
71. Perlmutter JS, Mink JW. Deep brain stimulation. Annu Rev Neurosci 2006;29:229–57.
72. Tharin S, Golby A. Functional brain mapping and its applications to neurosurgery. Neurosurgery 2007;60(Suppl 2):185–201.
73. Mayberg HS, Brannan SK, Tekell JL, et al. Regional metabolic effects of fluoxetine in major depression: serial changes and relationship to clinical response. Biol Psychiatry 2000;48(8):830–43.
74. Mayberg HS, Liotti M, Brannan SK. Reciprocal limbic-cortical function and negative mood: converging PET findings in depression and normal sadness. Am J Psychiatry 1999;156(5):675–82.
75. Nobler MS, Oquendo MA, Kegeles LS. Decreased regional brain metabolism after ECT. Am J Psychiatry 2001;158(2):305–8.
76. Mayberg HS, Lozano AM, Voon V, et al. Deep brain stimulation for treatment-resistant depression. Neuron 2005;45(5):651–60.
77. Eidelberg D. Metabolic brain networks in neurodegenerative disorders: a functional imaging approach. Trends Neurosci 2009;32(10):548–57.
78. Mure H, Hirano S, Tang CC, et al. Parkinson's disease tremor-related metabolic network: characterization, progression, and treatment effects. Neuroimage 2011;54(2):1244–53.
79. Fishman PS. Paradoxical aspects of parkinsonian tremor. Mov Disord 2008;23(2):168–73.
80. Kim DS, Garwood M. High-field magnetic resonance techniques for brain research. Curr Opin Neurobiol 2003;13(5):612–9.
81. Pfeuffer J, Adriany G, Shmuel A. Perfusion-based high-resolution functional imaging in the human brain at 7 Tesla. Magn Reson Med 2002;47(5):903–11.
82. Baliki MN, Chialvo DR, Geha PY, et al. Chronic pain and the emotional brain: specific brain activity associated with spontaneous fluctuations of intensity of chronic back pain. J Neurosci 2006;26(47):12165–73.
83. Fox MD, Raichle ME. Spontaneous fluctuations in brain activity observed with functional magnetic resonance imaging. Nat Rev Neurosci 2007;8(9):700–11.
84. Baria AT, Baliki MN, Parrish T, et al. Anatomical and functional assemblies of brain BOLD oscillations. J Neurosci 2011;31(21):7910–9.
85. Baliki MN, Baria AT, Apkarian AV. The cortical rhythms of chronic back pain. J Neurosci 2011;31(39):13981–90.
86. Barkhoudarian G, Klochkov T, Sedrak M, et al. A role of diffusion tensor imaging in movement disorder surgery. Acta Neurochir (Wien) 2010;152(12):2089–95.
87. Apkarian AV, Sosa Y, Sonty S, et al. Chronic back pain is associated with decreased prefrontal and thalamic gray matter density. J Neurosci 2004;24(46):10410–5.

Creating the Feedback Loop
Closed-Loop Neurostimulation

Adam O. Hebb, MD, FRCSC[a,*], Jun Jason Zhang, PhD[b], Mohammad H. Mahoor, PhD[b], Christos Tsiokos, MS[c], Charles Matlack, MS[d], Howard Jay Chizeck, ScD[d], Nader Pouratian, MD, PhD[e]

KEYWORDS

- Deep brain stimulation • Closed-loop • Local field potentials • Oscillations • Subthalamic nucleus • Control systems • Machine learning

KEY POINTS

- Closed-loop stimulation may be superior to open loop therapy by reducing the impact of DBS on cognitive processes that depend on coordinated neuronal oscillations.
- Understanding the relationship between the gross patient behavior (or severity of disease) and a neuronal signal that is under the influence of external stimulation is fundamental to using the signal in a control system.
- A closed loop system extracts a particular feature of a biological signal that has a desired reference value associated with a desired therapeutic state. The system attempts to bring the feature closer to the desired reference value to induce the desired therapeutic state.
- Reference values for biosignal features are expected to vary over time in the same patient, and vary over behavioral goals of the patient. Thus, systems must be designed to update with time and cover a range of behavioral situations, such as walking, talking, or writing.

INTRODUCTION

Implantable devices for electrical stimulation of the brain have been in routine clinical use since 1997, when the first commercial deep brain stimulation (DBS) system was approved for the treatment of tremor.[1] These DBS devices provide an invariant train of stimulatory pulses at a fixed frequency. This open-loop mode (meaning unidirectional signal generated from the device and delivered to the brain) of DBS therapy has proved to be effective for treatment of essential tremor,[2] Parkinson disease,[3,4] and dystonia.[5,6] As understanding of the neurophysiologic mechanisms of both DBS and movement disorders expands, the shortcomings of open-loop therapy DBS are evident and are discussed in this review. The design of a closed-loop implantable pulse generator (IPG) to sense and respond to physiologic signals (closed-loop meaning bidirectional signals moving in both sensing and responding directions, allowing sensor signals to provide feedback modulation of stimulation) within or outside the brain is considered the next frontier in brain stimulation research and will likely broaden the field to include new applications for neuromodulation.

[a] Colorado Neurological Institute, Department of Electrical and Computer Engineering, University of Denver, 499 E Hampden Ave Ste, 220 Englewood, CO 80113, USA; [b] Department of Electrical and Computer Engineering, University of Denver, 499 E Hampden Ave Ste, 220 Englewood, CO 80113, USA; [c] Department of Biomedical Engineering, University of California, Los Angeles, California, USA; [d] Electrical Engineering, University of Washington, Seattle, Washington, USA; [e] Department of Neurosurgery, University of California, Los Angeles, California, USA
* Corresponding author.
E-mail address: adam.hebb@aoh.md

Neurosurg Clin N Am 25 (2014) 187–204
http://dx.doi.org/10.1016/j.nec.2013.08.006
1042-3680/14/$ – see front matter

Implantable closed-loop stimulation systems are well established in the treatment of cardiac arrhythmias. Cardiac pacemaker devices capable of sensing and responding to atrial activity are closed-loop mode cardiac stimulation devices and have been in clinical use since 1963.[7] Despite the precedent for an IPG with dual sensing and stimulating functionality set 50 years ago, efforts to bring similar concepts to DBS devices[8,9] have been delayed 50 years in part because of the complexity of brain signals. Whereas cardiac pacemakers detect the P-wave signal of the atrial pacemaker, brain-generated signals are statistically complex. Perhaps more importantly, the clinical meaningfulness of recordable brain signals is not immediately obvious.

Strategy development for interpreting neuronal signals in closed-loop neurostimulation applications is underway. In broadest terms, an understanding of the relationship between a patient's clinical state and a neuronal signal under the influence of external stimulation is fundamental to any future use of the signal as a surrogate marker for clinical states. Clinical states are disease specific but collectively can be categorized by pathologic expressions of the disease (eg, the magnitude of tremor) and behavioral intentions (ie, attempting a task at hand such as walking, talking, or writing). Therefore, closed-loop neurostimulation relates available neuronal recording to meaningful clinical states and uses the surrogate measurements to update neurostimulation as the device is operating.

Recordable neurophysiologic signals are available from multiple levels of the brain, including a single neuron, multiple individual neurons, a localized population of neurons, or a large-scale population of neurons. Single-neuron recordings have been shown to be related to certain specific aspects of movement[10] and cognition.[11] Technical challenges of chronic recording from single neurons exist, such as increased sampling rate requirements, difficulty maintaining recordings from the same neuron for extended periods of time, and degradation at the neuron-electrode interface. These challenges contribute to the overall difficulty in maintaining sustained recordings from a single neuron. Recording from large populations of neurons, or local field potential (LFP) recordings, are much more stable over time. Oscillatory components of LFP recordings from highly specialized cortex, such as motor cortex or visual cortex, have been successfully related to clinical states such as movement and visual percepts.[12–14] However, recordings from these specialized cortical regions of the brain are limited because these regions are not typically accessed during routine surgery for neurostimulation.

This review presents current developments in closed-loop neurostimulation and strategies for manipulation of recordable signals to relate this information to a patient's clinical state (**Figs. 1** and **2**). Specifically, this review covers the rationale for closed-loop stimulation, meaningful categories of clinical patient states, brain signals available for recording, signal processing for prediction of patient states, and interventional DBS patterns aimed at restoring a desired state, or facilitating a desired state. Parkinson disease is a primary focus; however, principles can be applied to other movement disorders, as well as epilepsy, mood disorders, and other neuropsychiatric diseases. This review is intended as an introduction to engineering issues for clinicians and clinical issues for engineers.

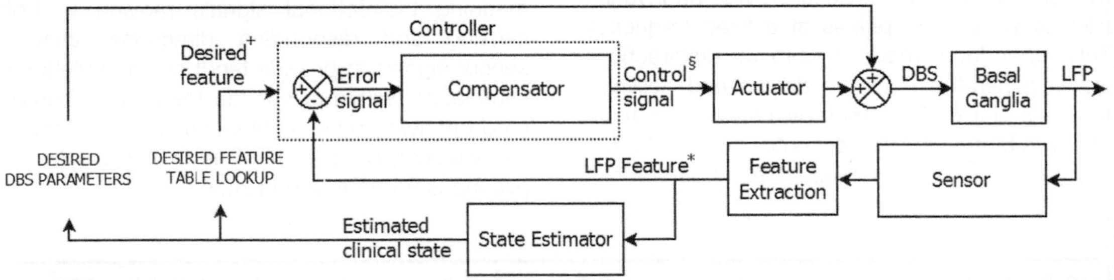

Fig. 1. General control system diagram representing a conceptualized closed-loop neurostimulation system for DBS. In this diagram, the reference signal (LFP Feature*) is the feature extracted from the basal ganglia local field potential. This reference signal* is used to predict a meaningful clinical state of the patient (estimated or predicted clinical state) and these states subsequently direct the selection of desired DBS parameters and appropriate reference values (Desired⁺ feature). The controller compares (and calculates an error signal) the reference signal* and value⁺, and calculates the controlled variable (Control§ signal). The control signal§ and actuator, together with the selection of desired DBS parameters, influence the DBS feedback to the basal ganglia, ultimately affecting the LFP and extracted features*. This impact on the LFP serves as a surrogate marker for the beneficial effect of DBS on the patient, bringing the reference signal* and value⁺ closer together.

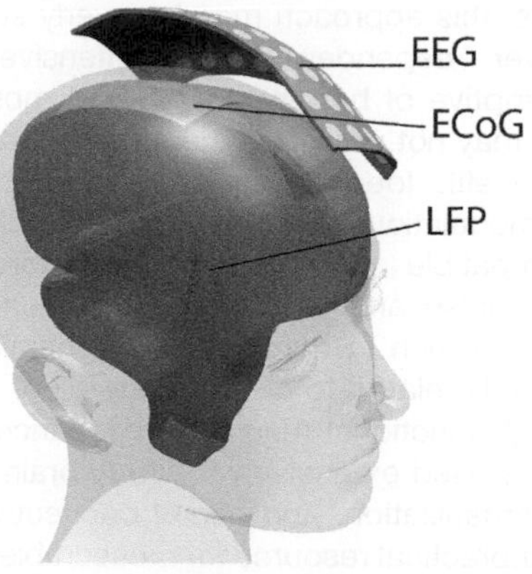

Fig. 2. Candidate neural signals for closed-loop neurostimulation systems include noninvasive electroencephalography (EEG), or invasive electrocorticography (ECoG), or local field potentials (LFP). In addition to these brain signals, the system could use electromyography (EMG), or physical sensors such as accelerometry (not shown).

RATIONALE FOR CLOSED-LOOP STIMULATION: PARKINSON DISEASE

Open-loop DBS is effective for treating the motor signs of Parkinson disease, but the side effects of this therapy and its inefficiencies may be diminished within a closed-loop system. Side effects of open-loop DBS experienced by some patients include impaired cognition, speech, gait, and balance.[15] Open-loop DBS could potentially disrupt decision making, learning, and cognitive association through its effect on LFP oscillations of the brain. Open-loop DBS therapy was developed before an understanding of how LFP oscillations influence the precise timing of neuronal action potentials (integral to the mechanism of Hebbian learning[16,17]), and influence communication between distant neuronal ensembles (the basis of cognitive association[18,19]). Studies have demonstrated that open-loop DBS impairs learning and object naming during stimulation of the pulvinar,[20] and impairs verbal fluency and reactive inhibition during stimulation of the subthalamic nucleus. These impairments may be caused by disruption of cortico-cortical or cortico-subcortical oscillatory synchronization between LFPs of connected brain regions.[20]

As a result of dopaminergic depletion in Parkinson disease, the basal ganglia are characterized by radical changes at the level of a single neuron and above. Neuronal firing patterns change significantly in animal models and in humans with Parkinson disease. In the pathologic state, neuronal pairs within and across boundaries of basal ganglia nuclei fire together with increased synchrony.[21] This phenomenon is reflected in the abnormal oscillatory activity revealed by LFPs within and between those structures.

The method by which high-frequency stimulation influences cortico-basal ganglia circuits and leads to a therapeutic outcome is under debate.[22,23] DBS effects are likely a combination of a local inhibitory effect and an excitatory effect on distal connected nuclei. The local inhibitory effect of DBS may be evident by the fact that both stimulation and lesioning of the globus pallidus lead to similar therapeutic effects in the clinical treatment of Parkinson disease. For the treatment of essential tremor, clinical effects of stimulation and lesioning of the thalamus are roughly equivalent. The distal excitatory effect of subthalamic nucleus DBS is evident by its observed effect of increasing the firing rate of neurons in the globus pallidus, a distal connected nucleus.[24]

Although the mechanism of DBS therapeutic benefit is poorly understood, an end result of open-loop DBS may be a neuronal network that is able to retain partial functionality despite insufficient dopaminergic innervation. If this is true, the present therapeutic methods may not be restoring basal ganglia functionality to the fullest extent possible, because of limitations of the static approach of open-loop DBS in an inherently dynamic system. It is therefore compelling to seek a treatment that could enhance surviving functionality in the basal ganglia. Dynamic restoration of neuronal rhythms by the integration of responsive signal processing might be an advantage of a closed-loop system. Conversely, damage to the basal ganglia may be the result of irreversible loss of neuronal circuitry involved in highly specialized information processing.[25] In this case, dynamic and responsive signal processing may not present an advantage compared with current open-loop DBS, especially if a damaged neuronal network generates faulty signal outputs.

RESTORING THE DESIRED STATE: A ROLE FOR CLOSED-LOOP STIMULATION

A central challenge for closed-loop therapy is the definition of a therapeutic or optimal state that neurostimulation attempts to maintain or restore. Therefore, closed-loop systems incorporate a single or multiple set points, that is, reference values corresponding to the desired state. Returning to the example of optimizing behavioral goals, each of these set points could correspond to a different behavioral intention, such as walking, talking, or writing.

The goal of closed-loop DBS in Parkinson disease is to restore lost functionality by stimulating the target nucleus. Stimulation of the basal ganglia is based on a state-space model of the basal ganglia dynamics. Stimulation is intended to force a certain feature that leads to some desired LFP reference value associated with the desired therapeutic state (see **Fig. 1**). The compensator attempts to bring the controlled variable closer to the desired reference value. The state-space model relies on the assumption that a disease symptom is attributable to 1 or more features (often just 1) that is constant at some reference value level in a nondiseased physiologic state. A second assumption is that restoring the value of the LFP output feature to the desired value is sufficient to restore basal ganglia functionality. These assumptions may be implausible if the pathologic cause of Parkinson disease is characterized more by loss of neuronal organization (precluding signal processing of normal neuronal signals) than by a disturbance of LFP oscillations.

A model for a closed-loop system that contains multiple modes of compensation could be useful in an attempt to replicate the nonlinear characteristics of the basal ganglia system and subcortical motor network facilitating a wide range of motor and cognitive tasks.[26] Such a model would address the need to generate a variety of concurrent signal patterns corresponding to multiple desired reference values. For example, before movement initiation, a desired reference value could constitute high suppression of the beta (13–30 Hz) oscillatory power of the LFP signal, whereas continuous execution of movement might call for concurrent beta suppression with an increase in high-frequency gamma (>30 Hz) oscillatory power. The advantage of multiple modes of compensation compared with a single set-point closed-loop compensation system is that therapy could be tailored to an individual patient's goals. First, desired reference values for normal corticobasal ganglia activity must be defined to later dynamically adjust the controlled variables. Those values could be obtainable by recording from motor-planning cortical areas[10] or sites in the basal ganglia, including those at the stimulation site.[27]

AVAILABLE SIGNALS

The availability of reliably detectable biosignals capable of driving feedback is essential to a closed-loop neuromodulation system. In current open-loop systems, the patient's clinical status and the provider's assessment of the clinical status via physical examination provides the feedback to regulate neuromodulation. Although effective and the basis for newer neuromodulation models, this approach may be overly subjective/observer dependent, time intensive, overly consumptive of battery power, and most importantly, may not provide patients with optimal clinical benefit. Ideally, biosignals for closed-loop neuromodulation would be easily detectable in a biocompatible manner, reliably recorded with limited noise and error, over an extended time (ie, years), rich in content, and dynamically and accurately related to clinical states. For example, although functional magnetic resonance imaging (fMRI) is used extensively to study brain function, brain organization, and neural connectivity, fMRI is an impractical resource for measurable neuronal activity on an ongoing basis. On the other hand, invasive and implantable electrophysiologic sensors that can detect neuronal signals on an ongoing basis would improve signal detection and feedback within closed-loop systems. Current research is focused primarily on neuroelectrophysiologic signal processing; however, biochemical, optical, electromyographic, and mechanical signals are other potentially useful resources.

Depending on the location of neuroelcotrophysiologic signal recording, signals may represent the activity of 1 neuron or an aggregate of cortical or subcortical neurons.[28] In general, the further away parenchymal recordings are from the brain, the poorer the temporal and spatial resolution and the higher the noise content in the measurements, but the better the perceived safety of each signal source (See **Fig. 2**).

Single-unit recordings, performed with invasive high-impedance (0.4–1.0 MΩ) penetrating microelectrodes such as those used for microelectrode recording in DBS surgery or those used with the Utah microelectrode array, detect action potentials from neighboring neurons (single or multiple). The action potential is considered the core unit of communication between neurons and therefore is extremely appealing as a potential data source for driving closed-loop systems. Recordings of single-unit and multi-unit neuronal activity have provided insight into patterned activity within the subthalamic nucleus and globus pallidus,[29] and for cognitive processing and memory.[30] Despite the potential appeal of microelectrode recording, the practicality of recording action potentials for long-term use are hindered by the requirement for repeated recalibration and difficulty in maintaining the fidelity of recordings over extended periods.[31,32] Moreover, because the measurement of unit activity requires penetrating microelectrodes, spatial sampling is inherently limited (although spatial resolution is outstanding), and necessitates precision when selecting a cortical or subcortical region for recording. Nevertheless, an ongoing trial, the BrainGate trial, is making use of Utah arrays as a signal source for prosthetic control, underscoring the potential of single-neuron recordings.[33,34]

Unlike measurement of individual action potentials, LFPs provide a measure of integrated population level activity, which is believed to be a combination of action potential activity, subthreshold membrane voltage changes, and changes in glial potentials. LFP can be measured with an array of electrodes, including the same microelectrodes that are used for the detection of unit activity as well as standard DBS leads and subcortical electrocorticographic strips and grids.[35–37] LFPs are less susceptible to drift over time and therefore provide higher fidelity and more reliable long-term recordings, which is a desirable characteristic for a control signal. Moreover, because LFPs measure population level oscillatory activity, the data are very rich in content, both in the temporal and the frequency domain, providing several potential bands of interest (eg, alpha, theta, beta, gamma, high gamma). Because signals are recorded using invasive probes, spectral content includes very high frequencies. These high-frequency bands may be critical to the control of closed-loop systems.[38,39] For example, within subthalamic nuclei and globus pallidus, very-high-frequency bands in the 200 to 300 Hz range and greater than 300 Hz range have been described and correlate with degree of Parkinson disease motor states.[38,39] Investigations of LFP measured via electrocorticographic arrays in patients with Parkinson disease have noted increased beta band activity and synchronization within the motor cortex in patients with Parkinson disease compared with other patients.[35] These studies have also shown that therapeutic stimulation in patients with Parkinson disease specifically modulates aberrant beta band activity.[40] Adaptations of DBS devices already in clinical use for invasive recording or stimulation have simplified the development of biocompatible probes for a closed-loop system.[8] The only closed-loop neuromodulation trial to date (NeuroPace) used recordings made by penetrating macroelectrodes and subdural electrocorticographic arrays.[41] Although there have been concerns regarding potential limitations of spatial resolution, studies using LFPs have so far concluded that LFP recording allows for sufficient specificity and functional localization, suggesting LFP recording is usable in closed-loop systems.[13,27]

Although measurement of unit activity and LFPs involves invasive recording approaches, noninvasive measurement of neuroelectrophysiologic activity using electroencephalography (EEG) is also a consideration. A model of the brain-computer interface, the P300 speller, uses EEG detection of evoked cerebral electrophysiologic activity to restore communication to locked-in patients.[42] In patients with Parkinson disease, EEG has detected aberrant patterns of cortical activity that are potential biomarkers of the disease state.[43] EEG essentially measures the same neuronal signals measured by electrocorticography (ECoG). However, because EEG signals are measured noninvasively, the recording electrode is further away from the electrical source and much of the higher frequency spectra (ie, >70–100 Hz) is filtered by the scalp and skull. Both of these factors contribute to a significant loss of spatial resolution. In addition, because EEG sensors are not implanted, they must be affixed to the scalp or skull and this may or may not be acceptable to the patient. Care must be taken in the sampling and recording process to avoid inadvertent creation of artifacts (such as aliasing).[44]

Aside from recording neuronal electrophysiologic signals, a closed-loop system might also use nonneuronal biological signals. For example, the biochemical state of various deep brain regions may be detected in real time using cyclic voltometry.[45] Given the dopaminergic-related origins of Parkinson disease and the biochemical basis of other neuropsychiatric diseases, the concept of integrating real-time biochemical assessments may be useful for managing dynamic fluctuations in medication effects. The groundwork for such models has begun with efforts to develop a wireless nonneuronal feedback system.[46] This approach would have potential limitations related to sampling error and would require additional implantation of penetrating electrodes, which might impart greater risk than other approaches. Other nonneuronal biosignals given serious consideration are recording of peripheral signals by electromyogram (EMG) and noninvasive accelerometers, because such signals indicate patient movement and clinical status in real time. Hilliard and colleagues[47] have reported the use of accelerometers attached to patients' wrists for determining effective stimulation sites within the subthalamic nucleus for treatment of tremor, bradykinesia, and gait disturbance. Such kinesthetically rich information derived from noninvasive peripheral measurement of clinical states might soon drive a successful closed-loop system.

The various biosignals available for incorporation within a closed-loop system each have distinct advantages and disadvantages with respect to invasiveness, resolution, signal content, and clinical relevance (**Table 1**). It is unlikely that

Table 1
Available signals for signal-based neurostimulation: the following table summarizes recent studies, experiments, and device development regarding brain signal–based neurostimulation

Feedback Signal	Stimulation Type	Feedback Mechanism	Application	Subject	Reference
Arm and hand EMG and acceleration sensors	DBS (STN, VIM)	Features of EMG and acceleration signals are used to predict tremor onset, regulating DBS not implemented	ET, PD	Human	48
EMG	DBS (VIM)	Features of EMG signals measure tremor and regulate DBS system via remote programmer	Intention tremor	Human	49
Cortical ECoG/LFP	Cortical stimulation via cortical depth electrodes or ECoG	Abnormal phase synchrony of cortical signals triggers stimulation	Epilepsy, seizure detection	Animal model (online) and human (offline)	50
Skull-mounted EEG	Cortical stimulation via skull-mounted EEG (F3)	Stimulation triggered by reduced EEG phase synchronization across multiple electrodes	Epilepsy	Rats	51
ECoG	Pharmacologic	Voltage window detectors and frequency analysis parameters matching patient's specific seizures trigger drug delivery system	Epilepsy	Rat model and offline human ECoG	52,53
Single-unit recording of spinal dorsal horn neurons	DBS periaqueductal gray	Stimulation triggered by user-defined clustering of interspike intervals used to classify physical stimuli	Pain	Rats	54
Neuronal firing rate	DBS	Adaptive algorithm adjusts DBS to maintain a stimulus to firing frequency ratio	Epilepsy	Computational model	55
Skull-mounted EEG over frontal barrel cortex	DBS (zona incerta)	Linear least squares was used to classify seizures based on entropy and spectral power	Epilepsy	Rats	56
Single-unit recording of primary motor cortex	DBS (GPi)	DBS pulse train delivered at fixed latency following M1 spike detection	PD	Primate model of PD	57
LFP recording (hippocampus)	DBS (hippocampus)	DBS and LFP recording via distinct contacts on macroelectrode. Seizures detected during stimulation with machine learning. Seizure modeled by afterdischarge potentials induced by hippocampal stimulation	Seizure	Sheep	58

Abbreviations: DBS, deep brain stimulation; ECoG, electrocorticography; EMG, electromyography; ET, essential tremor; GPi, globus pallidus pars internus; LFP, local field potential; PD, Parkinson disease; STN, subthalamic nucleus; VIM, ventral intermedius nucleus of the thalamus.

any single signal source will be appropriate for all closed-loop neuromodulation approaches. The selection of appropriate source will ultimately depend on the design of the entire system and is intimately related to the feature extraction and signal classification, as described in the subsequent sections.

PREDICTION METHODS

Feature Extraction

The purpose of feature extraction is to transform the time series data for successive processing and/or improved computational efficiency. For example, time series data could be transformed from the time domain into the frequency domain, thus changing the meaning of the data stream from when an event occurs to how frequently an event occurs. Neuronal ensembles may use frequency coding to communicate, and therefore transformation of data into the frequency domain can be considered translation of data into the language of neuronal networks.

To improve computational efficiency and increase processing speed, data are compressed, transformed, or otherwise reduced in dimension to remove redundancy and condense overall data size. After signal features are extracted, an additional processing component or feature selection/dimensionality reduction may be required to further reduce the number of features and/or dimensions, or remove noise/outlier features. As a result, the features that are meaningful in the learning and classification stage are identified and chosen, and outliers and artifacts are excluded from the data.

Time Domain

Time domain features of EEG or LFP signals such as event-related potentials may be extracted by splicing long (eg, 10 minutes) time series data recordings into shorter time segments/epochs (eg, 500 milliseconds), before and after an event. By averaging many event-aligned epochs, features of the data related to the event are emphasized and those features unrelated to the event cancel out through averaging. This technique is used to identify visual evoked potentials, somatosensory evoked potentials, and the cognitive oddball response, the P300.

Quantified temporal information derived from action potentials includes neuronal firing rates, peristimulus time histograms, and interspike time intervals. These measures are useful for interpreting neural information from cerebral neurons that are responding to external influences such as visuospatial memory,[59] visual presentation of faces,[60] or passive joint movements.[61] Firing rates are modulated by neurons responding to these external influences and encode motor plans. An example of this is seen in the motor cortex by the cosine tuning of neuronal firing rates in a manner corresponding to the direction of arm reach.[62] The timing of an electrophysiologic spike relative to the previous spike provides other specific information useful for decoding neural information.[63] The timing of the neuronal spikes is further influenced by the phase of low-frequency LFPs, as demonstrated by spike clustering at the trough of beta frequency LFP oscillations in the subthalamic nucleus.[64]

Time-Frequency Domain

Several power spectral estimation methods are used to transform recorded time domain data into time-frequency domain data and allow quantification of neuronal electrical oscillations. Common techniques to estimate spectral power include variations of short-time Fourier transform, wavelet transformation, and autoregressive models.[65–67] Frequency bands of interest within neuronal signals have historically been defined by their visual appearance and spatial distribution on EEG tracings. These include delta (<4 Hz), theta (4–8 Hz), alpha (8–13 Hz), mu (7–11 Hz), beta (13–30 Hz), and gamma rhythms (>30 Hz).[68] These definition terms are also applied to equivalent frequency signal ranges recorded invasively by ECoG and LFP. Unlike synchronous processes, which are band frequency limited, asynchronous processes have been shown to produce broad band spectral power, whereby power exponentially decreases at increasing frequencies.[69] Such changes in relative power within frequency bands have been correlated to movement and speech in both cortical and subcortical recordings,[13,27] and thus show promise for use in neural decoding within closed-loop neurostimulation paradigms.

Phase Domain

Features of amplitude, frequency, and phase can describe a sinusoidal function infinite in time. Phase can be interpreted as a shift or offset in time of that wave from some arbitrary reference time point. Valid phase values vary from $-\pi$ to $+\pi$, or $-\lambda/2$ to $\lambda/2$, where λ is the wavelength ($\lambda = 1/\text{frequency}$). Simple signal processing techniques such as filtering can change the phase of a signal in a frequency-dependent fashion. Phase analysis is inherently more difficult than simple signal processing because of the absence of a clear zero-phase reference point and the presence of artifacts resulting from signal processing techniques. Neural oscillations are finite in time and statistically nonstationary signals. For these reasons, no definitive method has been demonstrated to measure the phase of neural oscillations.[70–72] Furthermore, there is no clear interpretation for the instantaneous phase of a neural signal.[72] Despite these limitations, phases of neural oscillations have been shown to influence spike timing,[64] and are particularly relevant to mechanisms of cognitive processes like memory.[18]

Oscillations in the motor network are related to each other through nonlinear interactions. In particular, the phase of slower oscillations in the theta, alpha, and beta bands modulates the amplitude of faster rhythms in the beta, gamma, and very high gamma ranges,[38,73,74] a phenomenon referred to as phase-to-amplitude cross-frequency coupling (PA-CFC). PA-CFC indicates the extent to which the phase of 1 oscillation extracted from an LFP determines the amplitude of another oscillation. Hierarchical relationships between oscillations might play a significant role in a variety of cognitive and motor tasks[73,74] and could be applied as parameters in the design of a closed-loop DBS system. Despite accumulating evidence for PA-CFC's ubiquity and functional importance in the nervous system, PA-CFC has not received much attention as a potential closed-loop system parameter for indicating motor task selection and planning.

Studies have shown that PA-CFC is correlated with the pathologic state of the basal ganglia in movement disorders. For example, PA-CFC in the motor cortex (beta-gamma) is exaggerated in patients with Parkinson disease compared with patients with epilepsy who do not have a movement disorder.[35] Therapeutic stimulation of the subthalamic nucleus and dopaminergic therapy reduce the magnitude of coupling between beta phase and gamma amplitude,[35,38] highlighting the potential of PA-CFC as a biomarker of disease.

A current goal in the development of closed-loop DBS systems is to discover reference points to which a controlled variable converges and thereby leads to enhancement of motor capacity. Feature extraction is truly limitless in its potential for abstract manipulation of raw data. **Table 2** highlights the techniques and approaches for a subset of major approaches.

Pattern Classification

The objective of pattern classification is to learn a mathematical model (a classifier) that can recognize and segregate novel patterns. Pattern classification algorithms are powerful in that they can be applied naively to data. These machine-learning algorithms may be applied to recordings of the human voice for speech recognition,[116] images of handwriting for association with personality,[117] fMRI to decode emotion evoked by facial expressions,[118] and scalp EEG to allow communication.[119] For instance, in the case of brain-computer interfaces, a classifier given a segment of recorded brain signal is able to associate the neural signal with a given state, such as emotion, thought, behavior, or intention (a class label). During the training phase, subjects perform activities for which the corresponding class label is known (eg, motor activities class label) and the algorithm learns the corresponding pattern. **Table 3** summarizes several classification methods used for brain signal classification, including support vector machines (SVMs), artificial neural networks (ANNs), K-nearest neighbor (KNN), Bayesian classification, and the hidden Markov model (HMM). Two well-known techniques for pattern classification, KNN (a nonlinear classifier) and SVM (a linear classifier) are described and presented in **Fig. 3**.

KNN[121] is a simple but effective nonlinear classification technique. After a training phase using samples with known corresponding class labels in the feature space, KNN predicts the class label of a novel sample based on the label of its K closest (neighbor) samples. For example, if K is set to 3, KNN first finds the 3 neighbor samples closest to the test sample and then chooses the label of the novel sample based on the majority label of those 3 neighbor samples (**Fig. 3**A). Techniques for finding the nearest neighbors include calculations for Euclidean distance and Manhattan distance. The parameter K is usually selected empirically and can affect the sample recognition rate. In this KNN algorithm, the training data sets do not need to be linearly separable, as illustrated in **Fig. 3**.

SVM is another common method for pattern classification and regression[122] introduced by Cortes and Vapnik.[123] SVMs are used in many applications including isolated handwritten digit recognition,[123,124] brain signal classification,[125,126] face recognition in images,[127] and text categorization.[128] A linear binary SVM classifier technique uses 2 parallel hyperplanes to separate the margin between 2 different classes of data in the feature space (see **Fig. 3**B). The SVM selects directions for the hyperplanes via an optimization problem algorithm where the objective is to maximize the margin between the separating hyperplanes. SVM solves the optimization problem using training samples, called support vectors, that lie on the margin. Two classes of data are often not able to be separated by a plane in the original

Table 2
Feature extraction: this table summarizes the signal processing techniques for feature extraction that appear in several recent publications

Domain	Method	Reference
Time domain	Linear filtering	75–78
	Linear combination and regression	76,77
	Blind source separation (BSS)	76,77
	Matched filter	76,79,80
	Autoregressive model parameters	76,80–84
	Independent component analysis (ICA)	76,80,83,85,86
	Karhunen-Loeve transform (KLT)	87,88
	Kalman filtering, unscented Kalman filter	76,80,89
	Correlation of temporal average of stimulus locked response with template	76,79,80,90
	Size of temporal average of stimulus locked response	76,80
	Covariate shift adaptation	91
	Neural time series prediction preprocessing	92
	Barlow-based and Hjorth-based feature	76,92
	Neural firing rate	62,76,80,93,94
	Signal amplitude differences	76,80
	Event-related potential	80,93–105
	P300, steady-state visual evoked potential (SSVEP)	
	Lateralized readiness potential (LRP)	99
	Slow cortical potentials (SCP)	94,96,99,100
	Cross-correlation	90
Frequency domain	Spectral parameters, frequency band power	27,75,76,80,83,87,88,93,96,97,106–110
	Event-related (de)synchronization (ERD, ERS)	27,75–77,80,81,95,98,99,102
	Sensorimotor activity power spectral density (PSD)	94
	Motor imagery	84,93
	Neural time series prediction preprocessing	92
Time-frequency domain	Wavelet transform	76,80,83,111
	Short-time Fourier transform (STFT)	27,107
	Matching pursuit decomposition	112
Spatial Domain	Common spatial patterns (CSP)	76,83,106,113
	Beamforming	114
	Surface Laplacian derivation	75,81
	Linear minimum mean squared error (LMMSE) spatial filter	115
	Spatial filtering	75
Subspace domain	Principle component analysis (PCA)	76,77
Phase domain	Coherence or phase calculation	76,80

space (see **Fig. 3**C) and require mapping into a higher dimensional space to become linearly separable (see **Fig. 3**D). SVM uses kernel functions to project feature vectors onto a more discriminative space by representing data with a higher dimensionality, allowing the separation of data groups using nonlinear functions (eg, separating curves). The use of several different types of kernel mappings, such as radial basis function[129] and the polynomial function,[130] is reported in the literature.

Classification techniques such as KNN and SVM are directly applicable to closed-loop neurostimulation, and DBS devices with these algorithms embedded within the system hardware is in the near future.[131] With the appropriate choice of neural signals and feature extraction techniques, machine-learning algorithms have the potential to classify behavior and would allow the DBS system to adapt to dynamic patient requirements.

CLOSING THE LOOP: DBS PARAMETER INTERVENTIONS

Current DBS system neurostimulation consists of delivering a train of biphasic pulses with adjustable

Table 3
Prediction methods: this table summarizes several feature processing techniques, including feature modeling, detection, and classification reported in several recent publications

Method	Reference
Support vector machines (SVM)	76,80,82,86,95, 102,105,111
K-nearest neighbors (KNN)	76,80,87,95
Thresholding	75,76,79,80,90
Bayesian classification	76,80,104,106
Linear discriminant analysis (LDA), Fisher linear discriminant (FLD), Mahalanobis linear distance (MLD)	76,80,82,84,87,92,95, 102–105,109,115
Quadratic discriminant analysis (QDA)	82,84
Hidden Markov model (HMM)	76,80
Linear/nonlinear continuous transformation	76,80
Classifier adaptation	91
Gaussian process	110
Decision tree	81,97
Gaussian mixture model	78,84
Genetic algorithm	88,102
Logistic regression linear classifier	114
Neural network	82,92
Common spatial patterns (CSP), multiple-class CSP	84,106,113
Filter bank common spatial patterns (FBCSP)	84
Iterative spatiospectral patterns learning (ISSPL)	108
Fuzzy inference	120

parameters (amplitude, pulse width, and frequency). This train is spatially applied across a cathode and an anode that are adjusted according to the size of the stimulation electrode array. The charge is deposited at the cathode, the negative pole, and the current flows from the cathode to the anode.[132] Safety of the DBS is ensured because of a net zero current application across the biphasic waveform of each pulse of the train of stimulation,[133–135] use of platinum-iridium electrode material,[136] and limiting the charge density and charge per phase to 26 $\mu C/cm^2$/phase and 0.018 μC/phase, respectively.[136] The exact threshold for neural injury is unknown, however, neural injury has been noted at charge density of 50 $\mu C/cm^2$/phase and charge per phase of 1.0 μC/phase with platinum electrodes,[137] and at considerably lower values for stainless steel electrodes.[136] Although the spatial and pulse parameters of stimulation may be variably controlled in a closed-loop system, early closed-loop systems have used only an on/off control[49] for these parameters, or have used variable control of amplitude only.[138]

There are a limited number of published studies demonstrating mature closed-loop stimulation systems for essential tremor, Parkinson disease, and epilepsy. Therefore, individual reports of human and animal closed-loop neurostimulation systems are reviewed here.

Case Study 1: Pathologic Tremor Prediction Using Surface Electromyogram and Acceleration

Population

Humans with Parkinson disease and essential tremor, open-label feasibility trial.[48]

Objective

To develop a closed-loop neurostimulation system to switch DBS on/off using a tremor prediction algorithm. Tremor was predicted using a surface electromyogram (sEMG) and acceleration from tremor-affected extremities.

Approach

Signal features were extracted from recorded EMG and acceleration signals. These features included spectral parameters from Fourier and wavelet transforms, and nonlinear time series, such as sample entropy and recurrence quantification analysis. Features are used to classify and predict Parkinson disease and essential tremor states using a simple thresholding classifier, to turn the DBS on and off.

Main results

The resulting algorithm predicted tremor onset for all 91 trials recorded in 4 patients with Parkinson disease and for all 91 trials recorded in 4 patients with essential tremor. The predictor achieved 100% sensitivity for all trials considered, with an overall accuracy of 80.2% for Parkinson disease and 85.7% for essential tremor.

Case Study 2: Validation of a Bidirectional Pulse Generator for Neural State Classification

Study design

Ovine model of acute epilepsy, feasibility trial.[131]

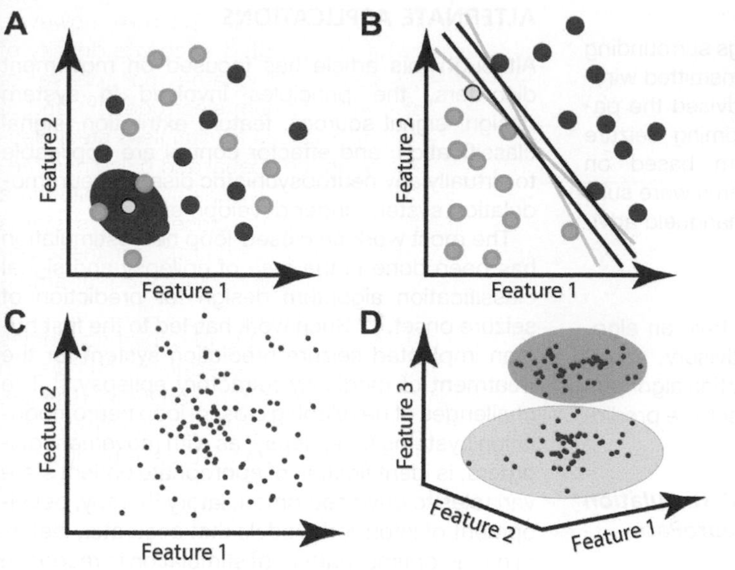

Fig. 3. Graphical representations of pattern classification algorithms. (*A*) KNN. In this case, the yellow (unknown) sample will be classified by polling its 3 nearest neighbors, and will be classified as a member of the green group. (*B*) SVM. If 2 groups of data can be separated by a line or plane in feature space, SVM will provide the plane that defines the widest gap between the 2 data sets. The group members that lie on (support) the parallel planes are called support vectors. (*C*) In this example, the 2 classes of data are not linearly separable in the depicted feature space. (*D*) Here, kernel functions add additional dimensions, or features to data sets. By adding a third feature to the data set in (*C*), the 2 groups are now separable and an SVM algorithm can classify new data.

Objective
To determine the feasibility of the use of an implantable bidirectional sensing and recording pulse generator to create a closed-loop neurostimulation system. Specific objectives were to measure disease-related neural data to detect a desired neural state and to update neurostimulation parameters in real time based on the detection state of the embedded algorithm.

Approach
Hippocampal stimulation-induced seizures were induced with concurrent sensing and recording. SVM pattern classification was used to categorize the 30-s stimulation train induced as a seizure, visible as after discharges on raw LFP tracing and visible in the frequency domain as increased low-frequency power in the 5 to 20 Hz band.

Main results
It is feasible to use LFPs recorded during ongoing stimulation to classify neural states such as an acute seizure. Attention must be given to the stimulation and recording electrode selection, as well as the stimulation frequency to minimize contamination of LFP with stimulation artifact.

Case Study 3: Spike Triggered Closed-Loop DBS for Parkinson Disease

Study design
Nonhuman primate 1-methyl-4-phenyl-1,2,3,6-tetrahydropyridine Parkinsonian model, feasibility trial.[57]

Objective
To compare the effectiveness of open-loop and closed-loop neurostimulation paradigms for globus pallidus pars internus (GPi) DBS.

Approach
A single-pulse or a short-pulse train (7 pulses at 130 Hz, biphasic, 80 μA, 200 microseconds) was delivered through a pair of GPi electrodes at a predetermined and fixed latency after action potential detection in either primary motor cortex or GPi. The open-loop paradigm consisted of 130 Hz continuous stimulation.

Main results
A 7-pulse train after an M1 spike significantly reduced the GPi firing rate and eliminated oscillatory firing patterns characteristic of Parkinson disease and improved limb akinesia. Standard DBS had a lesser effect on GPi neuronal firing, with greater maintenance of oscillatory properties and less improvement in limb akinesia.

Case Study 4: Prediction of Seizure Likelihood with an Implanted Seizure Advisory System

Study design
Humans with medically refractory epilepsy, open-label feasibility trial.[41]

Objective
To demonstrate the feasibility of implanting devices to predict an oncoming seizure, and advise the patient using a handheld device.

Approach

Sixteen channels of ECoG recordings surrounding known seizure onset zones were transmitted wirelessly to a handheld device that advised the patient of the likelihood of an upcoming seizure based on a proprietary algorithm based on patient-specific data. These algorithms were subsequently installed in the patient's handheld advisory device.

Main results

Eleven of 15 patients were able to train an algorithm for seizure prediction and advisory, and 8 of the 11 patients had a stable prediction algorithm over time. Five patients achieved a seizure prediction sensitivity greater than 60%.

Case Study 5: Responsive Cortical Stimulation for the Treatment of Epilepsy (NeuroPace Trial)

Study design

Humans with medically refractory epilepsy, a randomized pivotal clinical trial with a 12 week blinded, randomized on/off stimulation period.[139–141]

Objective

To demonstrate the effectiveness of a closed-loop neurostimulation system to detect and react to seizures. The trial included 191 patients; 50% had mesial temporal lobe onset, and 73% had bilateral temporal lobe epilepsy.

Approach

The research group implanted a responsive neurostimulator with intracranial depth and surface electrodes at known seizure onset zones. The device was capable of 3 seizure detection algorithms: line length,[142] half wave decomposition,[143] and integrated area under the ECoG signal in a sliding time window. Responsive stimulation parameters included frequency (1–333 Hz), current amplitude (0.5–12 mA), pulse width per phase (40–1000 microseconds), and burst duration (10–5000 milliseconds). Initial programing recommendations were provided. Maximum charge density was hardware limited at 25 $\mu C/cm^2$/phase.[141] Responders were defined as patients with 50% or greater reduction in seizure frequency.

Main results

In the randomized pivotal study, there was a statistically significant difference in mean seizure count per month between sham and stimulation groups. During the blinded period, the reduction in seizures in the stimulation arm was 38%, compared with a 17% reduction in the sham group ($P = .012$). The responder rate was 43% at 1 year.

ALTERNATE APPLICATIONS

Although this article has focused on movement disorders, the principles involved in system design, signal sources, feature extraction, signal classification, and effector control are applicable to virtually any neuropsychiatric disease neuromodulation system under development.

The most work on closed-loop neurostimulation has been done in the area of epilepsy and signal classification algorithm design for prediction of seizure onset.[144] Such work has led to the first human implanted seizure prediction system for the treatment of medically refractory epilepsy.[41] The challenges of developing closed-loop neuromodulation systems for epilepsy, as with movement disorders, is identification of appropriate patient state variables to drive neuromodulatory therapy; development of informed models that accurately determine the optimal pattern of stimulation in response to patient states; and detection of reliable biomarkers indicating response to therapy. Although the NeuroPace trial is seen as a success by some, the inability to precisely address all of these challenges of closed-loop systems may have, in part, contributed to suboptimal results.[140]

One can foresee the application of closed-loop systems to other neuropsychiatric diseases, particularly to diseases with cyclical symptom patterns, such as depression. Identification of neurophysiologic biomarkers that indicate a diseased or pathologic state could theoretically drive therapy parameters on demand. Similarly, a system for closed-loop neuromodulation can be envisaged that delivers therapies coincident with memory acquisition states to reinforce learning.

CLOSING REMARKS

Closed-loop neurostimulation is an interdisciplinary science incorporating disciplines of clinical neurosciences and electrical engineering. Given the importance of neuronal oscillations in the cooperative functioning of brain ensembles, the appeal for a neurostimulation system with a small electrical footprint is evident. Thus, closed-loop stimulation is preferable to open-loop stimulation for its less disruptive impact on cognitive processes that depend on coordinated neuronal oscillations.

Fundamentally, closed-loop stimulation strategies must target certain desirable neural states that can be restored, such as an optimal state for walking, talking, or writing. Closed-loop neurostimulation systems may use physiologic signals available at the site of the stimulation (eg, LFP data), or signals that are geographically removed from the site of stimulation (eg, ECoG or EEG data). Non–central nervous system signals are also available for use in closed-loop systems, such as EMG signals, or signals from internal and external sensors (eg, accelerometers, timing devices, or audio devices). Once these signals are measured and digitized, they must be compressed or transformed into features suitably efficient for processing by pattern classification algorithms for accurate prediction of neural patient states. These algorithms may be preembedded in the device,[131] or first explored within a high-power computer cluster before downloading a lightweight patient-customized version into the device's memory.[41] The algorithm must intelligently manipulate stimulation parameters in the domains of time, frequency, or space to optimize the patient's neurologic condition.

REFERENCES

1. FDA. Medtronic activa tremor control system P960009. 1997. Available at: http://www.accessdata.fda.gov/cdrh_docs/pdf/p960009.pdf. Accessed November 21, 2003.
2. Pahwa R, Lyons KE, Wilkinson SB, et al. Long-term evaluation of deep brain stimulation of the thalamus. J Neurosurg 2006;104:506–12.
3. Deuschl G, Schade-Brittinger C, Krack P, et al. A randomized trial of deep-brain stimulation for Parkinson's disease. N Engl J Med 2006;355:896–908.
4. Weaver FM, Follett K, Stern M, et al. Bilateral deep brain stimulation vs best medical therapy for patients with advanced Parkinson disease. JAMA 2009;301:63–73.
5. Kiss ZH, Doig-Beyaert K, Eliasziw M, et al. The Canadian multicentre study of deep brain stimulation for cervical dystonia. Brain 2007;130:2879–86.
6. Vidailhet M, Vercueil L, Houeto JL, et al. Bilateral, pallidal, deep-brain stimulation in primary generalised dystonia: a prospective 3 year follow-up study. Lancet Neurol 2007;6:223–9.
7. Nathan DA, Center S, Wu C, et al. An implantable synchronous pacemaker for the long term correction of complete heart block. Am J Cardiol 1963;11:362–7.
8. Rouse AG, Stanslaski SR, Cong P, et al. A chronic generalized bi-directional brain–machine interface. J Neural Eng 2011;8:036018.
9. Priori A, Foffani G, Rossi L, et al. Adaptive deep brain stimulation (aDBS) controlled by local field potential oscillations. Exp Neurol 2013;245:77–86.
10. Shanechi MM, Hu RC, Powers M, et al. Neural population partitioning and a concurrent brain-machine interface for sequential motor function. Nat Neurosci 2012;15:1715–22.
11. Ojemann GA, Schoenfield-McNeill J, Corina D. Different neurons in different regions of human temporal lobe distinguish correct from incorrect identification or memory. Neuropsychologia 2004;42:1383–93.
12. Flint RD, Lindberg EW, Jordan LR, et al. Accurate decoding of reaching movements from field potentials in the absence of spikes. J Neural Eng 2012;9:046006.
13. Miller KJ, Zanos S, Fetz EE, et al. Decoupling the cortical power spectrum reveals real-time representation of individual finger movements in humans. J Neurosci 2009;29:3132–7.
14. Wang Z, Logothetis NK, Liang H. Decoding a bistable percept with integrated time–frequency representation of single-trial local field potential. J Neural Eng 2008;5:433–42.
15. Hariz MI, Rehncrona S, Quinn NP, et al, Multicentre Advanced Parkinson's Disease Deep Brain Stimulation Group. Multicenter study on deep brain stimulation in Parkinson's disease: an independent assessment of reported adverse events at 4 years. Mov Disord 2008;23:416–21.
16. Johnson LA, Blakely T, Hermes D, et al. Sleep spindles are locally modulated by training on a brain-computer interface. Proc Natl Acad Sci U S A 2012;109:18583–8.
17. Masquelier T, Hugues E, Deco G, et al. Oscillations, phase-of-firing coding, and spike timing-dependent plasticity: an efficient learning scheme. J Neurosci 2009;29:13484–93.
18. Fell J, Axmacher N. The role of phase synchronization in memory processes. Nat Rev Neurosci 2011;12:105–18.
19. Fries P. A mechanism for cognitive dynamics: neuronal communication through neuronal coherence. Trends Cogn Sci 2005;9:474–80.
20. Hebb AO, Ojemann GA. The thalamus and language revisited. Brain Lang 2013;126:99–108.
21. Quiroga-Varela A, Walters JR, Brazhnik E, et al. What basal ganglia changes underlie the parkinsonian state? The significance of neuronal oscillatory activity. Neurobiol Dis 2013;58:242–8.
22. Miocinovic S, McIntyre CC, Savasta M, et al. Mechanisms of deep brain stimulation. In: Tarsy D, editor. Deep brain stimulation in neurological and psychiatric disorders. Totowa (NJ): Humana Press; 2008. p. 151–77.
23. Montgomery EB, Gale JT. Mechanisms of action of deep brain stimulation (DBS). Neurosci Biobehav Rev 2008;32:388–407.
24. Hashimoto T, Elder CM, Okun MS, et al. Stimulation of the subthalamic nucleus changes the firing pattern of pallidal neurons. J Neurosci 2003;23:1916–23.
25. Surmeier DJ, Ding J, Day M, et al. D1 and D2 dopamine-receptor modulation of striatal

glutamatergic signaling in striatal medium spiny neurons. Trends Neurosci 2007;30:228–35.
26. Temel Y, Blokland A, Steinbusch HW, et al. The functional role of the subthalamic nucleus in cognitive and limbic circuits. Prog Neurobiol 2005;76: 393–413.
27. Hebb AO, Darvas F, Miller KJ. Transient and state modulation of beta power in human subthalamic nucleus during speech production and finger movement. Neuroscience 2012;202:218–33.
28. Makeig S, Kothe C, Mullen T, et al. Evolving signal processing for brain computer interfaces. Proc IEEE 2012;100:1567–84.
29. Lettieri C, Rinaldo S, Devigili G, et al. Deep brain stimulation: subthalamic nucleus electrophysiological activity in awake and anesthetized patients. Clin Neurophysiol 2012;123:2406–13.
30. Suthana N, Fried I. Percepts to recollections: insights from single neuron recordings in the human brain. Trends Cogn Sci 2012;16:427–36.
31. Perge JA, Homer ML, Malik WQ, et al. Intra-day signal instabilities affect decoding performance in an intracortical neural interface system. J Neural Eng 2013;10:036004.
32. Simeral JD, Kim SP, Black MJ, et al. Neural control of cursor trajectory and click by a human with tetraplegia 1000 days after implant of an intracortical microelectrode array. J Neural Eng 2011;8:025027.
33. BrainGate2: feasibility study of an intracortical neural interface system for persons with tetraplegia. Available at: http://clinicaltrials.gov/ct2/show/NCT00912041. Accessed July 13, 2013.
34. Hochberg LR, Bacher D, Jarosiewicz B, et al. Reach and grasp by people with tetraplegia using a neurally controlled robotic arm. Nature 2012;485: 372–5.
35. De Hemptinne C, Ryapolova-Webb ES, Air EL, et al. Exaggerated phase-amplitude coupling in the primary motor cortex in Parkinson disease. Proc Natl Acad Sci U S A 2013;110:4780–5.
36. Ince NF, Gupta R, Arica S, et al. High accuracy decoding of movement target direction in non-human primates based on common spatial patterns of local field potentials. PLoS One 2010;5:e14384.
37. Wander JD, Blakely T, Miller KJ, et al. Distributed cortical adaptation during learning of a brain-computer interface task. Proc Natl Acad Sci U S A 2013;110(26):10818–23. Available at: http://www.pnas.org/cgi/doi/10.1073/pnas.1221127110. Accessed June 25, 2013.
38. Lopez-Azcarate J, Tainta M, Rodriguez-Oroz MC, et al. Coupling between beta and high-frequency activity in the human subthalamic nucleus may be a pathophysiological mechanism in Parkinson's disease. J Neurosci 2010;30:6667–77.
39. Tsiokos C, Hu X, Pouratian N. 200–300Hz movement modulated oscillations in the internal globus pallidus of patients with Parkinson's Disease. Neurobiol Dis 2013;54:464–74.
40. Whitmer D, de Solages C, Hill B, et al. High frequency deep brain stimulation attenuates subthalamic and cortical rhythms in Parkinson's disease. Front Hum Neurosci 2012;6:155. Available at: http://www.frontiersin.org/Human_Neuroscience/10.3389/fnhum.2012.00155/abstract. Accessed June 25, 2013.
41. Cook MJ, O'Brien TJ, Berkovic SF, et al. Prediction of seizure likelihood with a long-term, implanted seizure advisory system in patients with drug-resistant epilepsy: a first-in-man study. Lancet Neurol 2013; 12(6):563–71. Available at: http://www.sciencedirect.com/science/article/pii/S1474442213700759. Accessed June 25, 2013.
42. Mak JN, McFarland DJ, Vaughan TM, et al. EEG correlates of P300-based brain–computer interface (BCI) performance in people with amyotrophic lateral sclerosis. J Neural Eng 2012;9:026014.
43. Sarnthein J, Jeanmonod D. High thalamocortical theta coherence in patients with Parkinson's disease. J Neurosci 2007;27:124–31.
44. Matlack C, Moritz C, Chizeck HJ. Applying best practices from digital control systems to BMI implementation. Conf Proc IEEE Eng Med Biol Soc 2012; 2012:1699–702.
45. Lee KH, Chang SY, Jang DP, et al. Emerging techniques for elucidating mechanism of action of deep brain stimulation. Conf Proc IEEE Eng Med Biol Soc 2011;2011:677–80. Available at: http://ieeexplore.ieee.org/xpls/abs_all.jsp?arnumber=6090152. Accessed June 25, 2013.
46. Griessenauer CJ, Chang SY, Tye SJ, et al. Wireless instantaneous neurotransmitter concentration system: electrochemical monitoring of serotonin using fast-scan cyclic voltammetry-a proof-of-principle study: laboratory investigation. J Neurosurg 2010; 113:656–65.
47. Hilliard JD, Frysinger RC, Elias WJ. Effective subthalamic nucleus deep brain stimulation sites may differ for tremor, bradykinesia and gait disturbances in Parkinson's disease. Stereotact Funct Neurosurg 2011;89:357–64.
48. Basu I, Graupe D, Tuninetti D, et al. Pathological tremor prediction using surface electromyogram and acceleration: potential use in "ON–OFF" demand driven deep brain stimulator design. J Neural Eng 2013;10:036019.
49. Yamamoto T, Katayama Y, Ushiba J, et al. On-demand control system for deep brain stimulation for treatment of intention tremor. Neuromodulation 2013;16:230–5.
50. Abdelhalim K, Jafari HM, Kokarovtseva L, et al. 64-Channel UWB wireless neural vector analyzer and phase synchrony-triggered stimulator SoC. In: ESSCIRC (ESSCIRC), 2012 Proceedings of

the. 2012. Bordeaux, September 17–21, 2012. p. 281–4. Available at: http://ieeexplore.ieee.org/xpls/abs_all.jsp?arnumber=6341340. Accessed June 22, 2013.

51. Wang L, Guo H, Yu X, et al. Responsive electrical stimulation suppresses epileptic seizures in rats. PLoS One 2012;7:e38141.
52. Salam MT, Mirzaei M, Ly MS, et al. An implantable closedloop asynchronous drug delivery system for the treatment of refractory epilepsy. IEEE Trans Neural Syst Rehabil Eng 2012;20:432–42.
53. Salam MT, Mounaïm F, Nguyen DK, et al. Low-power circuit techniques for epileptic seizures detection and subsequent neurostimulation. J Low Power Electron 2012;8:133–45.
54. Farajidavar A, Hagains CE, Peng YB, et al. A closed loop feedback system for automatic detection and inhibition of mechano-nociceptive neural activity. IEEE Trans Neural Syst Rehabil Eng 2012;20:478–87.
55. Beverlin B II, Netoff TI. Dynamic control of modeled tonic-clonic seizure states with closed-loop stimulation. Front Neural Circ 2013;6:126. Available at: http://www.frontiersin.org/Neural_Circuits/10.3389/fncir.2012.00126/abstract. Accessed June 22, 2013.
56. Liang SF, Liao YC, Shaw FZ, et al. Closed-loop seizure control on epileptic rat models. J Neural Eng 2011;8:045001.
57. Rosin B, Slovik M, Mitelman R, et al. Closed-loop deep brain stimulation is superior in ameliorating parkinsonism. Neuron 2011;72:370–84.
58. Stanslaski S, Cong P, Carlson D, et al. An implantable bi-directional brain-machine interface system for chronic neuroprosthesis research. Conf Proc IEEE Eng Med Biol Soc 2009;2009:5494–7. Available at: http://ieeexplore.ieee.org/xpls/abs_all.jsp?arnumber=5334562. Accessed June 22, 2013.
59. Holmes MD, Ojemann GA, Lettich E. Neuronal activity in human right lateral temporal cortex related to visuospatial memory and perception. Brain Res 1996;711:44–9.
60. Fried I, Cameron KA, Yashar S, et al. Inhibitory and excitatory responses of single neurons in the human medial temporal lobe during recognition of faces and objects. Cereb Cortex 2002;12:575–84.
61. Sierens D, Kutz S, Pilitsis J, et al. Stereotactic surgery with microelectrode recordings. In: Bakay RA, editor. Movement disorder surgery: the essentials. New York: Thieme; 2008. p. 83–114.
62. Georgopoulos AP, Kalaska JF, Caminiti R, et al. On the relations between the direction of two-dimensional arm movements and cell discharge in primate motor cortex. J Neurosci 1982;2:1527–37.
63. Reich DS, Mechler F, Purpura KP, et al. Interspike intervals, receptive fields, and information encoding in primary visual cortex. J Neurosci 2000;20:1964–74.
64. Kühn AA, Trottenberg T, Kivi A, et al. The relationship between local field potential and neuronal discharge in the subthalamic nucleus of patients with Parkinson's disease. Exp Neurol 2005;194:212–20.
65. Avestruz AT, Santa W, Carlson D, et al. A 5 uW/channel spectral analysis IC for chronic bidirectional brain machine interfaces. IEEE J Solid State Circ 2008;43:3006–24.
66. Costa AH, Hengstler S. Adaptive time–frequency analysis based on autoregressive modeling. Signal Process 2011;91:740–9.
67. Semmlow JL. Biosignal and biomedical image processing: MATLAB-based applications. New York, London: Marcel Dekker, Taylor & Francis; 2004.
68. Chatrian G, Bergamini L, Dondey M, et al. A glossary of terms most commonly used by clinical electroencephalographers. Electroencephalogr Clin Neurophysiol 1974;37:538–48.
69. Miller KJ, Sorensen LB, Ojemann JG, et al. Power-law scaling in the brain surface electric potential. PLoS Comput Biol 2009;5:e1000609.
70. Le Van Quyen M, Foucher J, Lachaux JP, et al. Comparison of Hilbert transform and wavelet methods for the analysis of neuronal synchrony. J Neurosci Methods 2001;111:83–98.
71. Le Van Quyen M, Bragin A. Analysis of dynamic brain oscillations: methodological advances. Trends Neurosci 2007;30:365–73.
72. Denker M, Roux S, Linden H, et al. The local field potential reflects surplus spike synchrony. Cereb Cortex 2011;21:2681–95.
73. Canolty RT, Edwards E, Dalal SS, et al. High gamma power is phase-locked to theta oscillations in human neocortex. Science 2006;313:1626–8.
74. Tort AB, Kramer MA, Thorn C, et al. Dynamic cross-frequency couplings of local field potential oscillations in rat striatum and hippocampus during performance of a T-maze task. Proc Natl Acad Sci U S A 2008;105:20517–22.
75. Bai O, Lin P, Vorbach S, et al. A high performance sensorimotor beta rhythm-based brain–computer interface associated with human natural motor behavior. J Neural Eng 2008;5:24–35.
76. Bashashati A, Fatourechi M, Ward RK, et al. A survey of signal processing algorithms in brain–computer interfaces based on electrical brain signals. J Neural Eng 2007;4:R32–57.
77. Fatourechi M, Bashashati A, Ward RK, et al. EMG and EOG artifacts in brain computer interface systems: a survey. Clin Neurophysiol 2007;118:480–94.
78. Schalk G, Brunner P, Gerhardt LA, et al. Brain–computer interfaces (BCIs): detection instead of classification. J Neurosci Methods 2008;167:51–62.
79. Levine SP, Huggins JE, BeMent SL, et al. Identification of electrocorticogram patterns as the basis for

a direct brain interface. J Clin Neurophysiol 1999; 16:439–47.

80. Mason SG, Bashashati A, Fatourechi M, et al. A comprehensive survey of brain interface technology designs. Ann Biomed Eng 2006;35:137–69.
81. Bento VA, Cunha JP, Silva FM. Towards a human-robot interface based on the electrical activity of the brain. In: Humanoid robots, 2008. Humanoids 2008. 8th IEEE-RAS International Conference on. 2008. Daejeon (South Korea), December 1–3, 2008. p. 85–90. Available at: http://ieeexplore.ieee.org/xpls/abs_all.jsp?arnumber=4755936. Accessed June 22, 2013.
82. Faradji F, Ward RK, Birch GE. Plausibility assessment of a 2-state self-paced mental task-based BCI using the no-control performance analysis. J Neurosci Methods 2009;180:330–9.
83. Hoffmann U, Vesin JM, Ebrahimi T. Recent advances in brain-computer interfaces. In: IEEE 9th Workshop on Multimedia Signal Processing (MMSP'2007). 2007. p. 17–9. Available at: http://www.researchgate.net/publication/37452383_Recent_Advances_In_Brain-Computer_Interfaces/file/70e1160ed5c483a00e.pdf. Accessed June 22, 2013.
84. Lotte F, Guan C, Ang KK. Comparison of designs towards a subject-independent brain-computer interface based on motor imagery. Conf Proc IEEE Eng Med Biol Soc 2009;2009:4543–6. Available at: http://ieeexplore.ieee.org/xpls/abs_all.jsp?arnumber=5334126. Accessed June 22, 2013.
85. Kachenoura A, Albera L, Senhadji L, et al. ICA: a potential tool for BCI systems. IEEE Signal Process Mag 2008;25:57–68.
86. Ming D, Sun C, Cheng L, et al. ICA-SVM combination algorithm for identification of motor imagery potentials. In: Computational Intelligence for Measurement Systems and Applications (CIMSA), 2010 IEEE International Conference on. 2010. Taranto, Italy. September 6–8, 2010. p. 92–6. Available at: http://ieeexplore.ieee.org/xpls/abs_all.jsp?arnumber=5611755. Accessed June 22, 2013.
87. Bashashati A, Ward RK, Birch GE. Towards development of a 3-state self-paced brain-computer interface. Comput Intell Neurosci 2007; 2007:1–8.
88. Fatourechi M, Bashashati A, Ward RK, et al. A hybrid genetic algorithm approach for improving the performance of the LF-ASD brain computer interface. In: Acoustics, Speech, and Signal Processing, 2005. Proceedings (ICASSP'05). IEEE International Conference on. 2005. Philadelphia (PA). March 18–23, 2005. p. v–345. Available at: http://ieeexplore.ieee.org/xpls/abs_all.jsp?arnumber=1416311. Accessed June 22, 2013.
89. Li Z, O'Doherty JE, Hanson TL, et al. Unscented Kalman filter for brain-machine interfaces. PLoS One 2009;4:e6243.
90. Huggins JE, Levine SP, BeMent SL, et al. Detection of event-related potentials for development of a direct brain interface. J Clin Neurophysiol 1999; 16:448–55.
91. Krusienski DJ, Grosse-Wentrup M, Galán F, et al. Critical issues in state-of-the-art brain–computer interface signal processing. J Neural Eng 2011;8: 025002.
92. Coyle D, Prasad G, McGinnity TM. Faster self-organizing fuzzy neural network training and a hyperparameter analysis for a brain–computer interface. IEEE Trans Syst Man Cybern B Cybern 2009;39:1458–71.
93. Graimann B, Allison B, Pfurtscheller G. Brain–computer interfaces: a gentle introduction. In: Graimann B, Pfurtscheller G, Allison B, editors. Brain-computer interfaces. Berlin, Heidelberg (Germany): Springer; 2009. p. 1–27. Available at: http://www.springerlink.com/index/10.1007/978-3-642-02091-9_1; 2009. Accessed June 22, 2013.
94. Molina GG, Tsoneva T, Nijholt A. Emotional brain-computer interfaces. In: Affective Computing and Intelligent Interaction and Workshops, 2009. ACII 2009. 3rd International Conference on. 2009. Amsterdam, September 10–12, 2009. p. 1–9. Available at: http://ieeexplore.ieee.org/xpls/abs_all.jsp?arnumber=5349478. Accessed June 22, 2013.
95. Besserve M, Jerbi K, Laurent F, et al. Classification methods for ongoing EEG and MEG signals. Biol Res 2007;40:415–37.
96. Carabalona R, Castiglioni P, Gramatica F. Brain-computer interfaces and neurorehabilitation. Stud Health Technol Inform 2009;145:160–76.
97. Cecotti H. A self-paced and calibration-less SSVEP-based brain computer interface speller. IEEE Trans Neural Syst Rehabil Eng 2010;18:127–33.
98. Pfurtscheller G, Allison BZ, Brunner C, et al. The hybrid BCI. Front Neurosci 2010;4:30.
99. Plass-Oude Bos D, Reuderink B, Laar B, et al. Brain-computer interfacing and games. In: Tan DS, Nijholt A, editors. Brain-computer interfaces. London: Springer; 2010. p. 149–78. Available at: http://link.springer.com/10.1007/978-1-84996-272-8_10; 2010. Accessed June 22, 2013.
100. Stamps K, Hamam Y. Towards inexpensive BCI control for wheelchair navigation in the enabled environment–a hardware survey. In: Brain informatics. Springer; 2010. p. 336–45. Available at: http://link.springer.com/chapter/10.1007/978-3-642-15314-3_32; 2010. Accessed June 22, 2013.
101. Aloise F, Schettini F, Aricò P, et al. Advanced brain computer interface for communication and control. In: Proceedings of the International Conference on Advanced Visual Interfaces. Rome (Italy), May 25–29, 2010. p. 399–400. Available at: http://dl.acm.org/citation.cfm?id=1843076. Accessed June 22, 2013.

102. Bai O, Lin P, Huang D, et al. Towards a user-friendly brain–computer interface: initial tests in ALS and PLS patients. Clin Neurophysiol 2010;121: 1293–303.
103. Ikegami S, Takano K, Saeki N, et al. Operation of a P300-based brain–computer interface by individuals with cervical spinal cord injury. Clin Neurophysiol 2011;122:991–6.
104. Panicker RC, Puthusserypady S, Sun Y. Adaptation in P300 brain computer interfaces: a two-classifier cotraining approach. IEEE Trans Biomed Eng 2010;57:2927–35.
105. Salvaris M, Sepulveda F. Visual modifications on the P300 speller BCI paradigm. J Neural Eng 2009;6:046011.
106. Bobrov P, Frolov A, Cantor C, et al. Brain-computer interface based on generation of visual images. PLoS One 2011;6:e20674.
107. Kronegg J, Chanel G, Voloshynovskiy S, et al. EEG-based synchronized brain-computer interfaces: a model for optimizing the number of mental tasks. IEEE Trans Neural Syst Rehabil Eng 2007;15:50–8.
108. Wu W, Gao X, Hong B, et al. Classifying single-trial EEG during motor imagery by iterative spatio-spectral patterns learning (ISSPL). IEEE Trans Biomed Eng 2008;55:1733–43.
109. Zhang L, He W, He C, et al. Improving mental task classification by adding high frequency band information. J Med Syst 2008;34:51–60.
110. Zhong M, Lotte F, Girolami M, et al. Classifying EEG for brain computer interfaces using Gaussian processes. Pattern Recogn Lett 2008;29:354–9.
111. Sherwood J, Derakhshani R. On classifiability of wavelet features for EEG-based brain-computer interfaces. In: Neural Networks, 2009. IJCNN 2009. International Joint Conference on. 2009. Atlanta (GA), June 14–19, 2009. p. 2895–902. Available at: http://ieeexplore.ieee.org/xpls/abs_all.jsp?arnumber=5178939. Accessed June 22, 2013.
112. Jiang H, Zhang J, Hebb AO, et al. Time-frequency analysis of brain electrical signals for behaviour recognition in patients with Parkinson's disease. In: 47th Asilomar Conference on Signals, Systems and Computers. Pacific Grove (CA), November 3–6, 2013.
113. Wang H, Zheng W. Local temporal common spatial patterns for robust single-trial EEG classification. IEEE Trans Neural Syst Rehabil Eng 2008; 16:131–9.
114. Grosse-Wentrup M, Liefhold C, Gramann K, et al. Beamforming in noninvasive brain computer interfaces. IEEE Trans Biomed Eng 2009;56: 1209–19.
115. Gutiérrez D, Escalona-Vargas DI. EEG data classification through signal spatial redistribution and optimized linear discriminants. Comput Methods Programs Biomed 2010;97:39–47.
116. Han K, Wang D. A classification based approach to speech segregation. J Acoust Soc Am 2012;132: 3475–83.
117. Górska Z, Janicki A. Recognition of extraversion level based on handwriting and support vector machines. Percept Mot Skills 2012;114:857–69.
118. Mourão-Miranda J, Hardoon DR, Hahn T, et al. Patient classification as an outlier detection problem: an application of the one-class support vector machine. Neuroimage 2011;58:793–804.
119. Furdea A, Ruf CA, Halder S, et al. A new (semantic) reflexive brain-computer interface: in search for a suitable classifier. J Neurosci Methods 2012;203: 233–40.
120. Lotte F. Study of electroencephalographic signal processing and classification techniques towards the use of brain-computer interfaces in virtual reality applications. 2008. Available at: http://hal.archives-ouvertes.fr/tel-00356346/. Accessed July 7, 2013.
121. Duda RO, Hart PE, Stork DG. Pattern classification. 2nd edition. New York: Wiley; 2000.
122. Drucker H, Burges CJ, Kaufman L, et al. Support vector regression machines. In: Mozer MC, Jordan JI, Petsche T, editors. Neural information processing systems 9. Cambridge (MA): MIT Press; 1997. p. 155–61.
123. Cortes C, Vapnik V. Support-vector networks. Mach Learn 1995;20:273–97.
124. Schölkopf B, Burges CJ, Vapnik V. Extracting support data for a given task. In: Proceedings, First International Conference on Knowledge Discovery & Data Mining, Menlo Park. AAAI Press; 1995. p. 252–7.
125. Garrett D, Peterson DA, Anderson CW, et al. Comparison of linear, nonlinear, and feature selection methods for EEG signal classification. IEEE Trans Neural Syst Rehabil Eng 2003;11:141–4.
126. Hill NJ, Lal TN, Schröder M, et al. Classifying event-related desynchronization in EEG, ECoG and MEG signals. DAGM. Berlin, Heidelberg (Germany): Springer-Verlag; 2006.
127. Jennifer H, Volker B, Bernd H. Face recognition using component-based SVM classification and morphable models. Berlin, Heidelberg (Germany): Springer-Verlag; 2002.
128. Joachims T. Text categorization with Support Vector Machines: Learning with many relevant features. In: Nédellec C, Rouveirol C, editors. Machine Learning: ECML-98. Berlin Heidelberg (Germany): Springer-Verlag; 1998. p. 137–42.
129. Chapelle O, Haffner P, Vapnik VN. Support vector machines for histogram-based image classification. IEEE Trans Neural Netw 1999;10:1055–64.
130. Scholkopf B, Smola AJ. Learning with kernels: support vector machines, regularization, optimization, and beyond. Cambridge (MA): MIT Press; 2001.

131. Stanslaski S, Afshar P, Cong P, et al. Design and validation of a fully implantable, chronic, closed-loop neuromodulation device with concurrent sensing and stimulation. IEEE Trans Neural Syst Rehabil Eng 2012;20:410–21.
132. Montgomery EB. Deep brain stimulation programming: principles and practice. Oxford (United Kingdom), New York: Oxford University Press; 2010.
133. Butson CR, McIntyre CC. Differences among implanted pulse generator waveforms cause variations in the neural response to deep brain stimulation. Clin Neurophysiol 2007;118: 1889–94.
134. Lilly JC, Hughes JR, Alvord EC Jr, et al. Brief, noninjurious electric waveform for stimulation of the brain. Science 1955;121:468–9.
135. Pudenz RH, Bullara LA, Dru D, et al. Electrical stimulation of the brain. II. Effects on the blood-brain barrier. Surg Neurol 1975;4:265–70.
136. Harnack D, Winter C, Meissner W, et al. The effects of electrode material, charge density and stimulation duration on the safety of high-frequency stimulation of the subthalamic nucleus in rats. J Neurosci Methods 2004;138:207–16.
137. McCreery DB, Agnew WF, Yuen TG, et al. Charge density and charge per phase as cofactors in neural injury induced by electrical stimulation. IEEE Trans Biomed Eng 1990;37:996–1001.
138. Santaniello S, Fiengo G, Glielmo L, et al. Closed-loop control of deep brain stimulation: a simulation study. IEEE Trans Neural Syst Rehabil Eng 2011; 19:15–24.
139. Neuropace, Inc. RNS system for epilepsy. 2013. Available at: http://www.fda.gov/downloads/AdvisoryCommittees/CommitteesMeetingMaterials/MedicalDevices/MedicalDevicesAdvisoryCommittee/NeurologicalDevicesPanel/UCM340257.pdf. Accessed July 7, 2013.
140. Morrell MJ, On behalf of the RNS System in Epilepsy Study Group. Responsive cortical stimulation for the treatment of medically intractable partial epilepsy. Neurology 2011;77:1295–304.
141. Fountas KN, Smith JR. A novel closed-loop stimulation system in the control of focal, medically refractory epilepsy. In: Sakas DE, Simpson BA, editors. Operative neuromodulation. Vienna (Austria): Springer; p. 357–362. Available at: http://www.springerlink.com/index/10.1007/978-3-211-33081-4_41. Accessed July 13, 2013.
142. Esteller R, Echauz J, Tcheng T, et al. Line length: an efficient feature for seizure onset detection. In: Engineering in Medicine and Biology Society, 2001. Proceedings of the 23rd Annual International Conference of the IEEE. 2001. p. 1707–10. Available at: http://ieeexplore.ieee.org/xpls/abs_all.jsp?arnumber=1020545. Accessed July 13, 2013.
143. Gotman J. Automatic recognition of epileptic seizures in the EEG. Electroencephalogr Clin Neurophysiol 1982;54:530–40.
144. Carney PR, Myers S, Geyer JD. Seizure prediction: methods. Epilepsy Behav 2011;22:S94–101.

Index

Note: Page numbers of article titles are in **boldface** type.

A

Addiction, 137–141
Allodynia, in neuropathic pain, 3
Alzheimer disease, memory deficits in, 141–143
Amygdala, neuromodulation of, for posttraumatic stress disorder, 141
Anchors, for electrodes, 5
Anorexia nervosa, neuromodulation for, 151–153
Anterior cingulate cortex, in obsessive-compulsive disorder, 87–88
Artificial neural networks, in closed-loop neuromodulation, 194, 196
Avoidance learning theory, in obsessive-compulsive disorder, 86
Axial pain syndrome, 4, 6

B

Back pain, 4
Bariatric surgery, 148
Bayesian classification, in closed-loop neuromodulation, 194, 196
Biosignals, for closed-loop neuromodulation, 190–193
Bladder, disorders of, **33–46**
BOLD (blood oxygen level-dependent) MRI, 179–181
Boston Scientific PRISM Trial, 13
Botulinum injections, for overactive bladder, 38–39
Brain mapping, 179–181
Burk-Fahn-Marsden Dystonia Rating Scale Movement Score, 60–68

C

Capsulotomy, for obsessive-compulsive disorder, 90
Central neuromodulation, **77–83, 173–185**
Cephalgias, 4, 6
Cerebellum, in obsessive-compulsive disorder, 89
Cerebral palsy, dystonia in, 64
Ceretom-guided deep brain stimulation, 164
Cervical dystonia, 61
Chemical neuromodulation, for movement disorders, 47–49
Cingulate cortex, stimulation of, for depression, 105–109
Cingulate gyrus, neuromodulation of, for addiction, 139
Cingulotomy, for obsessive-compulsive disorder, 90
ClearPoint software, for imaging, 167
Closed-loop neuromodulation, **187–204**
  alternate applications of, 198
  for restoration of desired state, 189–190
  parameter interventions for, 195–198
  prediction methods for, 193–195
  rationale for, 189
  signals available for, 190–193
Cognitive behavioral therapy, for obsessive-compulsive disorder, 89
Cognitive function
  in dystonia, 68
  in neuromodulation, 70
Complex regional pain syndrome, 4
Computed tomography, for deep brain stimulation, 159–164, 170–171
Connectivity-based thalamic segmentation, 177–178
Cortex, neuromodulation treatment of, for dystonia, 70–71
Corticostriatothalamocortical circuits, in obsessive-compulsive disorder, 86–87
Craniocervical dystonia, 61
Craniofacial neuralgia, 3
Cryogenic neuromodulation, for movement disorders, 50, 54
Cystitis, interstitial, **33–46**

D

Deep brain stimulation, **159–172**
  advanced imaging techniques for, **173–185**
  Ceretom-guided, 164
  closed-loop systems for, **187–204**
  for depression, 105–106
  for dystonia, **59–75**
  for eating disorders, **147–157**
  for movement disorders, 51–55
  for obsessive-compulsive disorder, **85–101**
  for refractory pain, **77–83**
  for Tourette syndrome, **117–135**
  image-guided, **159–172**
  O-arm–guided, 160–163
  open-loop, 189
Depression, 109–111
  deep brain stimulation for, 105–106
  dystonia with, 68
  historical treatments for, 104
  transcranial magnetic stimulation for, 106–109
  trigeminal nerve stimulation for, 109–111
Diffusion imaging, 175–178

Neurosurg Clin N Am 25 (2014) 205–209
http://dx.doi.org/10.1016/S1042-3680(13)00128-9
1042-3680/14/$ – see front matter

Diffusion tractography, 176
Doro Halo Retractor System, 164
Dorsal lateral prefrontal cortex, in obsessive-compulsive disorder, 87–88
Dyskinesia, in neuromodulation, 70
Dystonia, neuromodulation for, **59–75**
age considerations in, 67
classification and, 59–60
cognitive function in, 68
disease duration and, 68
genetic factors in, 60, 65–66
heredodegenerative, 64
onset of, 59–60
patient selection for, 60–68
primary generalized, 60–61
psychiatric disease with, 68
secondary, 61–64
symptoms and, 67
target selection for, 68–71
with other disorders (dystonia-plus syndromes), 60
DYT mutations, in dystonia, 60, 65–66, 68

E

Eating disorders, neuromodulation for, **147–157**
anorexia nervosa, 151–153
obesity, 147–151
Electrical neuromodulation, for movement disorders, 51–55
Electrocorticography, in closed-loop neuromodulation, 192
Electrodes, for neuropathic pain, 4–7
Electroencephalography, in closed-loop neuromodulation, 191–192
Electromyography, in closed-loop neuromodulation, 191, 196
Emotional processing theory, in obsessive-compulsive disorder, 86
Entorhinal cortex, neuromodulation of, for memory deficit, 142
Epidural stimulation, for spinal cord injury, **15–23**
Epilepsy, 196–198
Essential tremor, neuromodulation for. *See* Movement disorders.
ESSIC (European Society for the Study of Bladder Pain Syndrome), 40

F

Facial neuralgia, 3
Fan-beam computed tomography, 159
Feature extraction, in closed-loop neuromodulation, 193
Feedback loop, in neurostimulation. *See* Closed-loop neuromodulation.
Fibromyalgia, 4
Flat-panel cone-beam computed tomography, 159–160
Fluoroscopy, for sacral neuromodulation, 36–37
Fornix, neuromodulation of, for memory deficit, 142–143
Frequency domain, in closed-loop neuromodulation, 193, 195
Frontal leukotomy, for obsessive-compulsive disorder, 90
Frontostriatal system, neuromodulation of, for anorexia nervosa, 151–153
Functional imaging, 178–181

G

Gangliosidosis, dystonia in, 64
Globus pallidus, neuromodulation treatment of, 52
for depression, 105–109
for dystonia, 68–69

H

Headache, 4, 6
migraine, **11–14**
Hemorrhage
in deep brain stimulation, 131
in globus pallidus stimulation, 69
Heredodegenerative dystonia, 64
Hidden Markov model, in closed-loop neuromodulation, 194, 196
Hippocampus, neuromodulation of, 142
Hypothalamus, obesity and, 148–151

I

Image-guided deep brain stimulation, **159–172**
computed tomography in, 159–164, 170–171
magnetic resonance imaging in, 164–171
Imaging, advanced techniques for, **173–185**
functional imaging, 178–181
structural imaging, 175–178
Implantable pulse generators, 5
Infections, in deep brain stimulation, 131
Inferior thalamic peduncle, stimulation of
for depression, 105–109
for obsessive-compulsive disorder, 94
Inguinal neuralgia, 3, 6
Insula, in obsessive-compulsive disorder, 89
Internal capsule, neuromodulation treatment of, for refractory pain, 79
Interstitial cystitis, sacral neuromodulation for, **33–46**
Ischemia, in peripheral vascular disease, spinal cord stimulation for, **25–31**

J

Joint pain, 6

Printed and bound by CPI Group (UK) Ltd, Croydon, CR0 4YY
03/10/2024
01040309-0005

K

K-nearest neighbor, in closed-loop neuromodulation, 194–196

L

Lateral area of hypothalamus, neuromodulation of, for obesity, 148–151
Lateral habenula, stimulation of, for depression, 105–109
Lesch-Nyhan disease, dystonia in, 64
Lidocaine, for movement disorders, 47–49
Limbic neuromodulation, **137–145**
  anatomic considerations in, 137
  for addiction, 137–141
  for memory deficits, 141–143
  for posttraumatic stress disorder, 141
Local field potentials, in closed-loop neuromodulation, 189–192
Lumbar spinal locomotor circuit, neuromodulation of, **15–23**

M

Magnetic neuromodulation, for movement disorders, 50–51, 54
Magnetic resonance imaging
  advanced techniques for, 174–181
  diffusion imaging, 175–178
  for deep brain stimulation, 164–171
  functional, 179–181
  ultrahigh field strength, 175
Mathematical models, in closed-loop neuromodulation, 194–195
Median forebrain bundle
  neuromodulation of, for addiction, 138–139
  stimulation of, for depression, 105–109
Medtronic ONSTIM Trial, 12–13
Memory deficits, neuromodulation for, 141–143
Microelectric recording, in deep brain stimulation, 160–161
Migraine headache, neuromodulation for, **11–14**
Mood disorders, in neuromodulation, 70
Morbid obesity, 147–151
Motor cortex stimulation, for refractory pain, 77–78
Movement disorders
  deep brain stimulation for, image-guided, **159–172**
  neuromodulation for, **47–58**
    chemical, 47–49, 54
    cryogenic, 50, 54
    electrical, 51–55
    magnetic, 50–51, 54
    modalities for, 54–55
    outcomes of, 53–54
    targets in, 52–53
    technique for, 51–52
    thermal, 50, 54
    ultrasound, 50, 54
MRI. *See* Magnetic resonance imaging.
Muscimol, for movement disorders, 49
Musculoskeletal pain, 4

N

Neck pain, 4
Nerve blocks, diagnostic, for neuropathic pain, 3
Neurodegeneration with brain iron accumulation, dystonia in, 64
Neuromatrix theory, 80
Neuromodulation. *See also* Deep brain stimulation.
  central, **77–83, 173–185**
  closed-loop, **187–204**
  for bladder disorders, **33–46**
  for depression, **103–116**
  for dystonia, **59–75**
  for eating disorders, **147–157**
  for migraine headache, **11–14**
  for movement disorders, **47–58**
  for neuropathic pain, **1–10**
  for obsessive-compulsive disorder, **85–101**
  for refractory pain, **77–83**
  for Tourette syndrome, **117–135**
  for vascular pathology, **25–31**
  of lumbar spinal locomotor circuit, **15–23**
  trial of, 2
NeuroPace Trial, 198
Neuropathic pain, peripheral nerve stimulation and field stimulation for, **1–10**
  complications of, 7
  indications for, 2–4
  programming of, 7
  surgical technique for, 4–6
Nexframe, for deep brain stimulation, 161, 164–165
Nucleus accumbens, neuromodulation of
  for addiction, 138–139
  for anorexia nervosa, 153
  for depression, 105–109
  for obsessive-compulsive disorder, 91, 93–94
Nucleus basalis of Meynert, neuromodulation of, for memory deficit, 143

O

O-arm–guided deep brain stimulation, 160–163
Obesity, 147–151
Obsessive-compulsive disorder, **85–101**
  cognitive models of, 86
  definition of, 85–86
  mechanisms of, 86–89
  treatment of, 89–95
Occipital Nerve Stimulation for the Treatment of Intractable Migraine (ONSTIM) Trial, 12–13
Occipital nerve stimulators, 5–6, **11–14**

Occipital neuralgia, 3
Open-loop deep brain stimulation, 189
Orbitofrontal cortex, in obsessive-compulsive disorder, 87–88
Orbitofrontal cortico-striato-pallido-thalamo-cortical system, neuromodulation treatment of, for refractory pain, 79
Oscillatory components, of local field potentials, 189–192, 194
Overactive bladder, **33–46**

P

Pain
  in dystonia, 67
  neuropathic, peripheral nerve stimulation and field stimulation for, **1–10**
  psychology testing for, 2
  refractory, **77–83**
Painful bladder syndrome, **33–46**
Parietal cortex, in obsessive-compulsive disorder, 89
Parkinson disease
  deep brain stimulation for, 196
  neuromodulation for. *See also* Movement disorders.
    closed-loop, 189–193, 196–197
Pattern classification, in closed-loop neuromodulation, 194–195
Pedunculopontine area, neuromodulation of, for memory deficit, 143
Pelvic pain, sacral neuromodulation for, **33–46**
Periaqueductal gray matter, neuromodulation treatment of, for refractory pain, 79–80
Peripheral nerve stimulation and field stimulation, for neuropathic pain, **1–10**
Peripheral neuromodulation, **11–14**
Peripheral vascular disease, spinal cord stimulation for, **25–31**
Periventricular gray matter, neuromodulation treatment of, for refractory pain, 79–80
Phase domain, in closed-loop neuromodulation, 193–195
Phase-to-amplitude cross-frequency coupling, in closed-loop neuromodulation, 194
Positron emission tomography, 178–179
Post-herpetic neuralgia, 3
Posttraumatic neuralgia, 3
Posttraumatic stress disorder, limbic neuromodulation for, 141
Precision Implantable Stimulator for Migraine (PRISM) Trial, 13
Prefrontal cortex, in obsessive-compulsive disorder, 88–89
PRISM (Precision Implantable Stimulator for Migraine) Trial, 13
Psychiatric disorders, dystonia with, 68
Psychotherapy, for obsessive-compulsive disorder, 89
Pudendal nerve stimulation, 37
Pulse generator, for sacral neuromodulation, 37, 42–43

R

Radiofrequency neuromodulation, for movement disorders, 50
Refractory pain, neuromodulation for, **77–83**

S

Sacral neuromodulation
  complications of, 39
  for bladder disorders, **33–46**
  technical aspects of, 36–37
St. Jude Medical Neuromodulation Trial, 13
Seizures, prediction of, 197–198
Selective serotonin reuptake inhibitors, for obsessive-compulsive disorder, 89
Sensory loss, in neuropathic pain, 2–3
Signals, for closed-loop neuromodulation, 190–193
SmartFrame, for neuromodulation, 165–169
Spatial domain, in closed-loop neuromodulation, 193, 195
Spinal cord injury, neuromodulation for, **15–23**
Spinal Cord Stimulation European Peripheral Vascular Disease Outcome Study, 26
Spinal cord stimulation, for vascular pathology, **25–31**
Stereotactic techniques
  for neuromodulation, 51–55, **159–172**
  for obsessive-compulsive disorder, 89–90
Striatum, in obsessive-compulsive disorder, 87–89
Subcaudate tractotomy, for obsessive-compulsive disorder, 90
Subspace domain, in closed-loop neuromodulation, 193, 195
Substantia nigra, neuromodulation of, for addiction, 138–139
Subthalamic nucleus, neuromodulation of, 52–54
  for addiction, 139
  for obsessive-compulsive disorder, 94
Supplementary motor area, stimulation of, for obsessive-compulsive disorder, 94
Support vector machines, in closed-loop neuromodulation, 194–196

T

Tardive dystonia, 61
Thalamus, neuromodulation treatment of, 52
  for dystonia, 70
  for refractory pain, 78–79
THAP1 mutations, in dystonia, 60, 66
Thermal neuromodulation, for movement disorders, 50, 54

Tibial nerve stimulation, for overactive bladder, 38
Time domain, in closed-loop neuromodulation, 193, 195
Time-frequency domain, in closed-loop neuromodulation, 193, 195
TOR1A mutations, in dystonia, 60, 65–66
Toronto-Western Spasmodic Torticollis Ratings Scale (TWSTRS), 61–64, 69
Tourette syndrome, deep brain stimulation for, **117–135**
  centromedian-parafascicular nucleus, 118–129
  complications of, 131–132
  dorsomedial nucleus, 129
  globus pallidus, 119–123, 125, 127
  internal capsule, 119, 121, 123–124, 129
  nucleus accumbens, 119, 122, 124–125, 129
  outcomes of, 130
  patient selection for, 132
  subthalamic nucleus, 119, 121, 123–124, 129
  ventro-oral internus of thalamus, 118–129
Tractography, 176, 178
Transcranial magnetic neuromodulation, for movement disorders, 50–51, 54
Transcranial magnetic stimulation
  for depression, 106–109
  for obsessive-compulsive disorder, 94–95
Transcutaneous electrical nerve stimulation, neuromodulation and, 3
Tremor
  deep brain stimulation for, 196
  dystonic, 70
  neuromodulation for. *See* Movement disorders.
Trigeminal nerve stimulation, for depression, 109–111
Trigeminal neuralgia, 3, 6
Tunnelers, for electrodes, 4–5
TWSTRS (Toronto-Western Spasmodic Torticollis Ratings Scale), 61–64, 69

U

Ultrahigh field strength MRI, 175
Ultrasound neuromodulation, for movement disorders, 50, 54

V

Vagus nerve, stimulation of
  for obsessive-compulsive disorder, 94
  for posttraumatic stress disorder, 141
Vascular pathology, spinal cord stimulation for, **25–31**
Ventral capsule, stimulation of
  for depression, 105–109
  for obsessive-compulsive disorder, 91
Ventral intermediate nucleus, neuromodulation treatment of, 52
Ventral posterior lateral nucleus, neuromodulation treatment of, for refractory pain, 78–79
Ventral posterior medial nucleus, neuromodulation treatment of, for refractory pain, 78–79
Ventral striatum, stimulation of
  for depression, 105–109
  for obsessive-compulsive disorder, 91
  for refractory pain, 79
Ventral tegmental area, neuromodulation of, for addiction, 138–139
Ventromedial nucleus, neuromodulation of
  for addiction, 139
  for obesity, 148–151

W

Weight gain, in neuromodulation, 70

X

X-linked dystonia-parkinsonism, 64